THE
Hospitalist Manual

Manish Mehta, MD

Assistant Professor of Medicine, Western University of Health Sciences
Hospitalist, Apogee Physicians
Chief of Credentialing, Providence Medford Medical Center
Medford, Oregon

Arun Mathews, MD

Chief of Clinical Research and Education
Apogee Physicians
Phoenix, Arizona

2010
PEOPLE'S MEDICAL PUBLISHING HOUSE
SHELTON, CONNECTICUT

People's Medical Publishing House
2 Enterprise Drive, Suite 509
Shelton, CT 06484
Tel: 203-402-0646
Fax: 203-402-0854
E-mail: info@pmph-usa.com

PMPH-USA

09 10 11 12/PMPH/9 8 7 6 5 4 3 2 1

ISBN 978-1-60795-019-6
Printed in China by People's Medical Publishing House
Copyeditor/Typesetter: Newgen

Sales and Distribution

Canada
McGraw-Hill Ryerson Education
Customer Care
300 Water St
Whitby, Ontario L1N 9B6
Canada
Tel: 1-800-565-5758
Fax: 1-800-463-5885
www.mcgrawhill.ca

Foreign Rights
John Scott & Company
International Publisher's Agency
P.O. Box 878
Kimberton, PA 19442
USA
Tel: 610-827-1640
Fax: 610-827-1671

Japan
United Publishers Services Limited
1-32-5 Higashi-Shinagawa
Shinagawa-ku, Tokyo 140-0002
Japan
Tel: 03-5479-7251
Fax: 03-5479-7307
Email: kakimoto@ups.co.jp

United Kingdom, Europe, Middle East, Africa
McGraw Hill Education
Shoppenhangers Road
Maidenhead
Berkshire, SL6 2QL
England
Tel: 44-0-1628-502500
Fax: 44-0-1628-635895
www.mcgraw-hill.co.uk

Singapore, Thailand, Philippines, Indonesia,
Vietnam, Pacific Rim, Korea
McGraw-Hill Education
60 Tuas Basin Link
Singapore 638775

Tel: 65-6863-1580
Fax: 65-6862-3354
www.mcgraw-hill.com.sg

Australia, New Zealand
Elsevier Australia
Tower 1, 475 Victoria Avenue
Chatswood NSW 2067
Australia
Tel: 0-9422-8553
Fax: 0-9422-8562
www.elsevier.com.au

Brazil
Tecmedd Importadora e Distribuidora
de Livros Ltda.
Avenida Maurilio Biagi 2850
City Ribeirao, Rebeirao, Preto SP
Brazil
CEP: 14021-000
Tel: 0800-992236
Fax: 16-3993-9000
Email: tecmedd@tecmedd.com.br

India, Bangladesh, Pakistan, Sri Lanka, Malaysia
CBS Publishers
4819/X1 Prahlad Street 24
Ansari Road, Darya, New Delhi-110002
India
Tel: 91-11-23266861/67
Fax: 91-11-23266818
Email:cbspubs@vsnl.com

People's Republic of China
PMPH
Bldg 3, 3rd District
Fangqunyuan, Fangzhuang
Beijing 100078
P.R. China
Tel: 8610-67653342
Fax: 8610-67691034
www.pmph.com

My family has been my inspiration
for every endeavor that I have undertaken.
Thanks for always being there.
—Manish

For Ramesh Navuluri,
who inspired myself and others
and will be missed.
—Arun

Contents

Preface

Hospitalist physician is a relatively new concept within modern healthcare. As this new field evolves, so too will the educational needs of internists who have chosen to practice this discipline. This work is aimed squarely at addressing this need. Internal medicine residency programs in this country strive to equip new graduates with a comprehensive set of skills for dealing with both inpatient and outpatient care. However, there remain practice management and workflow nuances that separate the traditional internist from the acute inpatient care physician, or hospitalist. These are the key areas this work hopes to shed light upon, in addition to acting as a quick reference for critical care and procedural elements that may arise in the practice of acute inpatient medicine. It is hoped that this text will enable a physician to respond to the patients' needs in real time, providing a service which was not possible for busy primary care doctors to perform in the recent past.

We hope you find this handbook informative and enjoyable. We value your feedback, and invite you to help us improve upon subsequent editions.

Manish Mehta, MD
Arun Mathews, MD

1

The Evolution of Hospitalist Medicine

Manish Mehta, MD
Arun Mathews, MD

Hospitalist medicine represents the fastest growing movement seen within modern health-care. As is the case with many emerging disciplines, necessity often drives their creation and governance until a process of formal accreditation occurs. Hospitalist medicine is cur-rently in this flux state, with limited resources available for new residents looking to start a career in this field, or for internists hoping to transition from traditional practice into the world of full-time acute inpatient medicine. This chapter serves to recap some of the salient events that brought about the emergence of this field, and concludes with delineating our responsibility to further hew its future role in healthcare.

In the mid-1970s, the average generalist physician had approximately 10 patients in the hospital, each staying for an average of 8 to 10 days. Consequently, these physi-cians spent up to 30% to 40% of their days visiting inpatients. When added to the demands of an office-based practice, physicians would be forced to round on their patients either extremely early or very late in the day.

As medical practice became more specialized and increasingly dependent on complex technology, caring for hospitalized patients changed. The acuity of illness increased, demanding greater physician presence and expertise throughout the typical workday. This was driven by a variety of factors, including the aging of the population, medical advances that allowed patients with chronic diseases to live longer, and the shifting of less complex cases to the outpatient setting.

At the same time, health care costs continued to escalate and payers moved to constrain reimbursement. In the 1990s, a new model of acute inpatient care emerged. The underlying concept was that a small number of inpatient-based phy-sicians, or *hospitalists*, would improve the quality and coordination of care while controlling health care costs. Wachter et al proposed the following definition for the term "hospitalist":

> Hospitalists are physicians who spend at least 25 percent of their professional time serving as the physicians-of-record for inpatients, during which time they

accept "hand-offs" of hospitalized patients from primary care providers, returning the patients back to the care of their primary care providers at the time of hospital discharge.*

As the success of these hospital medicine programs became more widely known, hospitalists began to proliferate rapidly throughout the health care system—from large academic health centers to small rural hospitals. In the mid-1990s, there were less than 1000 hospitalists in the United States. By 2004, nearly 13,000 hospitalists were practicing in almost 1800 hospitals, or 37% of all acute care hospitals in the United States. Projections indicate that by 2010, as many as 30,000 hospitalists may practice in this country. Hospital medicine is the fastest growing medical specialty in the history of medicine.

Hospitalists come from several medical disciplines, but general internal medicine is by far the most common (75%). This reflects the fact that residency training in internal medicine typically focuses on the care of acutely ill hospitalized patients, which leaves graduates well-suited to practice as hospitalists. At once both demanding and extremely gratifying, a dedicated inpatient practice allows a physician to respond to the hospitalized patient's needs in real time, providing a level of service not always possible for busy primary care doctors in the recent past. Such a system has the potential to grow into the backbone of any hospital inpatient service, with physicians dedicated to coordinating and co-managing care among the various hospital consultants and services, medical and surgical alike.

In summary, it is important to remember that the role of the hospitalist physician will continue to evolve with the backdrop of health care reform looming in the coming years. As a young field, we believe that this represents a tremendous opportunity to take a leadership role within our hospitals and communities, guiding our policy makers to legislate in favor of practical, efficient, and pro-active patient care. Working in concert with outpatient primary care providers, our charge, simply put, is to be the orchestrators of inpatient care, thereby shaping the delivery of hospital medicine locally, nationally and perhaps globally in the years to come. *Hospitium meditor excellentia.*

---

*Wachter RM, Goldman L. The emerging role of "hospitalists" in the American health care system. N Engl J Med 1996; 335:514–517.

2

Preparing for Your First Day

Arun Mathews, MD
Manish Mehta, MD

The commencement of a new job is ranked as one of the top three stressors that adults can face. While other vocations may have similar issues regarding learning nuances of co-workers, workflow layout, and information management systems, the acute care physician invariably also has to deal with the pressing issues of patient care throughout this experience. And, while there is no good way to suggest a fool-proof method for tackling this daunting task, certain principles come into play that can minimize adjustment pitfalls. Acknowledging that the first few weeks are going to be stressful, in addition to preparing for it, can actually alleviate anxiety.

INFORMATION GATHERING

As early as the interview, be sure to try to gather the following information.

Logistics
- The size of the hospital, but more specifically the number of medical/surgical and specialty beds
- Average census volumes, in addition to volume fluctuation through the "busy months"
- Average admission numbers both during the day and night
- Number of hospitalist physicians during the day and the night
- Admission autonomy: ie, who makes the final determination regarding a patient's admit status—the ED physician or the hospitalist physician?
- Expectations regarding critical care/procedures (in addition to the frequency and types of procedures)
- Size of the ICU
- Access to subspecialty consultation
- Access to tertiary care if the facility is a community hospital
- Average number of internal medicine/hospitalist consults per day: ie, the number of times Surgery or OB will request consultation
- Surgery/OB consultation and admission preferences: The hospitalist as primary or consultant?
- Rapid Response Team details: Hospitalist as first responder vs second responder?
- Code Team Responsibilities: Hospitalist as first responder vs ER physician?

Workflow Issues
- Hospital information management (HIM) system and training process
- Electronic medical records vs traditional paper chart vs hybrid systems
- Radiology (traditional vs digital)
- Physician work area size, comfort, and attentiveness of the unit secretary in both the ER, Critical Care, and General Medical floors
- Timely access to charts, labs, MARs, vitals flowsheets
- Nocturnal phlebotomy availability
- Proceduralist availability (PIC line specialists, anesthesiology, general medicine, vascular surgery, etc. on call)
- Transcription turnaround (speed of STAT dictations)
- Progress note dictation service (increases hospitalist efficiency and legibility of documentation)
- Nocturnalist services

■ Access to mid-levels
■ Care handoff (off shift/off service/discharge) process: Formalized vs ad-hoc?
■ Access to point of care information resources (UpToDate/eMedicine, etc.)

Communication
■ Beeper service, cell phone or both.
■ Redundant communication strategy: ie, what is the backup plan for contacting the hospitalist, should the first pathway fail?

Advancement Issues
■ Teaching responsibilities
■ Research opportunities

Life Issues
■ Quality of the cafeteria
■ Commute time
■ Nocturnal home call vs on site call
■ Access to a hospital gym and other amenities
■ Schedule autonomy or flexibility
■ Vacation (paid vs unpaid)
■ Benefits package

ACUTE CARE PHYSICIAN ATTIRE AND RATIONALE

A great deal may be written regarding the erosion of immaculate professional attire and the advance of "scrub culture." This discussion seeks to find a happy medium between the two and proffer some explanations for our perhaps controversial recommendations. It should be understood that these are merely recommendations and by no means hard and fast rules.

Regarding day attire, we would defer to the recommendations of the British Medical System or National Health Service:

- Short sleeve or rolled up, collared shirts (allow us this one vestige of decency) leaving the hands exposed from the mid-forearm down, allowing for proper CDC-determined handwashing technique.
- Avoidance of standard neckties (unless one can prove that these are laundered between each use). Bow ties are acceptable.
- Avoidance of white coats (once again, unless one can prove that these are laundered each day).

Scrub Attire Etiquette

- Daytime scrub use is frowned upon, but this is largely driven by patient/physician perception.
- Nocturnal scrub use is reasonable.
- Traveling *to* work with scrubs on: reasonable.
- Traveling *from* work with scrubs on: unreasonable and possibly a public health hazard. With community acquired MRSA and *Clostridium difficile* colitis rates on the rise, we recommend either changing out of scrubs altogether at the hospital prior to departure, or switching to a new pair prior to departure should stops in nonclinical areas be anticipated.

WHAT TO CARRY

If one were to liken the practice of medicine to a war, acute care internists would be the svelte strategists, coordinating and managing the various forces at their disposal in the battle against disease. Our advice is travel lightly, but understand what resources are available and where they are located at all times. Know for instance where the otoscope/ophthalmascope on each floor is. This saves the hassle of carrying around extra equipment and the inevitable cost of replacing the equipment that is destined to be lost within the first week of work. Advising one to travel light is not an excuse to be ill prepared. As you are well aware, the elicitation of signs (papilledema, acute otitis media, nonblanching petichiae) with equipment can be exhilarating, and usher one forward to a correct diagnosis. If your hospital doesn't have equipment readily available, make the request for it, if that doesn't work, build your own perfect kit and keep it in a safe place that you can easily access. The equipment list may include the following:

- Oto-/ophthalmascope
- Tuning fork (512 Hz to 1024 Hz)
- Sterile sharp object (fine touch/pin prick assessment)
- Reflex hammer
- Cotton swab
- Magnifying glass

These items we would recommend your keeping about your person:

- Hospital ID
- Pager
- Pen, preferably black or blue
- PDA or SmartPhone for pharma reference/medical equations
- Pharmacopoeia or pocket PDR if not carrying a PDA
- Rounding list
- Billing cards
- Pen light
- Stethoscope
- and finally, *The Hospitalist Manual*

The Stethoscope

Stethoscope owners from time to time fall prey to Mathew's Law: "The cost of the stethoscope is inversely proportional to the time prior to said device being lost or stolen." Admittedly somewhat flippant, the truth of the matter is that the vast majority of decisive clinical signs determined via a reasonably priced device are quite apparent. Larger diaphragms, micro-electronics, and other such malarky may help, but the subtle distinguishing features among various valvular maladies (rumbles vs snaps, crescendo vs decrescendo) are perhaps best left to the deft ears of a specialist, and are all inevitably confirmed by echocardiography.

Perhaps the most important point regarding this particular piece of equipment has nothing to do with its auditory prowess, but instead its potential for spreading infection. In a manner similar to unlaundered neckties and white coats, a stethoscope dragged from patient to patient circumvents hand hygiene and does nothing more than act as a microbiologic fomite. Picking up a new pan-systolic murmur in a hospitalized patient that has had a protracted hospital course and suddenly developed fevers? Well done, Doctor, you've diagnosed infective endocarditis with the very instrument that may have seeded the patient's anterior chest wall flora and subsequent subclavian central line from the patient in the previous room. This hypothetical scenario's perplexing irony is only overshadowed in magnitude by the tragedy of its avoidability.

Hypothetical cases aside, allow us to suggest the best practice of tying hand hygiene decontamination with scope decontamination. In short, consider using sterilizing wipes on your stethoscope as frequently as possible, and as a top-box practice, before and after every patient encounter.

Dictation Templates
Sound documentation is the cornerstone of care in the team setting that is hospitalist medicine. We have included a series of dictation templates that should help you organize your thoughts and provide complete comprehensive documentation in the form of dictated reports. Please refer to these templates in the Appendix to this book.

3

Coding and Billing

Manish Mehta, MD

Diligence in documentation translates into improved communication and fewer errors. We believe that billing and coding falls under the umbrella of documentation, supporting the physician's thought process and justifying the level of service provided for the patient. This is by no means an exhaustive guide, but instead meant to act as a quick reference for hospitalists in the field. Coding is based on the "patient diagnosis," while billing is the level and type of service that you provide.

COMMON ICD-9-CM (INTERNATIONAL CLASSIFICATION OF DISEASES) CODES

Cardiovascular
Chest pain 786.5
Unstable angina 411.1
Myocardial infarction (MI) 410
Supraventricular tachycardia (SVT) 427
Ventricular tachycardia 427.1
Atrial fibrillation 427.31
Congestive heart failure (CHF) 428.0
Hypertension (HTN) 401

Gastroenterology
GI bleed 578.9
Ascites 789.5
Cirrhosis 571.5
Acute pancreatitis 577.0
Hepatitis 573.3
Abdominal pain 789.0
Small bowel obstruction 560
Constipation 564.0

Renal
Acute renal failure 584.9
Chronic renal failure 585.9
Hyperkalemia 276.7
Hypokalemia 276.8
Hypernatremia 276.0
Hyponatremia 276.1
Acute tubular necrosis (ATN) 584.5
Nephrotic syndrome 581.9

Pulmonary
Acute respiratory failure 518.81
Acute respiratory distress syndrome (ARDS) 518.82
Chronic obstructive pulmonary disease (COPD) 491.21
Asthma 493.9
Pneumonia 486
Pneumothorax 512.8
Shortness of breath 786.05

Neurology
Transient-ischemic attack (TIA) 435.9
Intracranial bleed 432.9
Stroke 434.9
Altered mental status 438.6

Endocrine/ID

Diabetic ketoacidosis (DKA) 250.1
Hyperosmolar state 250.2
Hyperglycemia 790.6
Hypoglycemia 251.2
Urinary tract infection (UTI)... 599.0
Sepsis 995.91
Septic shock 785.52

Source: http://www.cms.hhs.gov

HOSPITALIST BILLING CODES

ADMISSION CODES

Observation
Initial Observation:

Low.. 99218
Moderate.. 99219
High 99220

Inpatient
Initial Inpatient:
Admit

Level 1.. 99221
Level 2.. 99222
Level 3.. 99223

ICU or Critical Care

First 75 min 99291
Each additional 30 min... 99292

Consult
Initial Consult:

Level 1.. 99251
Level 2.. 99252
Level 3.. 99253
Level 4.. 99254
Level 5.. 99255

FOLLOW-UP CODES

Observation

Level 1.. 99211
Level 2.. 99212
Level 3.. 99213
Level 4.. 99214
Level 5.. 99215

Inpatient
Inpatient Follow-Up:

Level 1.. 99231
Level 2.. 99232
Level 3.. 99233

ICU or Critical Care
First 75 min 99291
Each additional 30 min.. 99292

DISCHARGE CODES

Observation
Same 23-h discharge by same physician:
Level 1 99234
Level 2 99235
Level 3 99236
Next day discharge 99217

Inpatient
Discharge time less than 30 min.. 99238
Discharge time more than 30 min 99239

Source: http://www.cms.hhs.gov/transmittals/downloads/R1530CP.pdf; Beebe, M, et al. CTP 2009, professional edition. American Medical Association, 2009.

4

Medical Rounds

Manish Mehta, MD

In this chapter, we will discuss the most common cases encountered during ward rounds. It is always best to consider common etiologies first while admitting a patient. Again, we would like to emphasize that it is important to plan your day in advance. Start with the critical patients first, followed by discharges, and then the more stable patients. Eventually, you will have developed a plan that suits you best. A good bedside manner can take you a long way.

CARDIOVASCULAR DISEASES

CHEST PAIN

This can be multifactorial and the most commonly involved systems are cardiac, pulmonary, gastrointestinal, and musculoskeletal.

Etiology
■ Acute coronary syndrome (ACS), pneumonia, pneumothorax, pulmonary embolism (PE), aortic dissection, pericarditis, and esophageal spasm.

TRIAGING CHEST PAIN

Low Risk	Intermediate Risk	High Risk
Less than one or no cardiac risk factors	More than two cardiac risk factors or prior MI, CABG, PVD	More than two cardiac risk factors or prior MI, CABG, PVD
Reproducible pain	Typical cardiac pain >20 min either at rest or exertion relieved by nitroglycerin	Typical cardiac pain >20 min either at rest or exertion not relieved by nitroglycerin
Pleuritic pain		
Normal EKG and cardiac enzymes	Mildly positive cardiac enzymes	Positive cardiac enzymes
Disposition: CDU (observation unit)	Abnormal EKG	EKG suggestive of MI, ischemia
	Vital signs normal	Hemodynamically unstable
	Disposition: Telemetry	Disposition: CCU or Step Down Unit with goal of potential cardiac catheterization, if applicable

Abbreviations: CABG, coronary artery bypass graft; CCU, critical care unit; CDU, cardiovascular diagnostic unit; EKG, electrocardiogram; MI, myocardial infarction; PVD, peripheral vascular disease.

History
■ Do not forget PQRST as they might help differentiate the pain. Pleuritic nature would correlate with a pulmonary etiology. Association with food would relate to a gastrointestinal etiology and positional pain could be pericarditis.
■ ACS pain is typically "pressure-like," "squeezing," "sharp," and the most popular description is "as if an elephant is sitting on my chest." Commonly radiates to the left shoulder and lasts >20 minutes.

Physical Examination
■ *Lungs*: Dull to percussion, increased fremitus, and decreased breath sounds would signify pneumonia. Absent breath sounds could also signify pneumothorax.

- *Abdomen*: Epigastric discomfort or pain could be indicative of a GI etiology.
- *Heart*: S4, new pansystolic murmur, elevated jugular venous pulse (JVP), new crackles

Diagnosis

- *EKG*: ST elevation or T wave inversion is indicative of myocardial infarction or ischemia.
- S1-Q3-T3 with incomplete or complete right bundle branch block (RBBB) indicates pulmonary hypertension suggestive of pulmonary embolism.
- *Cardiac enzymes*: CK, CK-MB and troponin
- 2-D echocardiogram
- Chest x-ray
- Stress test if not having a MI or unstable angina and, if present, then a submaximal test can be done in about 4–7 days after a MI.

Treatment

- Give aspirin, high-dose statins, and beta blockers immediately while pending further workup if no contraindication to the above. Please refer to individual sections for further treatment details.

ST-ELEVATION MYOCARDIAL INFARCTION (MI)

This is an emergency. Signified by >1 mm ST elevation in at least two consecutive leads, with symptoms consistent with MI >30 minutes and <12 hours.

Etiology
■ Similar to the chest pain section

History
■ The history is critical in making the diagnosis of MI.
■ Chest pain, usually across the anterior precordium, is typically described as tightness, pressure, or squeezing.
■ Pain may radiate to the jaw, neck, arms, back, and epigastrium. The left arm is more frequently affected; however, a patient may experience pain in both arms.
■ Dyspnea, which may accompany chest pain, nausea, and abdominal pain, can present in infarcts involving the inferior or posterior wall.
■ Diaphoresis
■ Many MIs can be silent and patients with diabetes, women, and older patients can have vague, nonspecific symptoms.

Physical Examination
■ Hypotension may indicate ventricular dysfunction due to ischemia. Hypotension in the setting of MI usually indicates a large infarct secondary to either decreased global cardiac contractility or a right ventricular infarct.
■ *Heart*: New murmur can be a sign of acute valvular dysfunction. Valvular dysfunction usually results from infarction that involves the papillary muscle. Mitral regurgitation due to papillary muscle ischemia or necrosis may be present.
■ Elevated jugular venous distension could signify congestive heart failure (CHF). With right ventricular failure, cannon jugular venous *a* waves may be noted.
■ Third heart sound (S₃) may be present.
■ A fourth heart sound is a common finding in patients with poor ventricular compliance that is due to preexisting heart disease or hypertension.
■ *Lungs*: Rales may represent CHF.
■ *Extremities*: Pedal edema could be present.

Diagnosis
■ *EKG*: Peaked or inverted T waves can be an early sign of MI; ST elevation >1 mm in two consecutive leads and presence of new Q waves is diagnostic of new MI
■ *Cardiac enzymes*: CK, CK-MB, troponin I, myoglobin q6h × 3

■ *Chest x-ray*: Presence of pneumonia, pneumothorax can also mimic a MI
■ Echocardiogram shows wall motion abnormality, worsening LV function, and possible papillary muscle dysfunction.

Treatment

■ Primary PCI is the treatment of choice. Should be performed within 90 minutes by a skilled cardiologist in a well-established center: 27% decrease in mortality, 65% decrease in re-MI.
■ Should also be considered in the setting of septic shock, CHF, anterior MI
■ *Aspirin (ASA)*: 162–325 mg PO daily (23% decrease in mortality) ISIS-2
■ *High-dose statins like atorvastatin*: 80 mg PO daily (TIMI-22)
■ *Beta-blockers*: Metoprolol 25 mg PO q6h titrate to HR 55–60 bpm (15% decrease in mortality [ISIS-1]), contraindicated in decompensated CHF, 2nd or 3rd degree heart block, severe asthma
■ *Unfractionated heparin or low molecular weight Heparin at a therapeutic dose*
  ☐ *Unfractionated heparin*: 60–70 U/kg IV bolus then 12 U/kg/h. No mortality benefit
  ☐ *Low molecular weight heparin such as Enoxaparin*: 1 mg/kg SC bid (needs to be renal dosed), (25% decrease in mortality, ASSENT-3)
  ☐ *Glycoprotein 2b/3a inhibitors such as Eptifibate*: 180 µg/kg IV bolus, then 2 µg/kg/min infusion, 2nd 180 µg/kg IV bolus 10 minutes later if needed.
  ☐ *Abciximab*: 0.25 mg/kg IV bolus, then 0.125 µg/kg/min for 18–24 hours
  ☐ Also in unstable angina/NSTEMI treatment
■ *Heparin or low molecular weight heparin at a therapeutic dose*
  ☐ *UFH*: 60–75 U/kg IV bolus then 12–15 U/kg/hr (titrate to PTT 50–70 sec)
  ☐ *LMWH*: enoxaparin 1 mg/kg SC bid
  ☐ *Dalteparin*: 120 IU/kg SC bid
■ *Glycoprotein 2b/3a inhibitors based on the cardiologist's preference*:
  ☐ *Eptifibate*: 180 µg/kg IV bolus, then 2 µg/kg/min infusion × 72 hr
  ☐ *Abciximab*: 0.25/mg/kg IV bolus then 0.125 m/kg/min for 18–24 hr
■ *Clopidogrel (Plavix)*: 75 mg daily if stent placed or if aspirin allergy
■ *Nitroglycerin*: 0.4 mg SL q5min × 3 if chest pain and if persists may need IV infusion
■ *Oxygen*: Titrate via NC or other means to keep saturation >92% unless has history of chronic obstructive pulmonary disease (COPD)
■ Morphine could be used as needed as it helps to relieve pain and anxiety
■ *Angiotensin-converting enzyme (ACE) inhibitors*: Captopril 6.25 mg PO tid or lisinopril 5 mg PO daily (10% decrease in mortality at 4–6 weeks) (Class 1 indication within 24 hours after MI)
■ ARB can be an alternative if patient unable to tolerate ACE-I
■ Tight glycemic control with IV insulin

Fibrinolysis
Indications
- Signified by >1 mm ST elevation in at least two consecutive leads with symptoms consistent with MI >30 minutes and less than 12 hours
- New left bundle branch block
- *Age*: Patients greater than 75 years have less benefit from fibrinolysis

Contraindications
Absolute
- Prior intracranial hemorrhage
- Aortic dissection
- Nonhemorrhagic stroke within 3–6 months
- Intracranial neoplasm, aneurysm
- Active internal bleeding

Relative
- Trauma or major surgery within 2–4 weeks
- SBP >180 on presentation
- International normalized ratio (INR) >2
- Prolonged CPR >10 minutes
- Recent internal bleeding
- Prior streptokinase exposure
- Pregnancy

Fibrinolytics
- RPA 10 units IV over 2 minutes, repeat in 30 minutes × 1
- TNK single IV bolus over 5 seconds
  - ☐ <60 kg: 30 mg
  - ☐ 60–69 kg: 35 mg
  - ☐ 70–79 kg: 40 mg
  - ☐ 80–89 kg: 45 mg
  - ☐ 90 kg: 50 mg
- TPA 15 mg IV bolus, then 0.75 mg/kg (max 50 mg) over 30 minutes, then 0.5 mg/kg (max 35 mg) over 60 minutes
- SK 1.5 MU IV over 30–60 minutes

Consultation
- Cardiology

UNSTABLE ANGINA/NSTEMI

Unstable angina is defined as worsening angina and angina occurring even at rest, suggestive of myocardial ischemia without necrosis.

Etiology
■ Same as the chest pain section

TIMI CRITERIA FOR TREATMENT

Historical	Points
Age ≥65	I
≥3 CAD risk factors (FMHx, HTN, hyperlipidemia, DM, smoking)	I
Known CAD (stenosis ≥50%)	I
ASA in the past 7 days	I
Presentation:	
Recent severe angina ≤24 h	I
Elevated cardiac markers	I
ST elevation ≥0.5 mm	I

RISK OF CARDIAC EVENTS (%) BY 14 DAYS IN TIMI 11B

Risk Score	Death or MI	Death, MI or Recurrent Ischemia Requiring Urgent Revascularization
0–1	3	5
2	3	8
3	5	13
4	7	20
5	12	26
6–7	19	41

Source: Antman et al. *JAMA* 2000;284:835–842.

History
■ Increasing symptoms in the last 48 hours and pain lasting >20 minutes. Increasing shortness of breath and the description as "pressure like," "squeezing," "sharp," and the most popular description is "as if an elephant is sitting on my chest." Commonly this radiates to the left shoulder.

Physical Examination
■ *Heart*: S4, new pansystolic murmur, elevated JVP, new crackles, and/or hypotension

Diagnosis

■ *EKG*: ST changes >0.05 mm, TWI are indicative.

■ Cardiac enzymes like CK, CK-MB, troponin, and myoglobin may or may not be elevated.

■ Echocardiogram could show wall motion abnormality, worsening LV function, and possible papillary muscle dysfunction.

■ Chest x-ray could show pulmonary edema.

■ Monitor for Wellen syndrome: Preanterior wall infarction suggestive of critical proximal LAD stenosis as observed by deeply inverted T waves in V1-V3, biphasic T wave inversion

Treatment

■ *Aspirin (ASA)*: 81, 162, or 325 mg daily (mortality benefit with either dose)

■ *High-dose statins like atorvastatin*: 80 mg daily (TIMI 22)

■ *Beta blockers*: Metoprolol 25 mg PO q6h. Titrate to heart rate for 55–60

■ *ACE inhibitors*: Within 24 hours of acute MI (Class 1 indication), lisinopril 5 mg PO daily

■ *Clopidogrel (Plavix)*:75 mg daily (CURE)

■ *Heparin or low-molecular heparin*: At a therapeutic dose

■ *UFH*: 60–75 U/kg IV bolus, then 12–15 U/kg/h (titrate to PTT 50–70 sec)

■ *LMWH*: Enoxaparin 1 mg/kg SC bid

■ *Dalteparin*: 120 IU/kg SC bid

■ *Glycoprotein*: 2b/3a inhibitors based on the cardiologist's preference

■ *Eptifibate*: 180 µg/kg IV bolus, then 2 µg/kg/min infusion × 72 hours

■ *Abciximab*: 0.25 mg/kg IV bolus then 0.125 µg/kg/min for 18–24 hours

■ PTCA or DES placement within 1–2 days

Consultation

■ Cardiology

ATRIAL FIBRILLATION

When the atria beat out of synch with the ventricles in an irregularly irregular manner resulting in a rapid heart rate and impedence of blood flow to the body, we term that process as atrial fibrillation.

Etiology

■ Evaluate the cause and don't just treat atrial fibrillation.

Acute

■ *Cardiac*: MI, CHF, myocarditis/pericarditis, hypertensive crisis, cardiac surgery
■ *Pulmonary*: Pneumonia, COPD, PE
■ *Metabolic*: Electrolyte imbalances like hyperkalemia, hypomagnesemia, high catecholamine states (stress, infection, postoperative), thyrotoxicosis
■ *Drugs*: Alcohol, cocaine, amphetamines

Chronic

■ Older age, hypertension, ischemia, valvular heart disease, hyperthyroidism

Physical Examination

■ Evaluate if the patient is stable or unstable.
■ *Heart*: Irregularly irregular heart rate, murmurs may or may not be present.
■ *Lungs*: CHF, if present, may be indicated by rales, jugular venous distension, peripheral edema, and a gallop, which may be difficult to auscultate due to rapid rate.
■ It is necessary to look for any signs of embolization as would be seen in transient ischemic attack (TIA), stroke, or even peripheral arterial embolization.

Diagnosis

■ *EKG*: No P waves, irregularly irregular rhythm, can have rapid ventricular response
■ *Cardiac enzymes*: Underlying ischemia or MI could be a potential cause.
■ *CBC*: Infection can cause a high stress state leading to atrial fibrillation
■ *BMP with magnesium level*: Electrolyte abnormalities can be a potential trigger
■ *TSH, free T4*: Hyperthyroidism needs to be ruled out.
■ Chest x-ray
■ 2-D echocardiogram to look for LV hypokinesis, left atrial enlargement, LVH

Treatment

■ *If unstable atrial fibrillation*: Urgent cardioversion
■ *If stable atrial fibrillation*: First control the heart rate with either beta blockers or calcium channel blockers (CCBs).

■ *Recommended*: To start with diltiazem drip after initial bolus of 10 mg IV then titrate drip to HR 55–60. Can bridge with either metoprolol 25 mg PO q6h or diltiazem 30 mg PO q6h.

■ Spontaneous cardioversion occurs in 50–60% of patients with atrial fibrillation.

■ *If atrial fibrillation >48 hours*: There is a high risk of stroke. If planning cardioversion, then do transesophageal echocardiography (TEE) first to evaluate for left atrial thrombus. If present, then warfarin for 3–4 weeks and then cardioversion followed by another 4–12 weeks course of warfarin.

■ If thrombus absent, then proceed with the cardioversion followed by 6–12 weeks of warfarin.

■ *If atrial fibrillation <48 hours*: There is a low risk for stroke. Recommend use of pharmacological agents as most atrial fibrillation convert spontaneously.

■ Also the AFFIRM study (and similar findings from the smaller rate control vs electrical cardioversion [RACE] trial) has also recommended rate control for most patients and rhythm control for symptomatic patients.

Long-Term Prophylaxis

■ Long-term prophylaxis with warfarin is essential for patients with a high CHADS score. Most of these patients have two or more of the below risk factors:

  ☐ History of stroke or TIA, diabetes, HTN, CAD, valvular abnormalities, prosthetic valve, CHF, left atrial enlargement, and global LV dysfunction.

■ Recommendation regarding anticoagulation in atrial fibrillation:

  ☐ Patients who are 65 years and younger with risk factors receive warfarin therapy with a goal INR of 2–3.

  ☐ Patients who are 65 years and younger with no risk factors receive ASA therapy or no treatment.

  ☐ Patients who are older than 65 years receive warfarin therapy with a goal INR of 2–3.

  ☐ Patients who are older than 75 years with no risk factors receive ASA therapy.

  ☐ Patients with no structural heart disease and patients younger than 65 years have an extremely low risk for stroke. Generally, they do not need anticoagulation. Aspirin at 325 mg/d is recommended.

Surgical Therapies

■ Atrial compartmentalization with continuous ablation lines of block (MAZE procedure)

■ Catheter ablation of triggers of AF

■ Atrioventricular node ablation and eventual insertion of a permanent pacemaker

Consultation

■ Cardiology

SUPRAVENTRICULAR TACHYCARDIA (SVT)

The foci arise above the ventricles and cause a narrow QRS complex unless there is aberrant conduction or preexcitation

Etiology

- Sinus tachycardia (ST) is caused by fever, pain, hypovolemia, electrolyte imbalances, anemia, anxiety, beta agonists, etc.
- Multifocal atrial tachycardia (MAT) automaticity at multiple sites in the atria can be seen in COPD or asthma.
- Atrial flutter is reentry into the right atrium and can occur due to multiple causes such as MI, COPD, PE, electrolyte imbalances, hyperthyroidism, etc.
- Atrial fibrillation is irregular waves passing down the AV node and has multifactorial etiology similar to the above tachycardias.

Identifying the Rhythm

- *Sinus-tachycardia*: Upright P waves immediately before the QRS
- *Atrial tachycardias*: P different from sinus, could be inverted and before QRS
- *AV nodal reentrant tachycardia (AVNRT)*: Abrupt in onset, rate >150 bpm, has retrograde P waves that appear inverted in the inferior leads.
- *Atrioventricular reciprocating tachycardia (AVRT)*: Abrupt in onset, rate >150, has retrograde P waves but are distinct from the QRS.
- *Atrial flutter*: Usually regular but can be irregular in the presence of variable block. Ventricular rate >150, saw-toothed "F" waves at a rate of 300 bpm, can lead to atrial fibrillation.
- *Atrial fibrillation*: Absent P waves, rate 150–200, irregularly irregular rate, fine defibrillator waves are seen in atrial fibrillation.
- *Multifocal atrial tachycardia (MAT)*: Can be irregular. Rate is >100, P wave morphology may be very helpful in determining MAT, which has three different P wave morphologies.
- Response to vagal maneuvers (CSM, Valsalva) or rate control agents
- Rhythms due to increased automaticity such as ST, AT, MAT lead to slowing of rate or increased AV block.
- Rhythms due to reentry at AVN (AVNRT, AVRT) terminate quickly or have no response.
- Atrial flutter leads to increased AV block and appearance of "F" waves (fibrillatory waves).

Diagnosis

- CBC
- CMP, magnesium levels
- TSH, free T4

- Chest x-ray
- Cardiac enzymes every 6 hours × 3
- *EKG 12 lead*: Remember to obtain one in the A.M. as well.
- 2-D echocardiogram

Treatment

- *Unstable*: Cardioversion
- *Sinus tachycardia*: Observe and treat the underlying cause.
- *Atrial tachycardia*: Beta blockers or CCBs. May consider radiofrequency ablation (RFA) for long-term treatment.
- *Atrial fibrillation*: Beta blockers, CCB, digoxin. Warfarin for anticoagulation
- *Atrial flutter*: Treat like atrial fibrillation. Could consider ablation.
- *MAT*: CCB, treat underlying condition. AV nodal ablation can be considered.
- *AVNRT or AVRT*: Vagal maneuvers, adenosine, CCB, beta blockers. Consider RFA for long-term treatment (changed order).

Consultation

- Cardiology

VENTRICULAR TACHYCARDIA (VT)

Ventricular tachycardia (VT) originates from an ectopic focus in the ventricles. Since it is below the AV node, it is a wide QRS complex rhythm with a rate that exceeds 120 bpm. VT may be monomorphic (from a single focus with similar QRS complexes) or polymorphic (irregular rhythm, with varying QRS complexes). Nonsustained VT is defined as a run of tachycardia of less than 30 seconds duration; longer runs are considered sustained VT.

Etiology

- Coronary artery disease (CAD) causing myocardial scar. Chaga disease causing dilated cardiomyopathy among other causes such as ethanol alcohol (ETOH)
- Hypertrophic cardiomyopathy
- Electrolytes abnormalities
- Surgical incisions within the ventricle
- Arrhythmogenic RV dysplasia
- *Monomorphic*: When the same QRS electrocardiographic wave repeats itself, the VT is considered monomorphic. This means that the sequence of electrical activation is repetitive.
- *Causes for monomorphic VT*: Prior MI, cardiomyopathy, arrhythmogenic AV dysplasia, Brugada syndrome (pseudo-RBBB with ST elevation on resting EKG)
- *Polymorphic*: When the QRS complex varies from beat to beat, the rhythm is described as polymorphic VT and suggests a variable electrical activation sequence. The most dangerous form of polymorphic VT is torsade de pointes.
- *Causes for polymorphic VT*: The torsade de pointes form of polymorphic VT is related to acquired or congenital QT-interval prolongation. Acquired QT prolongation is seen with certain potassium channel-blocking medications. Drugs such as quinidine or erythromycin could potentially cause it. Even psychotropic agents like haloperidol are potential causes as they prolong the QT interval.
- *Monomorphic VT*: Can occur in patients who have no structural heart disease. That is termed idiopathic. Most commonly they arise from the right and left ventricular outflow tracts.

  Triggers of VT include ischemia and electrolyte abnormalities:
  - ☐ Hypokalemia and hyperkalemia can trigger VT or VF in patients with structural heart disease. Hypomagnesemia can also be a potential trigger.
  - ☐ Cocaine use can trigger VT.

History

- The main symptoms of VT are palpitation, lightheadedness, and syncope.
- Some patients describe a sensation of neck fullness, which may be related to increased central venous pressures and cannon A waves.
- Dyspnea can also be an important symptom.

■ Anxiety is often present, regardless of whether syncope occurs.

■ Risk factors include prior MI, structural heart disease, or a family history of premature sudden death. VT should be considered in a patient with syncope with similar family history or past medical history.

■ Any patient with a strong family history of premature or young deaths <35 yr should be evaluated for long-QT syndrome, short-QT syndrome, Brugada syndrome, arrhythmogenic right ventricular dysplasia, and hypertrophic cardiomyopathy.

Physical Examination

■ Hypotension and tachypnea can be present.

■ Signs of poor perfusion may be present such as altered mental status, diaphoresis, pallor, and hypotension.

■ Heart: Elevated JVP, cannon A waves may be observed. The first heart sound may vary in intensity, with displaced PMI, murmurs related to valvular heart disease or hypertrophic cardiomyopathy, and an S_3 gallop.

■ Lungs: Rales may be present during sinus rhythm if uncompensated CHF is present.

Diagnosis

■ All wide-complex tachycardias are VT, unless proven otherwise.

■ CBC

■ CMP with magnesium

■ EKG

■ Chest x-ray

■ Cardiac enzymes

■ 2-D echocardiogram

■ Signal-averaged EKG is a noninvasive test that often produces abnormal results in patients with VT who has a prior MI or RV dysplasia.

■ *Electrophysiologic study*: EP study is useful to determine if a focus is present in a patient presenting with nonsustained VT. A programmed electrical stimulation can reproduce the VT circuits.

Treatment

■ *Unstable/pulseless VT*: Will need cardioversion. Recently the American Heart Association revised the ACLS guidelines and gave more emphasis on CPR.

■ *Stable VT*: Amiodarone 150 mg IV bolus over 10 minutes, then 0.5 mg/min over 18 hours. Can be switched to PO eventually. Beta blockers can be used as well but are usually not the antiarrhythmics of choice.

■ RFA if isolated focus

■ ICD placement

Consultation

■ Cardiology (EP)

CONGESTIVE HEART FAILURE (CHF)

Definition

■ Failure of the heart to pump blood forward at a sufficient rate to meet the metabolic demands of the peripheral tissues, or ability to do so only at abnormally high cardiac filling pressures (Braunwald, Heart Disease, 6th ed., 2001).

Classification (New York Heart Association [NYHA])

■ *Class 1*: Symptomatic with greater than normal activity

■ *Class 2*: Symptomatic with ordinary activity

■ *Class 3*: Symptomatic with minimal activity

■ *Class 4*: Symptomatic at rest

Systolic dysfunction: Usually classified with an EF <40% (poor contractility)

Diastolic dysfunction: EF >50% associated with LVH (failure to relax and fill normally)

Etiology

Finding	Causes
Cardiac rhythm disorders	Complete heart block
	Supraventricular tachycardia
	Ventricular tachycardia
	Sinus node dysfunction
Volume overload	Structural heart disease (eg, VSD, PDA, AR, mitral regurgitation, complex cardiac lesions)
	Anemia
	Sepsis
Pressure overload	Structural heart disease (eg, AS, PS, aortic coarctation)
	Hypertension
Systolic ventricular dysfunction or failure	Myocarditis
	Dilated cardiomyopathy
	Malnutrition
	Ischemia
Diastolic ventricular dysfunction or failure	Hypertrophic cardiomyopathy
	Restrictive cardiomyopathy
	Pericardial or cardiac tamponade

History

■ *Left-sided failure*: Dyspnea on exertion or rest, orthopnea, and paroxysmal nocturnal dyspnea (PND)

■ *Right-sided failure*: Peripheral edema, RUQ discomfort

■ Unexplained weight gain

Physical Examination

- *Heart*: S3, Elevated JVP >10, PCWP >22
- *Lungs*: Crackles or dullness at base due to bilateral pleural effusions
- *Abdomen*: Hepatojugular reflex
- *Extremity*: Peripheral edema

Diagnosis

Apart from the clinical examination, which is very important to identify CHF, there are numerous other tests that are necessary to elaborate on the diagnosis.

- CBC
- CMP
- *Hyponatremia*: Suggestive of fluid overloaded states
- *Transaminitis*: Suggestive of hepatic congestion
- *Chest x-ray*: Showing pulmonary edema, congestion, cephalization for fluid or pleural effusion
- NT pro BNP >400 signifies CHF. It is important to know the patient's baseline value as well.
- Some patients with chronic CHF can have elevated BNP values, which can be misleading.
- 2-D echocardiogram (evaluate EF, chamber size, wall motion abnormalities, LVH)

Treatment

- Most patients with CHF exacerbations are admitted due to noncompliance with their medications. Before initiating new medications, it may be more useful to titrate the current medications to appropriate levels.
- *Diet*: Exercise, Na <2 g/d, fluid restriction; exercise training in ambulatory patients or monitoring weight gain or loss in a hospitalized patient is the best way to assess if the treatment is working.
- *ACE inhibitors*: 40% decrease in mortality in NYHA IV (CONSENSUS). It is the agent of choice for afterload reduction in systolic heart failure.
- High-dose ACE-I (>30 mg/d of lisinopril) more efficacious than low-dose (5 mg/d)
- Watch for azotemia, hyperkalemia with ACE-I
- *ATII receptor blocker*: Consider in patients with low EF and symptoms, in addition to ACE-I or as an alternative if cannot tolerate ACE-I due to cough
- *Hydralazine + nitrates*: Consider if cannot tolerate ACE-I or ARB for afterload reduction
- *Beta blocker*: Indicated in both types of CHF but should be avoided in decompensated CHF
- A decrease of 35% in mortality in NYHA II-IV (U.S. Carvedilol trial)
- Carvedilol superior to metoprolol (COMET)

■ *Digoxin*: An excellent agent to assist with symptomatic heart failure. Goal level is between 0.5 and 0.8; 23% decrease in CHF hospitalizations.

■ *Diuretics*: Start with furosemide; dose can be adjusted based on the patient's prior experience with furosemide and renal function. Usually start at 40 mg IV bid, adjust dose after 6 h if needed. Goal, 1–2 liters negative in I/O over 24 h initially. Again, make changes based on the patient.

■ *Aldosterone antagonists*: Should be considered in severe heart failure NYHA Class III-IV. Need to monitor for hyperkalemia.

☐ *Spironolactone*: 25–50 mg PO bid initially, and then can titrate with cardiology input and assistance. Decrease in mortality is 30% in NYHA Class III-IV (RALES).

■ *Biventricular pacing*: Consider if refractory CHF and prolonged QRS (MIRACLE)

■ *ICD*: Consider as primary prevention if CAD and EF less than 30% (MADIT II, DEFINITE)

■ *Anticoagulation*: Can be considered if there is severe systolic dysfunction with LV hypokinesis (EF <30%), LV thrombus, or in the setting of atrial fibrillation.

Consultation

■ Cardiology

BRADYCARDIA

Sinus bradycardia is defined as sinus rhythm with a rate of 60 bpm or less. Patients usually become symptomatic when their heart rate drops to less than 50 bpm.

SINUS BRADYCARDIA/HEART BLOCKS

Etiology
- *Medications*: Beta blockers, CCB, amiodarone
- *Electrolyte imbalances*: Hyperkalemia, hypokalemia, hypomagnesemia, acidosis
- Increased vagal tone
- Sepsis
- Myxedema
- Myocardial infarction
- Myocarditis

Treatment
- *Mild to moderate bradycardia*: Stop the offending agent if any. Monitor the patient for improvement or potential heart blocks
- *Moderate to severe bradycardia:* Can start with atropine 0.5 mg IV while waiting for an IV pacemaker. If the bradycardia is severe, a permanent pacemaker should be placed eventually. If atropine was not successful, consider epinephrine 1 mg IV push or epinephrine 2–10 µg/min infusion or dopamine 2–10 µg/min infusion in anticipation of an IV pacemaker

1st Degree
- AV block prolonged PR >200 msec but all impulses conducted. No treatment needed.

2nd Degree Mobitz Type I
- Progressive increase in PR until impulse not conducted (Wenckebach). Usually AV nodal in origin and transient. Seen in IMI, myocarditis
- Often no treatment is required.

2nd Degree Mobitz Type II
- Occasional or repetitive blocked impulses without increase in PR interval
- His-Purkinje in origin, can lead to a complete heart block.
- Seen in anteroseptal MI, degeneration of conduction system. This block worsens with atropine.
- Intravenous pacer should be placed initially followed by permanent pacemaker.

3rd Degree AV block or Complete Heart Block
- No conduction. Must distinguish from other forms of AV dissociations. Needs intravenous pacer and eventual permanent pacemaker.

Consultation
- Cardiology, emergency physician

HYPERTENSIVE CRISIS

- *Hypertensive emergency*: Elevated blood pressure, SBP >210, DBP >120 with end organ damage
- *Hypertensive urgency*: SBP >210 or DBP >120 without end organ damage
- This is an actual emergency as the elevated blood pressure is causing organ damage and will continue to do so until the blood pressure is controlled quickly.

Etiology
- *Cardiac*: MI, CHF, aortic dissection
- *Renal*: Acute renal failure
- *Neurologic*: Encephalopathy, visual changes, papilledema
- *Endocrine*: Pheochromocytoma, primary hyperaldosteronism
- Preeclampsia and eclampsia

History
- Patients might complain of headaches, blurred vision. In severe situations they can have end organ damage when presenting with severe chest pain from an MI, neurologic symptoms from a stroke or TIA. Severe chest pain radiating to the shoulder blades should make you think about aortic dissection.

Physical Examination
- *HEENT*: Look for papilledema on fundus exam, features of hypertensive retinopathy
- *Heart*: Murmurs might be present
- *Abdomen*: Hepatomegaly possible
- *Neuro*: Look for focal deficits, encephalopathy; mini mental exam needed, coma can occur.

Diagnosis
- CBC
- *CMP*: Evaluate renal failure
- *Cardiac enzymes*: CK, CK-MB and troponin q6h × 3
- CT scan of the chest with IV contrast if looking for aortic dissection
- Renal ultrasound
- Captopril renal scan
- Evaluate for endocrine disorders like pheochromocytoma, hyperadrenalism
- *EKG*: Look for LVH
- 2-D echocardiogram

Treatment

- ■ Reduce blood pressure over several hours in the case of hypertensive urgency using PO agents.
- ■ Hypertensive emergency is a real emergency; we need to decrease the BP by 25% within minutes to 2 hours by the IV route.

Intravenous agents:

- ■ *Nitroprusside*: 0.25–4 µg/kg/min
- ■ *Nitroglycerin*: 5–200 mcg/min
- ■ *Labetelol*: 20–80 mg bolus IV over 10 minutes or 2–4 mg/min drip
- ■ *Hydralazine*: 10–20 mg IV q2–4h
- ■ *Phentolamine*: 5–15 mg IV bolus prn (not the first agent of choice)

Oral agents:

- ■ *Captopril*: 25–50 mg PO tid
- ■ *Labetelol*: 200–400 mg PO q6–12h
- ■ *Clonidine*: 0.2 mg PO load then 0.1 mg q h
- ■ *Hydralazine*: 10–50 mg PO q6h

Consultation

- ■ Cardiology

EKG REVIEW

- EKG is an integral part of hospital medicine and is read for almost every patient. A hospitalist needs to be proficient in the art of reading an EKG.
- *P wave*: Atrial depolarization
- *QRS complex*: Ventricular depolarization
- *T wave*: Ventricular repolarization

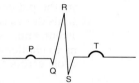

P wave : Atrial Depolarization
QRS complex: Ventricular Depolarization
T wave : Ventricular Repolarization

STEP I

Rate
Locate the QRS *complex* and then count either forward or backward to the next QRS complex. Count each large box in a forward or backward fashion as shown "300–150-100–75-60–50" to estimate the rate in *beats per minute*.

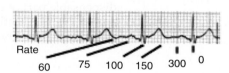

STEP 2

Rhythm
It is important to know whether the rhythm is regular or irregular. Look for a P wave before every QRS. It is sinus rhythm if there is a P wave before every QRS complex.

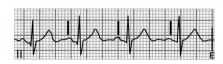

There should only be one P wave before each QRS. The P wave should be in only one direction, and not biphasic (except for leads V1 and V2).

STEP 3

Axis

A wave that is traveling **toward** the positive (+) lead will inscribe an upward deflection of the EKG; conversely a wave traveling **away** from the positive lead will inscribe a downward deflection. Waves that are traveling at a **90° angle** to a particular lead will create no deflection and are called **isoelectric** leads. First, determine if leads I and AVF are mostly positive, mostly negative, or isoelectric to determine your quadrant. Next, find your most isoelectric limb lead. Now, determine what lead is perpendicular to that biphasic lead and that is the axis vector.

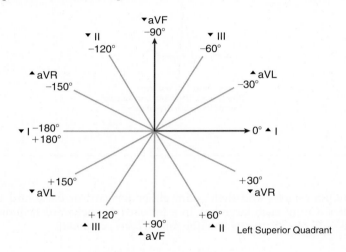

STEP 4

Intervals

Always measure the intervals and look for blocks.

PR Interval

- Represents atrial depolarization plus the normal delay at the AV node.
- Normally = 0.12–0.20 seconds. (No longer than one large box.)
- Increased in length if AV conduction is prolonged (first-degree AV block).

PR Segment

- Begins at the end of the P wave and ends with the onset of the QRS complex.

QRS Complex

- Represents depolarization of the ventricular myocardium.

Normal QRS Characteristics
- 0.07–0.11 seconds in width. QRS widths often vary in different leads. Commonly measured in lead I, II, and V1
- Should not be smaller than 6 mm in leads I, II, and III and nor should it be taller than 25–30 mm in the precordial leads

QT Interval
- Measurement of the refractory period or the time during which the myocardium would not respond to a second impulse; measured from the beginning of the QRS complex to the end of the T wave.
- Best measured in V_2 or V_3.
- *QT interval should be roughly less than half the preceding RR interval.*
- It is longer with slower rates and shorter with faster rates. Normal rates also vary with age and gender.
- If a QT table is not available, the QT interval can be corrected for heart rate using Basset's formula:

$$QTc = \frac{QT \text{ interval (secs)}}{\sqrt{RR \text{ interval (secs)}}}$$

STEP 5

Precordial leads/ ischemia or infarction:
- Inferior: II, III, and aVF, supplied by the right coronary artery
- Anterior/septal: V1-V4: Supplied by the LAD (left anterior descending artery)
- Lateral: I, aVL, V5-V6: Supplied by the circumflex artery

Transmural Ischemia
Acute transmural ischemia extends from the endocardium to the epicardium and causes the elevation of the ST segment of the EKG. This is visualized by the ST-segment being raised above the isoelectric baseline.

ST-SEGMENT ELEVATION

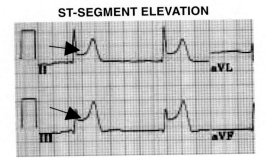

It is important to differentiate pathologic ST segment elevation from non-pathologic **J-point** elevation. J-point elevation is identified by an elevation of the terminal portion of the QRS which then *dips back down* toward the baseline before rising back up to the ST segment.

J-POINT ELEVATION

After the ischemia has progressed to an infarct, and the tissue has scarred, the EKG will show an inverted T wave. Eventually Q waves will also be formed.

Q WAVES WITH INVERTED T WAVES

Subendocardial Ischemia
ST-segment depression can signify an acute ischemic event or submyocardial infarction.

ST-SEGMENT DEPRESSION IN SUBENDOCARDIAL ISCHEMIA

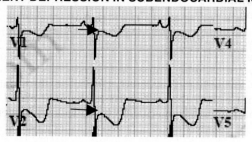

STEP 6

Blocks

When there is an interruption of electrical impulses traveling from the SA node to the ventricles. The blocks can occur in the SA and AV nodes as well as in the bundles.

SA Node Block

This consists of a failure of the SA node to transmit an impulse, and is usually seen as a "skipped beat." This block can occur occasionally in normal patient.

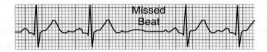

AV Node Block

This occurs when there is delay in the conduction of an impulse from the atria to the ventricles in the AV node. The criterion for 1st degree AV node block is a PR interval greater than .2 seconds (200 msec or 1 large box). Below we see an example of 1st degree AV node block.

1ST DEGREE AV BLOCK: PR INTERVAL >200 MS

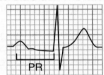

2nd Degree AV Block

This is a more advanced block. It is subclassified into Type I and Type II. Type I or Wenckeback block occurs at the AV node and is seen as a progressively increasing PR interval with an eventual skipped beat, whereas Mobitz Type II block can occur at the AV node or above it making it more advanced. In this type of block the PR interval is fixed with an eventual skipped beat. If more than 1 P wave preceding each QRS complex can be seen it is a 2:1 block. We see this below where there is a 2:1 ratio of P waves to each QRS.

2ND DEGREE AV BLOCK WITH A 2:1 P WAVE RATIO

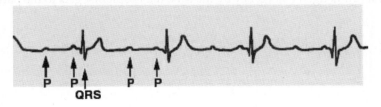

3rd Degree Block

This is a complete block of signals from the atria to the ventricles. It can present as AV dissociation. The P waves will be in a normal sinus rate, while the QRS will be either in a **nodal** rhythm (60 bpm) or a **ventricular** rhythm (30–40 bpm).

3RD DEGREE BLOCK OR COMPLETE HEART BLOCK

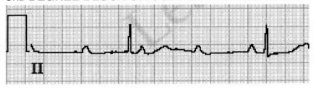

Bundle Branch Blocks (BBBs)

BBBs are blocks within the bundle of His, and normally consist of a left or right BBB. The key to recognizing a bundle block is to find an **R-R′** wave. The criteria consist of a QRS wider than .12 seconds (3 mm) and the 2 R waves. In left bundle branch block (LBBB) QRS >120 ms, monophasic R wave in I, V5, and V6, deflection of the ST and T wave in the opposite direction to the QRS deflection. In RBBB, QRS >120 ms, RSR′ pattern seen in the precordial leads and a wide S wave in I, V5, and V6.

Below we see examples of right and left BBBs.

RIGHT BUNDLE BRANCH BLOCK (LEAD V1)

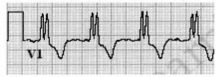

LEFT BUNDLE BRANCH BLOCK (LEAD V1)

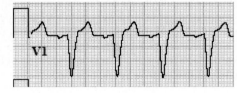

STEP 7

Other Important Rhythms
Ventricular Fibrillation
Ventricular fibrillation (**V-Fib or VF**) is the most life-threatening arrhythmia and is often the end rhythm before the **asystole** of death.

    The EKG pattern of V-Fib is recognized by a total lack of organized activity, ranging from **course** (large amplitude) to **fine** (close to asystole) in amplitude. This rhythm needs defibrillation. Below are examples of course and fine V-Fib.

COURSE AND FINE VENTRICULAR FIBRILLATION

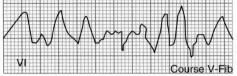 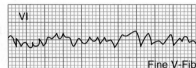

Supraventricular Tachycardias
Multifocal Atrial Tachycardia (MAT)
This arrhythmia is seen with an ectopic pacemaker somewhere in the atria. The abnormal pacemaker cell has stopped responding to the overdrive pacing from the sinus node. This causes there to be two or more asynchronous pacemakers for the heart. The hallmark of this form of SVT is the two or more P wave morphologies you see: one P wave from each pacemaker. Surprisingly this rhythm can often be broken by exercise or sinus tachycardia; the reason for this is that although the end result of MAT is tachycardia, each of the pacemakers is not tachycardia—it is the sum of their rates that produces the tachycardia. In exercise or other excitatory states, the sinus node will overdrive pace the ectopic cells.

MULTIFOCAL ATRIAL TACHYCARDIA

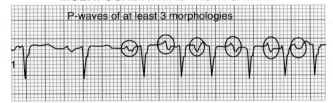

Atrial Flutter

The atria can also produce a flutter pattern, which is characterized by multiple, sawtooth-edged P waves before each QRS, called **flutter-waves**. This rhythm can progress to **atrial fibrillation**.

ATRIAL FLUTTER

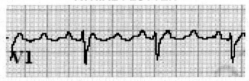

Atrial Fibrillation

Atrial fibrillation produces an irregularly irregular rhythm which is characterized by absence of P waves before every QRS complex. The rate of conduction is limited only by the AV node; in conditions of rapid conduction, such as Wolff-Parkinson-White (WPW) syndrome, where the conduction bypasses the node, the rate can approach 200–300 bpm.

ATRIAL FIBRILLATION

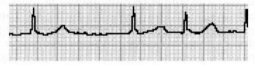

Ventricular Tachycardia

This originates from the ventricles and can be a life-threatening rhythm. It is a wide complex tachycardia. Below we see an example of V-Tach, with a ventricular rate of 150 bpm.

VENTRICULAR TACHYCARDIA

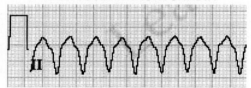

HYPERKALEMIA

This is a very important electrolyte abnormality that can cause some serious damage to the myocardium. It could potentially result in PEA or asystole. It is initially discovered on an EKG as peaked T waves that are more commonly seen with K levels >6. The other feature of the hyperkalemic EKG is a stretching of the entire waveform. Widening of the QRS, PR interval, and sine wave can be seen in severe hyperkalemia.

**PEAKED-T WAVES CONSISTENT
WITH HYPERKALEMIA**

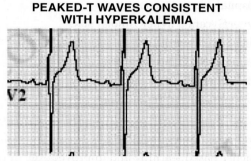

Adapted with permission from Feldman, Henry et al., A Guide to Reading and Understanding EKG, 1999; http://www.scribd.com/doc/6454322/Easy-ECG-Guide

PULMONARY DISEASES

ASTHMA

This is a chronic inflammatory disorder with airway hyperresponsiveness and airflow obstruction.

Etiology and Precipitants
- Allergens (house pets, carpets, dust mites, pollen)
- Respiratory irritants (perfumes, smoke, laundry detergents, strong odors)
- Respiratory infections such as pneumonia, bronchitis, URI
- Drugs such as ASA, beta blockers
- Noncompliance with asthma medications

History
- Clinical manifestations include the triad of wheezing, cough, and dyspnea.
- Patients would generally give a history of pollen allergy or other common precipitants. Also ask about new pets, detergents, or change of environment both at work and at home.
- During exacerbations it is important to note frequency, severity, duration, and required treatment.

Physical Examination
- *HEENT*: Presence of nasal polyps, rhinitis, rash, allergic component
- *Heart*: Tachycardia can be seen
- *Lungs*: Wheezing and prolonged expiratory phase
- Exacerbation may have pulsus paradoxus, use of accessory muscles of respiration

Diagnosis
- ABG
- CBC
- CMP
- Chest x-ray
- Blood culture if febrile or pneumonia suspected
- Sputum gram stain and culture

Pulmonary Function Test (PFT) in Asthma

■ Decrease in PEF rate

■ Spirometry shows low FEV1 and FEV1/ FVC

■ *Lung volumes*: Increased RV and TLC

■ A positive bronchodilator response (FEV1 >12%) strongly suggestive of asthma

■ If allergy suspected then consider serum IgE, eosinophils; skin testing/RAST should be ordered

Asthma Severity

■ *Mild*: Dyspnea on exertion but able to talk in full sentences, PEFR >80%, wheezing present. Less than two episodes per week.

■ *Moderate*: Dyspnea while talking, wheezing present, PEFR 50–80% and some use of accessory muscles of respiration. Greater than two episodes per week

■ *Severe*: Dyspnea at rest, diffuse wheezing, unable to talk, use of accessory muscles of respiration. Continuous symptoms. PEFR <50%.

Treatment of Asthma Exacerbation

■ Titrate oxygen to achieve saturation of >90%.

■ Albuterol MDl 4–8 puffs q20min or nebulizer 2.5–5.0 mg q20min and continuous if severe

■ Corticosteroids like prednisone 60 mg PO or methylprednisolone 80 mg IV q6–8h

■ Magnesium 2 mg IV over 20 minutes

■ Other agents that could be used:

  ☐ Epinephrine (0.3–0.5 ml SC of 1:1000 dilution): no advantage over inhaled B2-agonists

  ☐ Steroid inhalers can be added to optimize treatment.

  ☐ Montelukast 10 mg PO daily can be added to the asthma maintenance regimen.

■ Antibiotics have no role in the treatment of asthma unless associated pneumonia or other sources of bacterial infection are present.

Consultation

■ Pulmonary

CHRONIC OBSTRUCTIVE PULMONARY DISEASE (COPD)

Chronic obstructive pulmonary disease is a destructive process involving the large (central) airways, the small (peripheral) bronchioles, and the lung parenchyma.

Types
- Chronic bronchitis
- Emphysema

Etiology
- *Exposure to tobacco smoke*: Clinically significant COPD develops in 15% of cigarette smokers. It has been shown that passive inhalation of smoke (either second hand or environmental tobacco smoke) can increase the risk of respiratory infections.
- *Air pollution*: It plays a small role compared to cigarette smoking.
- Airway hyperresponsiveness
- *Alpha-1-antitrypsin deficiency*: AAT deficiency is the only known genetic risk factor for developing COPD and accounts for less than 1% of all cases in the United States.

History
- Shortness of breath is the main complaint with or without wheezing.
- Patients with COPD usually have a smoking history and sometime it takes several decades before the onset of symptoms.
- Fever, chills could represent an associated pneumonia. Cough could be present in both COPD and pneumonia.
- In severe situations cyanosis can occur.

Physical Examination
- Increased respiratory rate with or without use of accessory muscles of respiration.
- *Lungs*: Hyperinflation (barrel chest), wheezing, decreased breath sounds, hyperresonance on percussion, and prolonged expiration. Inspiratory crackles and rhonchi may be heard, and wheezes frequently are heard on forced and unforced expiration.
- In severe disease, cyanosis, elevated JVP, and peripheral edema are observed.

Diagnosis
- CBC
- CMP
- Chest x-ray
- CT scan of the chest if needed

- *PFT*: Obstructive disease, decreased FEV_1, decreased FEV_1/FVC ratio, decreased DLCO in emphysema, increased residual volume, total lung capacity ABG, EKG, could show right heart strain in the setting of cor pulmonale

Treatment of Acute Exacerbation

- *Oxygen*: Titrate to keep saturation 88–92%
- *Antibiotics*: Ceftriaxone 1 g IV q24h and azithromycin 500 mg IV q24h or levofloxacin 750 mg IV/PO daily. Goal is to cover typical and atypical organisms.
- *Ipratropium bromide*: First-line therapy, either MDI or nebulizers. Studies have not shown benefit of one over the other. Inhalation or nebulizer q4h as needed. Spiriva (tiotropium bromide) 18 mcg inhalation daily has been a recent advancement both in the acute and outpatient setting.
- Albuterol MDI or nebulizer 2.5–5 mg q4h as needed.
- *Corticosteroids*: No definite data on the mortality benefit of steroids in COPD but it has reduced hospital readmission rates. Studies have used methylprednisolone 125 mg IV q6h × 72 hours then transition to prednisone 60 mg PO daily × 4 days and taper over 10–12 days.
- Theophylline 100–300 mg PO bid. Not routinely used but just another option.
- *Noninvasive ventilation*: BiPAP; consider if retaining CO_2. If able to tolerate, can decrease the likelihood of intubation, improve mortality.
- Consider intubation if the above treatment fails.
- Once patient is stable, evaluate for home oxygen as that has proven to decrease mortality. It is usually indicated if $PaO_2 < 55$ or $SaO_2 < 89$.

Consultation

- Pulmonary

PULMONARY EMBOLISM (PE)

Embolism of thrombus from the venous system and migrates into the pulmonary arterial circulation. Can be fatal.

Etiology

■ *Hypercoagulable states*: Prolonged venous stasis or significant injury to the veins. Hypercoagulable states may be acquired or congenital. Most common genetic mutation in adults is "Factor V Leiden."

■ Deficiency of protein C, protein S, and antithrombin III; prothrombin gene mutation and antiphospholipid antibody syndrome.

■ *Risk markers*: The major risk factors for DVT and PE are a prior history of DVT or PE, recent surgery or pregnancy, prolonged immobilization, malignancy, long travel >4 h, and a history of hypercoagulable disorders.

History

■ PE should be considered in every patient who presents with any chest symptoms that cannot be proven to have another cause.

■ Symptoms of chest pain, chest wall tenderness, back pain, shoulder pain, upper abdominal pain, syncope, hemoptysis, shortness of breath, and painful respiration should heighten the suspicion of PE.

■ The classic triad of signs and symptoms of PE include hemoptysis, dyspnea, and chest pain.

■ Many patients with PE are initially completely asymptomatic and can have atypical presentation.

■ Pleuritic or sharp chest pain which might not be exertional chest pain is a particularly worrisome symptom.

Physical Examination

■ Hemodynamic instability can occur in a massive PE causing hypotension, chest pain, and severe hypoxia.

■ *Lungs*: Wheezing, pulmonary rub, chest wall tenderness without a good history of trauma, because patients with PE may have chest wall tenderness as the only physical finding.

■ Three most common signs in these patients are tachypnea, rales, and an accentuated second heart sound.

Diagnosis

■ CBC

■ CMP

■ *Chest x-ray*: Initial x-ray in PE is mostly normal but on occasion a Hampton's hump can be seen on an x-ray.

■ High resolution CT pulmonary angiogram has been found to be very sensitive and has a negative predictive value of greater than 99%.

- *V/Q scan of the lungs*: If unable to tolerate the dye required for pulmonary angiogram. High probability confirms PE, intermediate probability may require lower extremity Doppler studies to confirm the PE and low probability study almost rules out PE unless there is high clinical suspicion.
- *Echocardiogram*: To evaluate for RV dilation and hypokinesis. This can determine the prognosis of these patients.
- *Pulmonary angiography*: It's the gold standard but not routinely done.
- *EKG*: Tachycardia and nonspecific ST-T wave abnormalities. The finding of S1-Q3-T3 is nonspecific and insensitive in the absence of high clinical suspicion for a PE but signifies right heart strain.
- Hypercoagulable profile (Factor V Leiden, antithrombin III, homocysteine level, proteins C and S, antiphospholipid antibody, and prothrombin gene mutation)
- *D-Dimer*: Negative ELISA has higher negative predictive value than latex agglutination test

Treatment

- *Oxygen*: Titrate to keep saturation >92%
- *Anticoagulation*: Low molecular weight heparin such as enoxaparin at the full therapeutic dose of 1 mg/kg SC bid, overlap with warfarin 5 mg PO daily × 2 days or 10 mg PO daily × 2 days load followed by a maintenance dose. Please overlap for 1–2 more days once INR 2–3.
- *Fibronolysis*: Only indicated in massive unstable PE. Its indication for RV dilatation and hypokinesis is debated.
- Duration of treatment is usually 3–6 months but could be extended in the presence of high risk coagulable states.
- Such as idiopathic PE >6 months
- Cancer, nonmodifiable risk factor: 12 months to lifetime.

Consultation

- Pulmonary

COMMUNITY ACQUIRED PNEUMONIA (CAP)

This is the most common type of pneumonia. It can occur as a result of inhalation or aspiration of bacterial pathogen into the lungs.

Etiology

Typical Bacterial Pathogens in CAP (Approximately 85%)

- *Streptococcus pneumoniae*
  - ☐ Penicillin-sensitive *S pneumoniae*
  - ☐ Penicillin-resistant *S pneumoniae*
- *Hemophilous influenzae*
  - ☐ Ampicillin-sensitive *H influenzae*
  - ☐ Ampicillin-resistant *H influenzae*
- *Moraxella catarrhalis*

Atypical Respiratory Pathogens in CAP (Approximately 15%)

- *Legionella* species
- *Mycoplasma* species
- *C pneumoniae*

Other Bacterial Pathogens

- *Klebsiella pneumoniae*: Mostly in alcoholics and also in patients who stay heavily sedated.
- *Staphylococcus aureus*
- *Pseudomonas aeruginosa*: Only in patients with cystic fibrosis or bronchiectasis. Also seen if the patient was institutionalized.

History

- Patients with CAP can present with fever, chills, pleuritic chest pain, and productive cough. History of sick contacts should also be obtained.
- Clinical presentation in patients with CAP due to atypical pathogens usually is less acute than in those with typical bacterial pathogens but can have extra pulmonary features which can help differentiate them.
- *Legionella* species are the most important atypical pathogen causing CAP. Patients with *Legionella* infections may have a productive or nonproductive cough. It can also result in hepatic injury as seen with elevated transaminases.
- Blood-tinged sputum may be found with pneumococcal infections, *Klebsiella* pneumonia, or *Legionella* pneumonia.
- Vector-borne infections such as Q fever and psittacosis should be investigated if there is a known history of vector exposure. These pneumonias can cause bradycardia as well.
- Legionnaires disease can also cause bradycardia hence the above zoonotic pneumonias need to be eliminated from the history before that diagnosis is made.

Physical Examination

■ *Lungs*: Decreased breath sounds at the region of consolidation, increased fremitus, bronchial breathing, and E to A change may be present. Increased rales are heard upon auscultation of the chest over the involved lobe or segment. Patients with pleural effusion (usually due to *Haemophilus influenzae*) have signs of pleural effusion if it is large enough to be detected during the physical examination.

■ Patients with pleural effusion have diminished tactile fremitus and dullness upon chest percussion.

Diagnosis

■ CBC

■ *CMP*: LFT elevated in *Legionella* pneumonia

■ Blood culture × 2 prior to administration of antibiotics

■ Sputum gram stain and culture

■ ABG if needed

■ Oxygen

■ Chest x-ray

■ CT scan of the chest if needed

■ Urine *Legionella* antigen if suspected

■ Cold agglutinins ($\geq$1:64) for mycoplasma

Treatment

■ Oxygen to keep saturation >92% unless COPD

■ Empiric antibiotics should cover both typical and atypical organisms. Commonly used antibiotics are

■ *Ceftriaxone*: 1 g IV q24h and azithromycin 500 mg IV q24h

  or

■ *Levofloxacin*: 750 mg IV q24h

  or

■ *Doxycycline*: 100 mg IV bid

■ Once the organism is identified then the antibiotics can be narrowed.

■ Pseudomonas should be suspected for nosocomial pneumonias; if so, the agent of choice is piperacillin/tazobactam 4.5 g IV q6h.

■ Always calculate the dose of an antibiotic based on the creatinine clearance. Certain antibiotics like ceftriaxone do not need to be renal dosed.

Consultation

■ Pulmonary

GASTROENTEROLOGY

GASTROINTESTINAL (GI) BLEEDING

Gastrointestinal bleeding (GI bleed) signifies internal hemorrhage involving the upper or lower part of the GI tract and manifests as hematemesis, melena, or bright red blood per rectum.

Etiology
- *Upper GI bleed*: Erosive gastritis, peptic ulcer disease, esophageal varices, AVM, and Mallory-Weiss tears. Medications such as aspirin, NSAIDs, clopidogrel, and warfarin can cause or worsen an ulcer.
- *Lower GI bleed*: Diverticulosis, angiodysplasia, cancer, chronic constipation, and recent instrumentation.
- Coagulation disorders can exacerbate a GI bleed.

History
- Patients may complain of melena which can be a symptom of upper GI bleed, although right-sided colonic bleeds can also present as melena.
- Hematemesis or coffee-ground emesis signifies an upper GI source of bleeding.
- Bright red blood per rectum is usually a symptom of lower GI bleed but in certain situations an upper GI bleed can also present as bleeding per rectum. This could be very critical as hemodynamic compromise or shock could be present.
- Significant weight loss and anemia could be early signs of cancer.

Physical Examination
- Patients with active bleeding can be hypotensive or tachycardic suggesting hemodynamic compromise.
- *HEENT*: Pallor
- *Heart*: Tachycardia
- *Abdomen*: Epigastric or lower abdominal tenderness. Peritoneal signs can suggest a perforated ulcer.

Diagnosis
- NG aspiration to confirm an upper GI bleed.
- CBC
- CMP
- Coagulation profile
- Type and cross
- Hb and Hct q6–8h

Treatment

■ GI consult for either upper endoscopy or colonoscopy

■ Remember the ABCs.

■ Protect the airway.

■ Stabilize the patient first. Make sure the patient has two large bore IVs. Initiate isotonic saline or lactated Ringer solutions.

■ Packed red blood cell transfusion

■ Correct the coagulation abnormalities with fresh frozen plasma (FFP) and/or vitamin K. Initially 2–4 units of FFP may be needed. Based on the INR, the dose of vitamin K can be adjusted.

■ *Diet*: Either NPO if actively bleeding or clear liquids with no red or purple colors if not currently bleeding and endoscopy is planned the following day.

■ PPIs such as pantoprazole IV bid or as a drip.

■ Variceal bleed can be deadly. Octreotide 50–100 mcg bolus followed by 25–50 mcg/h infusion should be initiated while waiting for endoscopy for variceal banding or ligation. Nadolol or propranolol can help reduce portal hypertension. TIPS procedure could be needed to reduce portal pressures eventually.

■ Tagged RBC technetium-99 scan to locate the source of lower GI bleed.

■ Capsule endoscopy may be useful for those small bowel bleeds that cannot be reached by an endoscope.

■ Maintenance therapy for PUD, erosive gastritis: Gradually advance the diet at discharge. PPI such as pantoprozole 40 mg PO bid until seen by the gastroenterologist as outpatient.

Consultation

■ Gastroenterology

ACUTE PANCREATITIS

Acute pancreatitis refers to inflammation of the pancreas resulting in sudden onset of severe abdominal pain.

Etiology

- It is reported that nearly 60–75% of acute pancreatitis is caused by either alcohol or gallstones.
- *Gallstone pancreatitis*: It is one of the major causes of pancreatitis. Since the cystic duct and the pancreatic duct are connected by the common bile duct, any stone lodged in the common bile duct (CBD) can precipitate pancreatitis.
- *Alcoholic pancreatitis*: Alcohol is also a common cause of acute pancreatitis. Alcoholic pancreatitis is more common in men than women. Patients with long-standing alcohol abuse history are at higher risk.
- *Hereditary conditions*: Familial hypertriglyceridemia and hereditary pancreatitis.
- *Drug-induced pancreatitis*: Drugs such as DDI, 6-mercaptopurine, 6-MP, ACE inhibitors.
- *Post-ERCP*: Nearly 3–5% of patients can develop acute pancreatitis post-ERCP.
- *Severe triglyceridemia*: This can be a major cause of pancreatitis as well. When triglyceride values exceed 600, the patient can be at a higher risk for pancreatitis. This can be both acquired or hereditary.
- *Idiopathic*: Nearly 20% of pancreatitis might not have an etiology.

History

- Sudden, constant pain in the epigastric region is the most common symptom of acute pancreatitis.
- Right upper quadrant tenderness radiating to the back and the right shoulder can be mistaken for biliary colic but this pain is not intermittent as seen in biliary colic. It is constant.
- Acute pancreatitis caused by alcohol abuse usually occurs 2–3 days after a binge or the last alcoholic drink.
- A detailed history outlining the above etiologies is very important.

Physical Examination

- *Lungs*: Decreased breath sounds at the base could be due to pleural effusion.
- *Abdomen*: Evaluate for peritonitis, "Cullen's sign" and "Grey Turner's sign." These could be a sign of retroperitoneal hemorrhage. RUQ or epigastric tenderness.
- *Neurology*: Mental status changes can occur.

Diagnosis

- CBC
- CMP

- Amylase, lipase (more sensitive)
- LDH
- Triglycerides and lipid profile
- CT scan of the abdomen and pelvis with IV contrast to rule out necrotizing pancreatitis.
- *Ultrasound of the abdomen*: Evaluate the CBD for dilatation, pseudocyst.
- *KUB*: Sentinel loop of bowel
- *Serum triglyceride levels*: In patients with pancreatitis due to hypertriglyceridemia, the triglyceride levels are usually very high (>1000 mg/dL with normal being 150 mg/dL).

RANSON'S CRITERIA

At admission:
- Age in years >55 years
- White blood cell count >16,000 cells/mm^3
- Blood glucose >11 mmol/L (>200 mg/dL)
- Serum AST >250 IU/L
- Serum LDH >350 IU/L

At 48 hours:
1. Calcium (serum calcium <2.0 mmol/L (<8.0 mg/dL)
2. Hematocrit fall >10%
3. Oxygen (hypoxemia PO$_2$ <60 mm Hg)
4. BUN increased by 1.8 or more mmol/L (5 or more mg/dL) after IV fluid hydration
5. Base deficit (negative base excess) >4 mEq/L
6. Sequestration of fluids >6 L

Interpretation
- Score 0 to 2: 2% mortality
- Score 3 to 4: 15% mortality
- Score 5 to 6: 40% mortality
- Score 7 to 8: 100% mortality

Source: Ranson JH, Rifkind KM, Roses DF, Fink SD, Eng K, Spencer FC. Prognostic signs and the role of operative management in acute pancreatitis. *Surg Gynec Obstet* 1974;139(1):69–81.

Treatment
The goals are to identify and treat the underlying cause of pancreatitis thus improving the pancreatic inflammation. Patients are usually admitted as inpatients and require a few days of therapy. Always remember that pancreatitis can "kill." Be cautious when treating pancreatitis. A mild case of pancreatitis can very quickly turn to severe if the appropriate treatment is not started early.

■ *Mild pancreatitis*: Mild pancreatitis is self-limited, and requires supportive care such as monitoring, drugs to control the pain, and IV fluids. Keep NPO until pain resolves. IV fluid should be administered at a high rate unless the patient has CHF.

■ *Moderate to severe pancreatitis*: Moderate to severe pancreatitis requires more detailed monitoring and supportive care. Keep NPO, high rate of IV fluids, mainly isotonic saline. When necrotizing pancreatitis is suspected, antibiotics and surgery may be needed.

Monitoring

■ *Intravenous fluids*: IVF should be initiated early at a high rate to prevent dehydration as pancreatitis is a distributive process that can deplete the intravascular volume in severe cases.

■ *Feeding and eating*: Studies suggest that early enteral feeding through temporary tubes like "Dobhoff" may actually help prevent infections, and can reduce complications.

■ *Parenteral feeding*: Via PICC or central line is an alternative for people who cannot tolerate enteral feeding or who cannot get enough nutrients with enteral feeding.

■ *Antibiotics*: Goal is to cover gram negatives and anerobes. Should be initiated if necrotizing pancreatitis is suspected. Ampicillin-sulbactem or imipenem is recommended.

■ *Surgical debridement*: When acute pancreatitis is complicated by necrosis, timely debridement or necrosectomy might be needed. This is usually done at larger centers as prolonged surgical care might be needed.

■ *Specific treatments of gallstone pancreatitis*: Once the pancreatitis resolves, patient should get a cholecystectomy with intraoperative cholangiogram or an ERCP before the procedure.

Consultation

■ Surgery

■ Gastroenterology

ILEUS

Ileus is caused as a result of hypomotility of the gastrointestinal tract. The impaired propulsive action of the bowels can lead to an ileus or partial small bowel obstruction.

Etiology

Iatrogenic

- Medication such as opiods, anticholinergic agents
- Sepsis
- Constipation
- Electrolyte imbalances such as hypokalemia, hyperkalemia, hyponatremia, and hypomagnesemia
- Pneumonia
- MI biliary colic
- Peritonitis

Postoperative

- Intraabdominal or neurosurgical procedures

DIFFERENTIATING ILEUS, PSEUDO-OBSTRUCTION, AND SIMPLE MECHANICAL OBSTRUCTION

	Ileus	Mechanical Obstruction	Pseudo-obstruction
Symptoms	Abdominal pain, bloating, nausea, vomiting, obstipation, constipation	Crampy abdominal pain, constipation, obstipation, nausea, vomiting, anorexia	Crampy abdominal pain, constipation, obstipation, nausea, vomiting, anorexia
Physical examination findings	Abdominal, distension, tympanic, slightly diminished bowel sounds	Borborygmi, peristaltic waves, high-pitched bowel sounds, distension, localized tenderness	Borborygmi, tympanic, peristaltic waves, hypoactive or hyperactive bowel sounds, distension, localized tenderness
X-ray findings	Large and small bowel dilatation	Step-ladder pattern of bowel loops, air-fluid levels paucity of colonic gas distal to lesion, diaphragm mildly elevated	Mainly large bowel dilatation, diaphragm elevated

Source: Adapted with permission from Mukherjee, S. Ileus. eMedicine Journal [serial online]. 2008, available at http://emedicine.medscape.com/article/178948-overview.

History

Patients with ileus present with feeling of fatigue, mild abdominal pain, and a bloating sensation. Nausea and vomiting may or may not be present initially but are usually present in more advanced cases. Patients may or may not continue to pass flatus and stool.

Physical Examination

■ *Abdomen*: Distended, bowel sounds may be diminished or absent. It is important to differentiate them from the high-pitched bowel sounds of complete obstruction.

Diagnosis

■ CBC
■ CMP
■ Magnesium and phosphorus
■ If febrile, then blood cultures
■ *KUB flat and upright*: Ileus appears as gaseous dilatation of the small intestine and colon with or without air/fluid levels.
■ CT scan of the abdomen and pelvis with PO and IV contrast
■ Always keep mesenteric ischemia in the back of your mind.

Treatment

■ *Supportive treatment*: Most cases of postoperative ileus resolve with watchful waiting and supportive treatment.
■ IV fluids, mostly crystalloid.
■ If constipation is present, then appropriate laxatives or enema should be initiated.
■ Pain control with low dose opoids if at all. It can decrease the bowel motility, hence be careful.
■ NG suction, intermittent if small bowel obstruction suspected, no definite benefit for ileus
■ Mechanical obstruction should be excluded in patients with ileus unresponsive to supportive and conservative treatment with contrast imaging studies.
■ Correct any underlying electrolyte abnormality. Keep potassium level >4.
■ NSAIDs can replace the use of postoperative narcotics and can help in the setting of ileus by decreasing local inflammation. Care must be taken to avoid stress ulcers. Appropriate PPIs or H2 blockers should also be started.
■ *Diet*: Keep the patient NPO until flatus is passed or the patient starts having a regular bowel function. Enteral feeding can be initiated but residuals need to be checked diligently.
■ *Activity*: Ambulation may improve bowel motility but it has not been proven in studies.

■ Use of prokinetic agents has had moderate success.

■ Erythromycin, a motilin receptor agonist, can be used for postoperative gastroparesis or diabetic gastroparesis but has not been effective in ileus.

■ Metoclopramide (Reglan), a dopaminergic antagonist, has antiemetic and prokinetic properties. Some studies have shown that it may actually worsen ileus.

Consultation

■ Surgery

■ Gastroenterology

NEPHROLOGY

ACUTE RENAL FAILURE

Sudden decrease in renal function from an acquired cause.

Etiology
Prerenal Failure

■ *Diminished blood volume*: CHF, cirrhosis, acute blood loss, sepsis

■ *Renal artery obstruction*: Renal arterial stenosis (atherosclerotic, fibromuscular dysplasia)

Intrinsic Renal Failure

■ Acute tubular necrosis, toxins such as contrast dye, heme pigments, drugs such as antibiotics.

■ Interstitial nephritis caused by drug reactions, autoimmune diseases (eg, systemic lupus erythematosus [SLE])

■ Nephrotic and nephritic syndromes

■ *Vascular*: HTN, vasculitis

Postrenal Failure

■ Mostly obstruction can cause this type of renal failure.

■ Stones at the level of the renal pelvis such as calcium oxalate, struvite, uric acid stones, etc.

■ *Ureteral obstruction*: Tumor, retroperitoneal fibrosis urolithiasis, papillary necrosis

■ *Urethral obstruction*: BPH, tumor of the GU tract such as prostate, cervical, bladder, and even colorectal carcinomas, bladder hematoma, bladder stones.

History

■ Patients can present with symptoms related to dehydration, including thirst, decreased urine output, fatigue, and orthostasis. This type of presentation is mainly seen in prerenal failure.

■ Look for a history of excessive fluid loss via hemorrhage, GI losses, sweating, or renal sources. Also, obtain a detailed history to evaluate for intrinsic and postrenal failure as well. Accurate medication history is essential.

■ Patients with severe heart failure can also have poor renal function presenting with orthopnea and PND.

■ Poor urinary output or oliguria can be a symptom of all types of renal failure.

Physical Examination

▦ Patients will complain of fatigue and altered mental status. Hypotension and tachycardia can suggest decreased renal perfusion. Signs of dehydration can also be seen.

▦ *HEENT*: Keratitis, iritis, uveitis, dry conjunctivae; autoimmune vasculitis, band keratopathy (ie, hypercalcemia); multiple myeloma, diabetic or hypertensive retinopathy, icterus suggestive of hepatic disorders. Dry mucous membranes.

▦ *Heart*: Elevated JVP, arrhythmias due to electrolyte imbalances, rales, S3.

▦ *Lungs*: Rales: Goodpasture syndrome, Wegener granulomatosis, pulmonary edema

▦ *Abdomen*: Costovertebral angle tenderness can be seen in nephrolithiasis, papillary necrosis, pelvic and rectal masses; prostatic hypertrophy; distended bladder due to urinary obstruction.

▦ *Skin*: Livido reticularis, palpable purpura as a sign of vasculitis, maculopapular rash seen in allergic nephritis.

Diagnosis

▦ *CBC*: Elevated WBC count seen in SLE, leulopenia, and thrombocytopenia suggest SLE or TTP; anemia and rouleaux formation suggest multiple myeloma; eosinophilia suggests allergic interstitial nephritis, polyarteritis nodosa, etc.

▦ *BMP*: To evaluate renal failure with elevated creatinine/BUN.

▦ *Urine output*:

☐ Anuria (<100 mL/d): Rapidly progressive GN, urinary tract obstruction, and renal artery obstruction.

☐ Oliguria (100–400 mL/d): All causes of prerenal failure; hepatorenal syndrome

☐ Nonoliguria (>400 mL/d): Acute GN, acute interstitial nephritis, ATN, radiocontrast-induced ARF, and rhabdomyolysis

URINALYSIS

Normal urinary sediment without blood, protein, cells or casts is consistent with prerenal and postrenal failure, HUS/thrombotic thrombocytopenic purpura (TTP)

Granular casts: ATN, acute GN, interstitial nephritis

RBC casts: Acute GN, severe HTN

WBC casts: Acute interstitial nephritis, pyelonephritis

Eosinophiluria: Acute allergic interstitial nephritis

Crystalluria: Ethylene glycol toxicity, acyclovir, sulfonamides, methotrexate, contrast dyes

▦ *Cockcroft-Gault equation*: GFR mL/min = (140 − age years) (weight in kg) × (0.85 if female)/(72 × serum creatinine mol/L)

▦ Coagulation profile disturbances indicate liver disease or hepatorenal syndrome.

▦ Elevations in liver transaminases are seen in hepatorenal syndrome. Elevated CK in acute MI and rhabdomyolysis.

In Prerenal Failure
- Urine specific gravity >1.018
- Urine osmolality (mOsm/kg H_2O) >500
- Urine sodium (mEq/L) <15–20
- Plasma BUN/creatinine ratio >20
- Urine/plasma creatinine ratio >40

In Acute Tubular Necrosis (ATN)
- Urine specific gravity <1.012
- Urine osmolality (mOsm/kg H_2O) <500
- Urine sodium (mEq/L) >40
- Plasma BUN/creatinine ratio <10–15
- Urine/plasma creatinine ratio <20

Calculation of Fractional Excretion of Sodium (FeNa)
- FeNa = (urine Na/plasma Na)/(urine creatinine/plasma creatinine)
- FeNa <1% = prerenal ARF
- FeNa >1% = ATN

Imaging Studies
- Chest radiography
- *Renal*: Ultrasound if RAS suspected
- CT scan of the abdomen if nephrolthiasis suspected
- EKGs to look for manifestations of hyperkalemia and arrhythmias, such as atrial fibrillation

Procedures
- Renal biopsy to look for a specific cause of renal failure

Treatment
- *IV fluids*: Start with normal saline.
- *Urinary catheter placement*: Urinary obstruction often is an easily reversible cause of ARF. Caution when using urinary catheters in all patients as it has a tendency to cause infections of the urinary tract.
- *Dialysis*: The principal methods of renal replacement therapy (RRT) are intermittent hemodialysis (IHD), continuous venovenous hemofiltration (CVVH), and peritoneal dialysis (PD).
- Peritoneal dialysis is inexpensive, easily available, and does not result in hypotension. However, it is not capable of removing large volumes of fluid or solute.

- Indications for initiation of dialysis include the following:
  - ☐ Volume overload
  - ☐ Hyperkalemia (K+ >6.5 or rising)
  - ☐ Acid-base imbalance
  - ☐ Symptomatic uremia causing pericarditis, encephalopathy, bleeding dys-crasia
  - ☐ Uremia (BUN > 100)
  - ☐ Certain drug overdoses

Consultation
- Nephrology

HYPERKALEMIA

Elevation of serum potassium levels can be life threatening. It is difficult to diagnose without lab tests as patients might have vague symptoms.

Hyperkalemia is defined as a potassium level greater than 5.5 mEq/L. Ranges are as follows:

- 5.5–6.0 mEq/L: Mild
- 6.1–7.0 mEq/L: Moderate
- 7.0 mEq/L and greater: Severe

Etiology

- *Lab error*: Always rule that out first. It occurs due to hemolysis of the blood sample.
- *Redistribution*: Acidosis, insulin deficiency, acute digoxin intoxication or overdose, succinylcholine
- Hyperkalemic familial periodic paralysis
- *Excessive intravascular potassium*: Hemolysis, rhabdomyolysis, internal hemorrhage
- *Excessive intake of potassium*: Parenteral administration, potassium supplements
- *Diminished potassium excretion*: Acute or chronic renal failure, RTA type IV, decreased mineralocorticoid activity
- *Medications*: ACE inhibitors, NSAIDs, potassium-sparing diuretics.

History

- As always, a detailed history is very important as the complaints can be vague. Sometimes it is discovered incidently.
- Patients can present with cardiac arrhythmias, some of them can be life threatening. Weakness, fatigue, and body ache are common symptoms. Certain neurologic symptoms such as paresthesias, paralysis, and palpitations can also suggest the possibility of hyperkalemia.

Physical Examination

- Since patients can present with life-threatening arrhythmias, it is essential to get vital signs first.
- *Heart*: Extrasystoles, tachycardia, pauses, or bradycardia.
- *Neurology*: Altered mental status, diminished DTR, parasthesias, and decreased motor strength.
- In rare cases, muscular paralysis resulting in hypoventilation can also occur.
- *Skin*: Edema

Diagnosis

- *EKG*: This should be one of the first diagnostic tests that is needed. Initially peaked T waves are seen followed by widening of the QRS accompanied by bundle branch blocks, prolonged PR interval, disappearance of the P wave, widened QRS morphology resulting in a sine wave. This can eventually lead to V-Fib, asystole, or PEA.
- CBC
- BMP
- BUN and creatinine level: For evaluation of renal status
- *Calcium level*: Hypocalcemia can exacerbate arrhythmias.
- Glucose level
- *ABG level*: To evaluate acidosis
- *Urinalysis*: Important in the presence of renal failure
- Cortisol and aldosterone levels

Treatment

- ABCs
- Admit patient to telemetry: Indicated for evaluation of rhythm disturbances
- Discontinue medications such as ACE-I and any potassium-sparing drugs or dietary potassium.
- In mild hyperkalemia with K level 5.5–6 mEQ/L and no EKG changes, just kayexalate should be sufficient at 15–30 g PO as a one-time dose, but can be repeated if necessary. Remember that unless the patient has a bowel movement, the potassium bound to kayexalate cannot be excreted.
- If the hyperkalemia is severe (potassium >7.0 mEq/L) or the patient is symptomatic, begin treatment first.
- Calcium gluconate 1 ampule IV stat if EKG changes for hyperkalemia are seen.
- Regular insulin 10 units IV with D50 glucose stat but this effect is temporary.
- IV fluids also drive the K into the cells.
- Beta-2-agonist inhalation
- Bicarbonate 1–2 amps IV
- Furosemide 40 mg IV
- Kayexalate 30 g PO/PR
- Eventually, if still refractory to treatment, then hemodialysis

Consultation

- Nephrology

HYPOKALEMIA

- Reduction in the intravascular potassium level is termed hyopkalemia.
- Hypokalemia is defined as a potassium level less than 3.5 mEq/L.
- Moderate hypokalemia is a serum level of 2.5–3 mEq/L.
- Severe hypokalemia is defined as a level less than 2.5 mEq/L.

Etiology

- *Medications*: Loop diuretics, beta agonists, steroids, and aminoglycosides
- *Renal losses*: RTA I-III, hyperaldosteronism, hypomagnesemia, and leukemia
- *GI losses*: Vomiting or nasogastric suctioning, diarrhea, enemas, or laxative use
- Decreased dietary intake

History

- Similar to hyperkalemia, patients with hypokalemia can also present with vague symptoms such as weakness, fatigue, muscle ache, and certain neurological symptoms as parasthesias. GI symptoms also occur in hypokalemia such as nausea, vomiting, constipation, abdominal pain.
- Psychosis, delerium, hallucinations along with depression can be seen in severe cases.

Physical Examination

- *HEENT*: Dry conjunctiva
- *Lungs*: Tachypnea
- *Heart*: Arrhythmias, cardiac arrest, PAC, PVC, hypotension
- *Abdomen*: Signs of ileus
- *Neuro*: Delerium, decreased muscle tone and reflexes
- *Skin*: Edema

Diagnosis

- CBC
- CMP with serum potassium level <3.5 mEq/L (3.5 mmol/L), BUN, and creatinine level
- Digoxin level if patient is taking digoxin as hypokalemia can exacerbate digoxin-induced arrhythmias.
- *ABG*: Alkalosis can cause potassium to shift from extracellular to intracellular.
- CT scan of the adrenal glands is indicated if mineralocorticoid excess is noted.
- *EKG*: T-wave flattening or inverted T waves, prominent U wave with QT prolongation, ST-segment depression, ventricular arrhythmias, atrial arrhythmias (eg, premature atrial contractions [PACs], atrial fibrillation)

Treatment

- ABCs
- Admit to telemetry
- If patient has severe bradycardia or is manifesting other cardiac arrhythmias, appropriate pharmacologic therapy or cardiac pacing should be considered.
- For severe bradycardia, atropine 1 mg IV push can be administered first. This dose can be repeated if necessary. Transcutaneous pacing should be considered in such patients who are refractory to medications.
- Treat hypomagnesemia
- Potassium chloride: KCl 40 mEq PO q4–6h or KCl 10 mEq/h IV
- Patients with mild or moderate hypokalemia (potassium of 2.5–3.5 mEq/L), who are asymptomatic or have mild symptoms may only need oral K therapy.
- If the potassium level is less than 2.5 mEq/L, intravenous potassium should be given.

Consultation

- Nephrology, if needed

HYPERNATREMIA

■ Elevation of serum sodium level to >145 mEq/L.

Etiology

Hypovolemic Hypernatremia

■ *Extrarenal volume loss*: Vomiting, diarrhea, severe burns
■ *Renal volume loss*: Osmotic diuretics, postobstructive diuresis, intrinsic renal disease

Hypervolemic Hypernatremia

■ Hypertonic saline
■ Excessive sodium bicarbonate administration
■ Increased salt ingestion
■ Mineralocorticoid excess, eg, Cushing syndrome

Euvolemic Hypernatremia

■ Central DI, nephrogenic DI
■ In these patients, the volume loss is at the intracellular and interstitial level.

Central DI Differential Diagnosis

■ Head trauma
■ Suprasellar or intrasellar tumors
■ Granulomas such as TB and sarcoidosis
■ Histocytosis
■ Infections of the nervous system, such as encephalitis and meningitis
■ Vascular such as stroke, hemorrhage, cerebral aneurysm, Sheehan syndrome

Nephrogenic DI Differential Diagnosis

■ Chronic renal failure
■ *Electrolyte disturbances*: Hypokalemia, hypercalcemia
■ *Systemic diseases*: Amyloidosis, Fanconi syndrome, sickle cell disease, renal tubular acidosis
■ *Diet*: Increased salt intake. Poor water intake.
■ *Drugs*: Lithium, demeclocycline, vinblastine, amphotericin B
■ *Diuresis*: Medication induced, diabetes, diuretic phase of ATN

History

■ Patient presents with a history of nausea, vomiting, and diarrhea for several days. Patients with severe burns can also present with hypernatremia due to 3rd spacing. These symptoms are followed by altered mental status, lethargy, and eventually coma. Body aches, ataxia, and tremors can also be present.

Physical Examination
- *HEENT*: Dry conjunctiva
- *Heart*: Arrhythmias or hypotension.
- *Neuro*: Delerium, ataxia, or hyperreflexia. Rarely hemiparesis.
- *Skin*: Dry mucous membranes, poor skin turgor, or orthostatic vital signs.

Diagnosis
- CBC
- *CMP*: Serum sodium levels of more than 190 mEq/L are seen with long-term salt ingestion.
- Serum sodium levels of more than 170 mEq/L are seen in DI.
- Serum sodium levels of 150–170 mEq/L are seen in dehydration.
- UA/C+S
- Urine osmolality
- Hypotonic urine and polyuria are characteristic of DI.

Imaging Studies
- Head CT scan or MRI is suggested in all patients with severe hypernatremia. Dural sinus thrombosis can occur due to hypovolemia. Causes for central DI or other potential causes of hypernatremia can also be determined by imaging.

Other Tests
- *Water deprivation test*: This test induces dehydration and provides useful information when we check UA, urine output, and body weight. The body's normal response to dehydration is to concentrate urine and conserve water, so urine becomes more concentrated. Patients with DI are unable to do that and as a result, their urine is extremely dilute even in a state of induced dehydration.
- *ADH stimulation*: With nephrogenic DI, urine osmolality does not increase after ADH or desmopressin acetate administration, whereas it improves in central DI.

Treatment
- Supportive treatment
- ABCs
- Before initiating the fluids calculate the free water deficit:

$$\text{Free } H_2O \text{ deficit: TBW} \times [Na] \text{ serum} - 140/140$$

$$\text{Change in serum sodium} = ([Na] \text{ Infused} - [Na] \text{ Serum}) (TBW + 1)$$

Percentage of TBW should be as follows:
- Young men: 0.6%
- Young women and elderly men: 0.5%
- Elderly women: 0.4%

- *IVF*: Isotonic fluids initially to stabilize hypovolemic patients followed by D5W, D5 ½ NS, or D5 ¼ NS. It is important to volume replete the patient before correcting the free water deficit with hypotonic solutions, as isotonic saline remains intravascularly longer than the hypotonic agents. No need to use colloids in this case.

- Hypernatremia should not be corrected at a rate greater than 1 mEq/L/h. Overcorrection can result in cerebral edema.

- Strict I/O measurement is necessary.

- Euvolemic patients are treated with hypotonic fluids or free water either orally or IV, ie, D5W or ¼ NS.

- Hypervolemic patients are treated by combining diuretics and D5W infusion to remove excess sodium. Patients with acute renal failure may require dialysis.

- *If hypernatremia due to DI*: May need to give desmopressin (DDAVP) if central DI, but if nephrogenic need to stop the offending agent like lithium, salt restrictions, and thiazide diurectics.

Consultation

- Nephrology

HYPONATREMIA

■ Serum sodium concentration of less than 136 signifies hyponatremia. There are many mechanisms that can contribute to this.

Types

■ *Hypovolemic hyponatremia*: Total body water (TBW) decreases, and total body sodium also decreases.

■ *Euvolemic hyponatremia*: Total body water increases while total sodium remains normal.

■ *Hypervolemic hyponatremia*: Total body sodium increases, and TBW also increases. Edema is present.

■ *Pseudohyponatremia*: Dilution secondary to lipid, proteins, and glucose. The TBW and total body sodium are unchanged. This condition is seen with hypertriglyceridemia, hyperglycemia, and multiple myeloma.

Etiology

Hypovolemic Hyponatremia

■ Excess fluid losses (eg, vomiting, diarrhea)

■ Acute or chronic renal insufficiency

■ Salt-wasting nephropathy

■ Traumatic brain injury, subarachnoid hemorrhage, and intracranial surgery causing cerebral salt-wasting syndromes

■ Exposure to heat resulting in a heat stroke or exhaustion

Euvolemic Hyponatremia

■ Psychogenic polydipsia, often in psychiatric patients

■ SIADH

Hypervolemic Hyponatremia

■ Fluid overload states such as CHF, cirrhosis, nephrotic syndrome, etc.

■ Adrenal insufficiency, hypopituitarism

■ *Iatrogenic*: It can be euvolemic or hypovolemic.

■ Diuretics, SSRI, ACE-II receptor blockers, ACE-I, amiloride

History

■ Patients with hyponatremia can present in many ways depending on the degree of hyponatremia.

■ In milder cases when the sodium level is 125–136, patients can present with mild anorexia, headache, and muscle cramps.

■ In moderate or severe cases that range between sodium levels of 115–125, symptoms can be more severe such as altered mental status with altered mental status, seizures, or even coma.

- Hyponatremia can be seen in patients with pulmonary or neurologic diseases, most due to SIADH.
- The patient's medication list should be examined for drugs known to cause hyponatremia.
- Hyponatremia is present in patients who are malnourished and who abuse alcohol on a daily basis.
- A history of hypothyroidism or adrenal insufficiency is important as it can be with hypoosmolar hyponatremia.

Physical Examination

- *HEENT*: Dry conjunctiva
- *Heart*: Arrhythmias, S3 gallop, jugular venous distenstion, peripheral edema
- *Lungs*: Crackles due to CHF
- *Abdomen*: Hepatic congestion
- *Neuro*: Delerium, coma is a possibility, unilateral fixed dilated pupil, decorticate or decerebrate posture can be a sign of brain stem herniation.
- *Extremity*: Peripheral edema

Diagnosis

- Check the result, possible lab error CBC
- *CMP*: Pseudohyponatremia associated with hyperglycemia occurs due to redistribution of water from the intracellular space to the extracellular space. Serum sodium concentration is diluted by a factor of 1.6 mEq/L for each 100 mg/dL increase above normal serum glucose concentration.
- Hyponatremia may be noted in patients whose serum contains unusually large quantities of protein or lipid.
- Hyperproteinemia causing pseudohyponatremia is seen in multiple myeloma.
- *Serum osmolarity*: To diagnose hypoosmolar hyponatremia. Serum osmolarity is low in patients with hypoosmolar hyponatremia, but it is normal in patients with pseudohyponatremia due to hyperlipidemia or hyperproteinemia, and normal or elevated in patients with hypertonic hyponatremia due to serum hyperglycemia.
- *Urine osmolarity*: Useful in the diagnosis of SIADH. Patients with SIADH have inappropriately concentrated urine, with urine osmolarity in excess of 100 mOsm/L.
- *Urine sodium levels*: Patients with hypovolemic hyponatremia due to nonrenal causes (eg, vomiting, diarrhea, etc.) have urine sodium levels <20 mEq/L, whereas those with hypovolemic hyponatremia due to renal causes (eg, diuretics, salt-losing nephropathy, aldosterone deficiency) have elevated urine sodium levels >20 mEq/L.
- Patients with hypervolemic hyponatremia have low urine sodium levels of <20 mEq/L, whereas those with renal causes of hypervolemic hyponatremia have urine sodium levels >20 mEq/L.

- *TSH, Free T4*: To evaluate hypothyroidism
- Random cortisol levels for adrenal insufficiency
- ACTH stimulation test if needed

Imaging Studies
- Chest X-ray for CHF, pneumonia, and other potential causes of hypervolemic hyponatremia and euvolemic hyponatremia such as SIADH
- Usually, a head CT scan is indicated in the patient with altered mental status to ensure that no other underlying cause for the mental status is present.

Treatment
- ABCs
- Supportive care
- *Hypovolemic hyponatremia*: Fluid resuscitation with normal saline if dehydration is evident. Stop the offending agent, if a medication is suspected such as diuretics. Serum sodium level should increase no faster than 0.5 mEq/L/h or 12 mEq/L/d to prevent central pontine mylinolysis. For symptomatic patients the rate of correction can be 2 mEq/L/h but only until symptoms resolve. These patients have to be monitored closely with neurologic checks.
- *Euvolemic hyponatremia*: SIADH and psycogenic polydipsia. Free water restriction from 500 to 1000 mL with appropriate total volume restriction would be needed. In SIADH, urine will be extremely concentrated.
- *Hypervolemic hyponatremia*: Correct the underlying etiology.
- If seizures are present secondary to hyponatremia, treat the seizure first and stabilize it while correcting the sodium levels as they can take time to normalize.
- Hypotonic fluids can exacerbate cerebral edema.
- Patients with seizures, severe confusion, coma, or signs of brain stem herniation should receive hypertonic (3%) saline to rapidly correct serum sodium level toward normal but only enough to arrest the progression of symptoms. An increase in serum sodium level of 4–6 mEq/L is sufficient.
- Symptoms of CPM include altered mental status, seizures, dysarthria, and paraplegia, and in severe cases shock. These symptoms can occur 1–3 days after correction of serum sodium level.
- Further correction should proceed at an overall rate that is no greater than 0.5 mEq/L/h or 12 mEq/L/d.

Consultation
- Nephrology, if needed

NEUROLOGY

TRANSIENT ISCHEMIC ATTACK (TIA)

TIA is temporary loss of cerebral function which usually lasts between 15 minutes and 2 hours but should completely resolve within 24 hours.

Etiology
- Carotid vertebral artery disease are the major causes of TIA
- Cerebral embolism
- *Embolic sources*: Mural thrombus in the left atrium dislodged due to atrial fibrillation, ventricular thrombus, valvular disease, and atheroembolism
- Arterial dissection
- Vasculitis
- Drugs
- Intracranial masses or hemorrhage

History
- A TIA may last only several minutes. Detailed history should be obtained from the family members in addition to the patient, as there might be subtle symptoms that the family noticed while the patient was unaware of them.
- Family members are an invaluable source of information concerning symptoms of a TIA.
- By talking to the family, the examiner can not only discuss symptoms but also begin an assessment of the home environment.

Physical Examination
- *HEENT*: Cranial nerve exam, hearing, and EOM evaluation
- *Heart*: Irregularly irregular heart beat can signify atrial fibrillation, which could be a cause of the TIA.
- *Neurologic exam*: A patient with a suspected TIA requires a complete physical examination with attention to a detailed neurologic examination. Approach the patient who has had an apparent TIA with the goal of accurately diagnosing conditions that resemble a stroke. Overall health of the patient should be assessed giving attention to the following:
  - ☐ Attentiveness
  - ☐ Ability to interact with the examiner
  - ☐ Language and memory skills
  - ☐ Overall hydration status
  - ☐ Development

■ Identify signs of vasculitis, sinusitis, mastoiditis, and meningitis. Carotid arteries are examined for pulse upstroke, bruit, and presence of carotid endarterectomy scars.

■ Mental status can be assessed formally (eg, Mini-Mental Status Examination) or as part of the patient's overall response to questions and interactions with the examiner.

Diagnosis
■ CBC
■ BMP
■ Coagulation studies
■ Erythrocyte sedimentation rate (ESR)
■ Syphilis serology, RPR, VDRL
■ Complete blood count
■ Platelet count
■ Antiphospholipid antibodies
■ Glucose level
■ Drug screens
■ Cardiac enzymes
■ Anemia and elevated ESR (>100 mm/h): Hallmarks of temporal artery arteritis
■ Lipid profile

Imaging Studies
■ Location of the disease is very important for treatment and prognosis.
■ Noncontrast CT scan of the head: An area of infarction appropriate for the TIA symptoms has been identified in 29–34% of patients with TIA.
■ *MRI of the brain*: Acute infarcts are located more accurately using MRI than with CT scan. Abnormal vascular flow can be detected within minutes of onset of symptoms.
■ *Magnetic resonance angiography (MRA)*: Provides noninvasive images of carotid and vertebral arteries.
■ *Cerebral arterial imaging*: Carotid and vertebral artery ultrasound is required to identify the surgical candidate with high-grade carotid stenosis.

Treatment
■ ABCs
■ Administer supplemental oxygen.
■ Obtain a finger stick glucose level and treat accordingly.
■ Start aspirin 325 mg daily.
■ If patient is already on aspirin start clopidogrel 75 mg daily.

■ Obtain an EKG and initiate treatment for symptomatic rhythms or evidence of ischemia.

■ Blood pressure should be managed cautiously as it can decrease cerebral perfusion causing ischemia; hence permissive hypertension is allowed initially.

■ Even a modest reduction in BP can extend a fragile ischemic event. Recent studies have recommended treatment of SBP if greater than 220.

■ If atrial fibrillation is present then that could be the likely cause of TIA. Anticoagulation with heparin and eventually warfarin should be started to achieve an INR between 2 and 3. Consider each patient separately weighing the risks and benefits.

Consultation

■ Neurology (particularly if questioning whether the presentation is consistent with TIA)

ACUTE STROKE

Stroke is a term given to loss of cerebral function due to ischemia or hemorrhage in a certain vascular territory. Classified as either hemorrhagic or ischemic, strokes typically manifest with the sudden onset of focal neurologic deficits, such as weakness, sensory deficit, or difficulties with language. Ischemic strokes can be caused by thrombosis, embolism, and hypoperfusion, while hemorrhagic strokes can be either intraparenchymal or subarachnoid.

Mechanisms of Stroke/Etiology
Embolic Strokes
- Cardiac sources like atrial fibrillation, MI, mural thrombus, and valvular heart diseases
- Arterial sources from the arch of aorta, carotids, and vertebral arteries in the form of atheroemboli or cholesterol emboli

Thrombotic Strokes
- Thrombotic strokes can involve the smaller vessels as well as the larger ones. They mainly occur in the vertebrobasilar and cerebral artery distribution.

Lacunar Strokes
- Nearly 20% ischemic strokes are lacunar strokes. They generally occur in the distribution of the penetrating branches of MCA, vertebral artery, basilar artery, and along the circle of Willis.

Watershed Infarcts
- These infarcts, also known as border zone infarcts, can occur due to hypoperfusion in the most distal artery distribution.

History
- The American Stroke Association advises the public to be aware of the symptoms of stroke:
  - ☐ Sudden numbness or weakness of face, arm, or leg, especially on one side of the body
  - ☐ Sudden confusion, difficulty in speaking or understanding
  - ☐ Sudden deterioration of vision of one or both eyes
  - ☐ Sudden difficulty in walking, dizziness, and loss of balance or coordination
  - ☐ Sudden severe headache with no known cause
- A focused medical history aims to identify risk factors.
- In younger patients, elicit a history of recent trauma, coagulopathies, and cocaine abuse.
- Family members, bystanders, can provide invaluable information regarding the time and events surrounding the onset of symptoms or when the patient was last seen normal.

■ Establishing time of onset is especially critical when thrombolytic therapy is being considered. If the patient is unable to communicate and time is a major factor, a detailed history obtained from family members or bystanders could be crucial.

■ If the patient is a candidate for thrombolytic therapy, a thorough review of the inclusion and exclusion criteria must be performed. The absolute and relative contraindications are the same as in fibrinolysis for acute MI. The exclusion criteria largely focus on identifying risk of hemorrhage with using thrombolytics.

Physical Examination

■ *General status*: Patients comfort level, orientation, and speech

■ *Vital signs*: HTN may be present; O_2 saturation could be diminished.

■ *HEENT*: Pupils may or may not respond to light; EOM may not be intact. Auscultation of the neck may elicit a bruit, suggesting carotid disease as the cause of the stroke.

■ *Heart*: Irregularly irregular heart rate may be present, mumurs may be present.

■ *Lungs*: Signs of CHF

■ *Extremities*: Unequal pulses or blood pressures in the extremities signify the presence of aortic dissections.

■ *Neurology*: Do a complete neurologic exam to localize the area of the stroke.

■ A useful tool in measuring neurologic impairment is the National Institutes of Health Stroke Scale (NIHSS). This scale can be used easily, is reliable and valid, provides insight to the location of vascular lesions, and can be correlated with outcome in patients with ischemic stroke.

NIH STROKE SCALE

	Category	Description	Score
Ia	Level of consciousness (LOC)	Alert	0
		Drowsy	1
		Stuporous	2
		Coma	3
Ib	LOC questions (month, age)	Answers both correctly	0
		Answers 1 correctly	1
		Incorrect on both	2
Ic	LOC commands (open-close eyes, grip and release hand)	Obeys both correctly	0
		Obeys 1 correctly	1
		Incorrect on both	2
2	Best gaze (follow finger)	Normal	0
		Partial gaze palsy	1
		Forced deviation	2
3	Best visual (visual fields)	No visual loss	0
		Partial hemianopia	1
		Complete hemianopia	2
		Bilateral hemianopia	3

(Continued)

NIH STROKE SCALE (*Continued*)

4	Facial palsy (show teeth, raise brows, squeeze eyes shut)	Normal	0
		Minor	1
		Partial	2
		Complete	3
5	Motor arm left (raise 90°, hold 10 sec)	No drift	0
		Drift	1
		Cannot resist gravity	2
		No effort against gravity	3
		No movement	4
6	Motor arm right (raise 90°, hold 10 sec)	No drift	0
		Drift	1
		Cannot resist gravity	2
		No effort against gravity	3
		No movement	4
7	Motor leg left (raise 30°, hold 5 sec)	No drift	0
		Drift	1
		Cannot resist gravity	2
		No effort against gravity	3
		No movement	4
8	Motor leg right (raise 30°, hold 5 sec)	No drift	0
		Drift	1
		Cannot resist gravity	2
		No effort against gravity	3
		No movement	4
9	Limb ataxia (finger-nose, heel-shin)	Absent	0
		Present in one limb	1
		Present in two limbs	2
10	Sensory (pinprick to face, arm, leg)	Normal	0
		Partial loss	1
		Severe loss	2
11	Extinction/neglect (double simultaneous testing)	No neglect	0
		Partial neglect	1
		Complete neglect	2
12	Dysarthria (speech clarity to "mama, baseball, huckleberry, tip-top, fifty-fifty")	Normal articulation	0
		Mild to moderate dysarthria	1
		Near to unintelligible or worse	2
13	Best language (name items, describe pictures)	No aphasia	0
		Mild to moderate aphasia	1
		Severe aphasia	2
		Mute	3
	Total	—	0-42

Source: National Institutes of Health, available at www.ninds.nih.gov/doctors/NIH_Stroke_Scale.pdf

Diagnosis

■ *CBC*: CBC provides key information regarding hemoglobin and hematocrit, as well as platelet count, which is important in fibrinolytic candidates.

■ *CMP*: Hypoglycemia can mimic stroke along with some other electrolyte disorders such as those that cause altered mental status.

■ *PT/PTT*: Needed prior to starting antiplatelet agents or anticoagulation. Also in the setting of hemorrhagic stroke, the coagulation status of a patient is extremely important.

■ *Cardiac enzymes*: Can be elevated in the presence of demand ischemia or acute MI, which may coexist with an acute stroke.

■ Additional tests are patient specific, such as rapid plasma reagent (RPR), toxicology screen, fasting lipid profile, sedimentation rate, pregnancy test, antinuclear antibody (ANA), rheumatoid factor, and homocysteine.

■ In select patients with possible hypercoagulable states, protein C, protein S, antithrombin III, and Factor V Leyden may be tested. It is better to consult a neurologist prior to ordering these tests.

Imaging Studies

■ CT scan of the brain without contrast. It can detect strokes and intracranial bleeds. It is absolutely necessary before administration of any anticoagulant.

■ *MRI with MRA*: Diffusion-weighted MRI can detect subtle areas of ischemia in the brain than standard T1/T2-weighted MRI images or CT scan. MRA is very useful as it evaluates the patency of the cerebral arteries.

■ Carotid duplex scanning is one of the most useful tests in evaluating patients with stroke. Patients with symptomatic critical stenoses are at higher risk for a CEA. They need to be on clopidogrel or anticoagulation prior to the procedure.

Other Tests

■ *Echocardiography*: Transthoracic echocardiography (TTE) and TEE are needed to evaluate possible cardiac etiology for the stroke. TEE is more sensitive than TTE and can evaluate the aortic arch and thoracic aorta for plaques, dissections, or mural thrombus but is more invasive.

■ *EKG*: It is essential to exclude cardiac rhythm disorders such as atrial fibrillation that could potentially lead to a stroke.

■ *Chest X-ray*: If needed.

Treatment

■ Prehospital stroke assessment tools, such as the Cincinnati Prehospital Stroke Scale or Los Angeles Prehospital Stroke Scale, can identify patients with potential stroke.

■ If there is high suspicion of stroke in a patient, then depending on the hospital, a stroke team should be called and appropriate departments such as radiology should be notified.

■ O$_2$ via nasal cannula

■ ABCs are extremely important in the setting of a stroke.

■ *Immediate finger stick*: As hypoglycemia can present as a stroke.

■ The goal of acute stroke management in the Emergency Department is rapid and efficient care. Continuing from the assessment of the ABCs and stroke patient evaluation, if eligible, fibrinolytic therapy should be administered within 3 hours from presentation. Always consult a neurologist before administration of fibrinolytics.

■ Admit to telemetry as either an outpatient or inpatient depending on the severity of the stroke.

Medications

■ *Aspirin*: 325 mg PO daily

■ *Clopidogrel*: 75 mg PO daily if already on aspirin previously

■ Use of aggrenox is currently being debated.

■ In case of a cardioembolic stroke, IV heparin to warfarin with goal INR of 2–3 should be appropriate. Consider each patient separately, keeping in mind whether the patient would tolerate anticoagulation or not.

■ Avoid anticoagulation in a large ischemic stroke with potential of hemorrhagic conversion or a hemorrhagic stroke.

GENERAL MANAGEMENT

■ Physical therapy

■ Speech and swallow evaluation. Some patients with severe effects can loose their gag reflex and some are just unable to swallow and could easily aspirate. It is best to keep the patient NPO until seen for speech and swallow therapy.

■ Aspiration precautions, with the head of the bed elevated to 30°, need to be observed.

■ Physical therapy will test and suggest level of activity. This should be ordered as soon as possible based on the patient's clinical status.

■ If hypoglycemia is present, then treat with D50 depending on the severity as explained in the hypoglycemia section.

■ Strict glycemic control is needed in the setting of stroke. If blood glucose is >300, then it is reasonable to treat with IV insulin.

Blood Pressure Management in Acute Stroke

■ Emphasis should be given to permissive hypertension in ischemic stroke to prevent cerebral hypoperfusion. In hemorrhagic stroke, the blood pressure should be much lower.

■ Do not treat SBP unless >220 and DBP >120 for ischemic stroke but in cases of hemorrhagic stroke, blood pressure needs to be lower than 140 SBP.

Agents Commonly Used for Blood Pressure Management in Acute Stroke

■ *Sodium nitroprusside*: 0.5 mcg/kg/min; may reduce approximately 10–20%

■ *Labetalol*: 10–20 mg IVP over 1–2 minutes; may repeat and double every 10 minutes up to maximum dose of 150 mg or nicardipine 5 mg/h IV infusion and titrate

■ *Enalapril*: 1.25 mg IVP

■ *Hydralazine*: 10–15 mg IV q6h

■ *Fibrinolytic therapy*: Intravenous TPA for appropriate patients within 3 hours from the onset of symptoms. It is a Class I recommendation by the American Stroke Association.

■ *Diet*: Patients with acute stroke are at great risk of aspiration. All patients should remain NPO until a swallowing assessment is performed.

Consultations Needed

■ Neurology, PM&R, cardiology, or neurosurgery (depending on the type and extent of the stroke)

■ During hospitalization, arrangements need to be made for a rehab facility versus home stay with visiting nurses. A case manager should be consulted early in the process.

MENINGITIS

Meningitis is an inflammation of the leptomeninges. Patients with this illness can present with high-grade fever, and mental status changes within a day's duration.

Etiology

- Common organisms causing meningitis in adults: S. *pneumoniae*, (30–50%), *H. influenzae* (1–3%), *N. meningitidis* (10–35%), gram-negative bacilli (1–10%), staphylococci (5–15%), streptococci (5%), and *Listeria* species (5%).
- In adults older than 50 years or adults with disabling disease or alcoholism, the most common microorganisms are *S. pneumoniae*, coliforms, *H. influenzae*, *Listeria* species, *Pseudomonas aeruginosa*, and *N. meningitidis*.
- Persons aged 60 years or older are at higher risk.
- Immunosuppressed patients are at higher risk of acute bacterial meningitis.
- High incidence in military recruits and college dorm residents due to overcrowding, which increases risk of outbreaks of meningococcal meningitis.
- Splenectomy and sickle cell disease predisposes to meningitis, as it is an encapsulated organism.
- *Alcoholism and cirrhosis*: Multiple etiologies of fever and seizures in these patients make meningitis challenging to diagnose.
- Neoplasm
- Diabetes
- Recent exposure to a patient with meningitis
- Contiguous infection (eg, sinusitis)
- IV drug abuse
- Bacterial endocarditis
- Ventriculoperitoneal shunt
- Malignancy (increased risk of *Listeria* species infection)

History

- Patients can present with headache, fever, and altered mental status. Sometimes it is extremely vague. Hence, it is always said that if the change in mental status is unexplained then always evaluate for meningitis. About 25% of patients with bacterial meningitis present acutely within 24 hours of onset of symptoms. Symptoms for viral meningitis can occur over 1–7 days or longer for fungi or atypical bacteria such as *M. tuberculosis*. Meningitis due to TB and fungi can have similar symptoms but should be suspected in immunocompromised patients.
- Classic symptoms include the following:
  - ☐ Headache
  - ☐ Nuchal rigidity
  - ☐ Fever and chills

- ☐ Photophobia
- ☐ Vomiting
- ☐ Prodromal upper respiratory infection (URI) symptoms prior to current presentation
- ☐ Seizures
- ☐ Altered mental status

Physical Examination

- ■ Patients can sometimes present with shock.
- ■ *HEENT*: Papilledema is present in only one-third of meningitis patients with increased ICP; it takes at least several hours to develop.
- ■ *Neurology*: Signs of meningeal irritation, Nuchal rigidity or discomfort on neck flexion
    - ☐ *Kernig sign*: Passive knee extension in supine patient elicits neck pain and hamstring resistance
    - ☐ *Brudzinski sign*: Passive neck or single hip flexion is accompanied by involuntary flexion of both hips. CN III, IV, VI, VII can be affected in 10–20% of patients.
- ■ *Systemic findings*: Extracranial infection (eg, sinusitis, otitis media, mastoiditis, pneumonia, and urinary tract infection) may be noted.
- ■ Arthritis can be seen with *N. meningitides*.
- ■ *Skin*: Nonblanching petechiae and cutaneous hemorrhages are seen classically with *N. meningitidis* but can be seen with other bacterias as well.

Diagnosis

- ■ CBC
- ■ CMP
- ■ Coagulation profile and platelets if DIC is suspected.
- ■ Urinary electrolytes and osmolality if SIADH is suspected.
- ■ Serum cryptococcal antigen
- ■ Cultures should be obtained prior to starting antibiotics if possible.
- ■ Serum test for syphilis such as VDRL or RPR is indicated, if neurosyphilis is in differential diagnosis.

Imaging Studies

- ■ Head CT scan with contrast or MRI with gadolinium is useful to identify other causes of mental status change such as CNS bleed, stroke, or malignancy. Sometime infections with ring enhancing lesions can also be seen.
- ■ CT should be done prior to LP if papilledema is present. Blood cultures, LP should be obtained prior to initiating.
- ■ Brain abscess, sinus or mastoid infection, skull fracture, and congenital anomalies also need to be ruled out with imaging studies.

- *Chest x-ray*: Nearly half of the patients with *N. meningitidis* can also have evidence of pneumonia.
- Lumbar puncture (refer to our procedure section)
- Elevated opening pressure is seen in bacterial and fungal meningitis. These patients can have high morbidity and mortality.
- Tube #1, protein and glucose
- Tube #2, cell count with differential.
- Tube #3, gram stain, bacterial culture, acid-fast bacillus (AFB) stain and tuberculosis (TB) cultures, India ink stain and fungal cultures, VDRL, and cryptococcal antigen, if indicated, HSV PCR
- Tube #4, for repeat cell count with differential, if needed (or for other subsequent studies not initially ordered).

COMPARISON OF CSF FINDINGS BY TYPE OF ORGANISM

	Bacterial Meningitis	Viral Meningitis	Fungal Meningitis/TB
Pressure 5–15 cm H_2O	Elevated	Normal or mildly elevated	Variable: Might be increased
Cell count	Mainly PMN >1000. Rarely can be normal	Usually <500 cells, nearly 100% lymphocytes. Up to 48 h, significant PMN pleocytosis may be seen, which can be similar to bacterial meningitis	>100 lymphocytes but can be variable
Organisms	Gram stain 80% effective. Culture yield after administration of antibiotics decreases and is about 20%	No organism	India ink 80–90% effective for fungi; AFB stain 40% effective for TB
CSF-to-serum glucose ratio	Decreased/normal	Normal	Decreased. Lower in TB, parasitic meningitis
Protein	>150, may be >1000	Mildly increased/normal	Increased: >1000 can suggest fungal infection. Increased in TB as well

Source: Adapted from Arevalo CE, Barnes PF, Duda M, Leedom JM. Cerebrospinal fluid cell counts and chemistries in bacterial meningitis. *South Med J* 1989;82:1122–1127.

Treatment

■ ABCs

■ Evaluate and treat patient for shock or hypotension. Infuse crystalloid until euvolemic.

■ In acutely ill patients, perform an LP (if appropriate) and administer first dose(s) of antibiotics +/– steroids within 30 minutes of presentation.

■ Start empiric therapy if LP cannot be performed within 30 minutes.

■ Begin empiric therapy prior to head CT scan if a focal neurologic deficit is present. If no mass effect is present, perform LP

■ Monitor for signs of hydrocephalus and increasing ICP.

■ Hyperventilation in intubated patients, with a goal of $PaCO_2$ 25–30 mm Hg, may briefly lower ICP. These needs to be done under the guidance of a neurologist.

■ Place ICP monitor in comatose patients or in those with signs of increased ICP.

■ With elevated ICP, remove CSF until pressure decreases by 50%

■ *Seizure precautions*: Lorazepam 0.1 mg/kg IV and IV load with phenytoin 15 mg/kg or phenobarbital 5–10 mg/kg in the setting of active seizures

■ Administration of dexamethasone is controversial; it can be given with or just before antibiotics.

■ Administer first dose of dexamethasone (0.4 mg/kg IV q12h for 2 days or 0.15 mg/kg q6h for 4 days) 15–20 minutes before first dose of antibiotics.

■ In areas where prevalence of DRSP is >2%, primary treatment is either cefotaxime 2 g IV q4h or ceftriaxone 2 g IV q12h plus vancomycin (adult dose: 750–1000 mg IV q12h or 10–15 mg/kg IV q12h). Some add rifampin (600 mg PO qd). If *Listeria* species is suspected, add ampicillin (50 mg/kg IV q6h).

■ Alternative treatment (or if severely penicillin allergic) is chloramphenicol (12.5 mg/kg IV q6h) or clindamycin 900 mg IV q8h or meropenem 1 g IV q8h.

■ In areas with low prevalence of DRSP, use cefotaxime (2 g IV q4h) or ceftriaxone (adult: 2 g IV q12h) plus ampicillin (50 mg/kg IV q6h).

■ Alternative treatment (or if severely penicillin allergic) is chloramphenicol (12.5 mg/kg IV q6h) plus trimethoprim/sulfamethoxazole (TMP/SMX; TMP 5 mg/kg IV q6h) or meropenem 1 g IV q8h.

■ Administer first dose of dexamethasone (0.4 mg/kg q12h IV for 2 d or 0.15 mg/kg q6h for 4 d) 15–20 minutes before first dose of antibiotics. (Data regarding the use of steroids are limited.)

■ In HIV-positive/AIDS patients/immunocompromised, consider cryptococci, *Mycobacterium tuberculosis*, syphilis, HIV aseptic meningitis, *Listeria* species, and viral meningitis. Consider ampicillin + ceftazidime + vancomycin + acyclovir

■ In patients who have had trauma or neurosurgery, the most common microorganisms are *S. pneumoniae*, *S. taphylococcus aureus*, and *P. aeruginosa*. Primary treatment is vancomycin (1 g IV q12h) plus ceftazidime (2 g IV q8h).

■ Alternative treatment is meropenem (1 g IV q8h).

■ Aseptic meningitis (normal CSF glucose, negative bacteria on gram stain), is caused by enteroviruses, human herpesvirus-2 (HHV-2), lymphocytic chorio-meningitis virus (LCM), HIV, and other viruses. Other etiologies include drugs (NSAIDs, metronidazole, IV immunoglobulin)

■ *Complications*: Hypotension and shock in severe cases, hypoxemia, hypona-tremia (SIADH), cardiac arrhythmias and ischemia, cerebrovascular accident (CVA), and exacerbation of chronic diseases which need to be treated individu-ally.

■ Meningitis prophylaxis for close contacts of a suspected case of *N. meningitidis* who were in close contact with patient for at least 4 hours during the week before onset (eg, house mates, daycare center, and cell mates) or were exposed to patient's nasopharyngeal secretions (mouth-to-mouth resuscitation, intuba-tion, nasotracheal suctioning). Spread is via respiratory droplets.

■ At this time, flouroquinolones like ciprofloxacin are used primarily. Other antibiotics to be considered are rifampin and cephalosporins.

Consultation
■ Neurology
■ Infectious diseases

SEIZURES

Seizures occur as a manifestation of abnormal discharges from the cortical neurons

Classification

■ *Partial-onset seizures*
  ☐ *Simple partial seizures*: This type of seizure is short lived and has preserved consciousness.
  ☐ *Complex partial seizures*: The patient is unconscious of the event but has an aura prior to the episode. The aura could be sensory, motor, or autonomic.
■ *Secondarily generalized seizures* often begin with an aura which eventually converts into a complex partial seizure and then into a generalized tonic-clonic seizure. These patients may have a tonic-clonic seizure right after the aura as well.
■ *Generalized-onset seizures* are further classified as: (1) absence seizures, (2) myclonic seizures, (3) clonic seizures, (4) tonic seizures, (5) atonic seizures.
■ Absence seizures are short in duration and have no prior aura or postictal state. They are accompanied by automatisms such as repetitive blinking or twitching. These seizures usually last for 20 seconds or less.
■ Myoclonic seizures are characterized by brief jerking, motor movements that last only a few seconds. They can occur in clusters. They can also lead to a clonic seizure when the jerking movements are in rhythm.
■ Clonic seizures consist of rhythmic, motor, jerking movements with or without impairment of consciousness.
■ Tonic seizures are characterized by sudden tonic extension or flexion of the head, trunk, and the extremities for several seconds.
■ Tonic-clonic seizures are also termed as grand mal seizures. The patient has generalized tonic extension of the extremities lasting for several seconds to minutes proceeded by clinic movements. If this seizure is not controlled or does not resolve quickly, it could lead to status eplilepticus that is a medical emergency. Patients are usually postictal following this seizure.
■ Atonic seizures should be considered in patients with history of unprovoked falls. They occur as a result of loss of postural tone.

Etiology

Epileptic seizures can occur due to many reasons. Some of them are genetic, others can even be metabolic. Patients usually have no control over the onset of these events, as they are unprovoked. Seizures that occur as a result of direct injury or alcohol are not termed as epileptic seizures.

Remember VITAMINS:

V: Vascular: Stroke, TIA, aneurysm. See the appropriate section for details.

I: Infection: Do not miss UTI among others.

T: Trauma: Take appropriate history and definitely obtain a CT scan of the head.

A: Alcohol: A very common reason for altered mental status

M: Metabolic: Obtain basal metabolic panel

I: Iatrogenic: Also review medications as potential causes

N: Neoplasm

S: Seizures: Treat as per the seizure section

History

■ It is very important to get a detailed history when evaluating seizures. Clinical diagnosis of seizures is based on the history obtained from the patient and, most importantly, the observers.

■ Any warnings, loss of bowel or bladder control, loss of consciousness, postictal state, length of the seizure, and type of activity during the seizure helps differentiate the type.

Physical Examination

■ *HEENT*: Injury to the mouth, tongue bites, bruises due to falls.

■ *Heart*: Tachycardia

■ *Lungs*: Decreased breath sounds, possible crackles due to aspiration.

Diagnosis

■ Prolactin levels obtained shortly after a seizure have been studied with some success to assess the etiology of a suspected seizure episode. It can help to differentiate whether the episode was epileptic or nonepileptic.

■ The prolactin levels are usually twice the upper limit of normal if tested within 60–90 minutes of a seizure episode. They can be much higher with grand mal seizures.

■ Obtain serum levels of anticonvulsants that the patients may have been taking like phenytoin, carbamazepine, etc.

■ CBC

■ *CMP*: To evaluate for any metabolic derangements

Imaging Studies

■ *CT scan of the head*: Can help to determine any bleed, stroke, or infection that could have precipitated the seizure.

■ *MRI of the brain*: May or may not be needed immediately but if no other etiology is found, it should be done. It is a better test to locate strokes, specially the DWI (diffusion-weighted images), and neoplasm.

■ *EEG*: Needed after a seizure to confirm it. Video EEG can also help to characterize the type of seizure.

■ *Procedure*: Lumbar puncture for CSF examination is done in the patient with altered mental status or in patients in whom meningitis or encephalitis is suspected.

Treatment

■ The treatment is initiated promptly if the patient is actively seizing. If the seizure is secondary to alcohol withdrawal, the recommendation is to observe the patient while they are on an alcohol withdrawal protocol with benzodiazepines like lorazepam. If no further seizure occurs, then anticonvulsants are not necessary.

■ Treatment with anticonvulsants

    □ The mainstay of treatment is anticonvulsant medication.

    □ The type of seizure and the specific epileptic syndrome play a role in the selection of anticonvulsants, probably because of the different pathophysiologic mechanisms.

Anticonvulsive Treatments for Specific Types of Seizures

■ *Absence seizures*: If only absence seizures are present, most neurologists treat them with ethosuximide. If absence seizures are present with other types (eg, generalized tonic-clonic seizures, myoclonic seizures), the choices are valproic acid, lamotrigine, or topiramate. Do not use carbamazepine, gabapentin, or tiagabine because they might exacerbate absence seizures. Whether pregabalin, a medication related to gabapentin, might also exacerbate this type of seizure is uncertain.

■ *Tonic or atonic seizures*: Tonic or atonic seizures typically indicate clinically significant brain injury. Tonic seizures are best treated with broad-spectrum drugs (eg, valproic acid, lamotrigine, topiramate). Other modalities include the use of vagal nerve stimulation (VNS).

■ *Myoclonic seizures*: The best medications for myoclonic seizures are valproic acid, lamotrigine, and topiramate. Levetiracetam has been FDA-approved for adjunctive therapy.

■ *Primary generalized tonic-clonic seizures*: This seizure type responds to valproic acid, topiramate, or lamotrigine. Levetiracetam has gained recent FDA approval as adjunctive therapy.

■ *Generalized seizures*: Recent data obtained from SANAD suggest valproate to be the recommended drug for these types of seizures.

■ *Partial-onset seizures*: Carbamazepine is considered first-line therapy.

■ *Doses*:

    □ *Phenytoin*: IV load 20 mg/kg at 50 mg/min, maintenance dose 100 mg PO tid

    □ *Fosphenytoin*: 20 mg PE/kg IV infusion

    □ *Phenobarbital*: IV load 20 mg/kg × 1, maintenance dose PO 60–180 mg/d in divided doses

☐ *Carbamazepine*: 600–1200 mg/d PO in divided doses
☐ *Valproic acid*: 30–60 mg/kg/d in divided doses PO bid or tid
☐ *Ethosuximide*: 250 mg PO bid

Consultation

■ Consult a neurologist if recurrent spells have not been diagnosed or if they have not responded to conventional therapy with a first- or second-line anticonvulsant.

ALTERED MENTAL STATUS

This can arise due to various factors. The best course is to review each one with the help of the common pneumonic VITAMINS.

V: Vascular: Stroke, TIA, and aneurysm. See the appropriate section for details

I: Infection: Do not miss UTI among others.

T: Trauma: Take appropriate history and definitely obtain a CT scan of the head.

A: Alcohol: A very common reason for altered mental status

M: Metabolic: Obtain basal metabolic panel

I: Iatrogenic: Also review medications as potential causes

N: Neoplasm

S: Seizures: Treat as per the seizure section

Diagnosis

■ CBC
■ CMP
■ Chest x-ray
■ CT scan of the head noncontrast
■ EEG
■ LP
■ Blood culture if febrile
■ UA C+S
■ Urine toxicology screen/serum toxicology screen
■ TSH, free T4
■ VDRL, RPR

Treatment

■ Based on the diagnosis

HEMATOLOGY

ANEMIA

Anemia is defined as the decrease in red blood cell mass. In females, anemia is diagnosed with Hb levels less than 12.5 g/dL, and in males, with Hb levels less than 13.5 g/dL.

Etiology

Hematologic Abnormalities
- Hemoglobinopathies
- Thalassemias
- Enzyme abnormalities of the glycolytic pathways
- Defects of the RBC cytoskeleton
- Rh null disease
- Abetalipoproteinemia
- Fanconi anemia
- Thrombotic thrombocytopenic purpura
- Hemolytic uremic syndrome

Nutritional Deficiencies
- Nutritional
- Iron deficiency
- Vitamin B12 deficiency
- Folate deficiency
- Starvation and generalized malnutrition

Blood Loss
- *Acute hemorrhage*: GI, CNS, menstruation

Infections
- *Viral*: CMV, hepatitis, infectious mononucleosis
- *Bacterial*: Clostridia, gram-negative sepsis
- *Protozoal*: Malaria, leishmaniasis, toxoplasmosis
- *Medications*: Immunosupressive agents

Chronic Diseases
- Renal, cardiac, hepatic diseases

Immunologic
- Antibody-mediated abnormalities

Malignancies

History
- A detailed history and a thorough physical examination are essential in every patient with anemia because the findings usually provide important clues to the etiology of the underlying disorder.
- Obtain history of pregnancies, abortions, and menstrual loss. GI blood loss is an important part of the history. Melena or bright red blood per rectum could suggest upper or lower GI bleed. Changes in bowel habits can be useful in discovering neoplasms of the colon. Other gastrointestinal complaints that may suggest gastritis, peptic ulcers, hiatal hernias, or diverticula are also important.
- Hemorrhoidal blood loss should not be ignored as it can also cause significant anemia.
- Note the routine dietary intake of the patient. Explore the history to elicit details pertaining to the patient's cardiac, hepatic, or renal problems contributing to the anemia.

Physical Examination
- *HEENT:* Pallor, possible icterus, splinter hemorrhages, petechiae
- *Heart:* Systolic murmurs could be heard.
- *Abdomen:* Hepatomegaly and splenomegaly could be present.
- Rectal exam with stool to check for blood.
- *Neurology:* The neurologic examination should include tests of position sense and vibratory sense, examination of the cranial nerves, and testing for tendon reflexes.

Diagnosis
- CBC with peripheral smear, anemia is either microcytic (mean corpuscular volume [MCV] <84) or macrocytic (MCV >96) or normocytic.
- CMP
- Iron, ferritin (most sensitive), TIBC, and saturation
- Vitamin B12 and folate if macrocytosis present
- Coagulation profile
- Hemoglobin electrophoresis if thalasemia suspected
- Erythropoietin level useful in patients with chronic diseases such as chronic renal failure.
- Bone marrow aspiration can lead to a definitive histologic diagnosis of leukemias, lymphomas, myelomas, and metastatic carcinomas. Certain iron stains like Prussian blue can be used to identify sideroblastic anemia. Possible colonoscopy if guaiac positive or anemia in an elderly patient.

Anemia Classification

MICROCYTIC HYPOCHROMIC ANEMIA (MCV <83; MCHC <31)

Condition	Serum Iron	Total Iron-Binding Capacity (TIBC)	Bone Marrow Iron	Ferritin
Iron deficiency	Low	High	0	Low
Chronic disease	Low	Low	++	N/High
Thalassemia major	Low	N	++++	N
Thalassemia minor	N	N	++	N
Lead poisoning (basophilic stippling)	N	N	++	N
Sideroblastic (ring sideroblasts in marrow)	High	N	++++	High

MACROCYTIC ANEMIA (MCV > 95)

Megaloblastic bone marrow	Deficiency of vitamin B12, folate deficiency, medications, genetic disorders
	Hypoplastic and aplastic anemia
	Liver failure
	Hypothyroidism

- In microcytic hypochromic anemia, seek a source of bleeding. Serum iron level, TIBC, and ferritin levels should be obtained.

- In iron deficiency anemia, serum iron level is decreased, TIBC is increased, and a diagnosis of iron deficiency can be made. Therapy can then be initiated, and a search for the cause of the iron deficiency can be started.

- In magaloblastic anemia, vitamin B12, folate levels should be obtained. If necessary, a bone marrow aspirate should be done. Shillings test or intrinsic factor antibodies might be needed to evaluate vitamin B12 deficiency.

- Normocytic normochromic anemia could be because of blood loss, hemolysis, and decreased production. Anemia of chronic disease can be either microcytic or normocytic.

Imaging Studies

- Imaging studies are useful in the workup for anemia when a neoplastic etiology is suggested.

Treatment

- Transfusion of packed RBCs should be done only in symptomatic individuals with Hb <7 or Hct <21 unless actively bleeding or having an MI.

- Erythropoietin has become an extremely useful agent to treat anemia in chronic illnesses such as renal failure and avoid a blood transfusion.

■ In acute blood loss, the main treatment is to correct the underlying cause of bleeding. Once stable then oral iron therapy can be initiated with ferrous sulfate or gluconate. It might take weeks for the iron stores to be repleted but the initial blood transfusion expedites the process. Very rarely parenteral iron therapy may be needed.

■ Appropriate nutritional assessment need to be done to treat deficiency of iron, vitamin B12, and folic acid due to inadequate dietary habits.

■ In case of folate deficiency, do not start with therapy unless vitamin B12 levels are obtained as it could result in permanent neurologic damage. Folate deficiency can coexist and hence needs evaluation.

■ Folate is given as 1 mg PO daily for 3 weeks until improved.

Vitamin B12 is repleted as

1. Cyanocobalamin tablets
   a. Preparations: 25 mcg, 50 mcg, 100 mcg, 250 mcg tablet
   b. Initial: 2000 mcg PO daily for 2 weeks
   c. Maintenance: 1000 mcg PO daily
2. Cyanocobalamin nasal gel 500 mcg each week
   a. Preparations: 400 mg/0.1 ml nasal gel
   b. Initial: 1500 mcg weekly intranasally for 3–4 weeks
   c. Maintenance: 500 mcg weekly
3. Cyanocobalamin injection
   a. Initial: 1000 mcg IM daily for 2 weeks
   b. Maintenance: 1000 mcg IM every 1–3 months

■ Pyridoxine is used in the treatment of patients with sideroblastic anemia in addition to removing the offending agent such as ETOH, lead, or INH

■ Corticosteroids are used in the treatment of autoimmune hemolytic anemia.

■ Aplastic anemia can be treated by removing the offending agent. Splenectomy can provide some benefit for hypoplastic but possibly not for aplastic anemias.

■ Patients with beta-thalassemia major and sickle cell anemia require frequent medical attention.

Diet

■ Patients who are vegans or vegetarians need to supplement their diet with iron and vitamin B12. Iron deficiency can also be geographical based on dietary preferences.

Consultation

■ GI

■ Hematology/oncology

DEEP VEIN THROMBOSIS (DVT)

Blood clots that are formed in the deep veins such as the popliteal, femoral, or iliac veins are termed as deep vein thrombosis (DVT). Calf-vein thrombosis is less likely to cause significant thromboembolism; 80% resolve spontaneously.

Etiology

General: Age, pregnancy, and the postpartum period; major surgery in previous 4 weeks; long plane or car trips (>4 h) in previous 4 weeks; prolonged immobilization longer than 3 days

Medical: Cancer, previous DVT, stroke, acute myocardial infarction (AMI), CHF, sepsis, nephrotic syndrome, ulcerative colitis

Trauma: CNS/spinal cord injury, burns, lower extremity fractures, such as hip

Vasculitis: Systemic lupus erythematosus (SLE) and the lupus anticoagulant, Behçet syndrome, homocystinuria

Hematologic: Inherited disorders of coagulation/fibrinolysis, antithrombin III deficiency, protein C deficiency, protein S deficiency, prothrombin 20210A mutation, factor V leyden, dysfibrino-genemias and disorders of plasminogen activation, polycythemia rubra vera, thrombocytosis

Drugs/medications: Oral contraceptives, estrogens, heparin like agents causing HIT

History

■ Patient would mostly complain of calf tenderness. Details in the history are essential such as long trips >3–4 hours, surgery, and past history and family history of clotting conditions. Sometimes shortness of breath can accompany calf tenderness, which should signify a PE.

■ Patients might have a low-grade fever. If the fever grade is higher, then an infective process might be playing a role.

Virchow's Triad for Thrombogenesis

■ *Stasis*: Bed rest, inactivity. Mostly seen after surgery.

■ *Injury to endothelium*: Trauma, surgery

■ *Hypercoagulability*: Antithrombin III deficiency, APC resistance, protein C or S deficiency, prothrombin 20210A mutation, factor V leiden.

Physical Examination

■ *Extremity*: Edema, principally unilateral, tenderness, if present, is usually confined to the calf muscles or along the course of the deep veins in the medial thigh.

■ *Homans sign*: Discomfort in the calf muscles on forced dorsiflexion of the foot with the knee straight has been a time-honored sign of DVT. This sign is not very specific, its presence can add to the diagnosis as it is present in only 1/3 of the patients with DVT.

■ *Superficial thrombophlebitis*: Present superficially and can be diagnosed clinically due to the palpable, indurated, cord-like lesions along the venous distribution.

Diagnosis

■ CBC

■ CMP

■ Coagulation profile

■ D-Dimer

■ CT pulmonary angiogram to rule out PE if suspected

■ Lower extremity Doppler to confirm DVT

■ *Hypercoagulable workup if the cause of DVT not known*: Protein S, protein C, antithrombin III, Factor V Leyden, prothrombin 20210A mutation, antiphospholipid antibodies, and homocysteine levels can be measured prior to administration of anticoagulants.

Treatment

■ Acute anticoagulation is needed to prevent further worsening.

■ *IV UFH*: 80 U/kg bolus then 18 U/kg infusion titrate to goal PTT of 45–80

■ Low molecular weight heparin like enoxaparin 1 mg/kg SC bid

■ If treatment is done as an inpatient due to patient's clinical condition, intravenous heparin or subcutaneous low molecular weight heparin should be started as soon as possible. Warfarin should be initiated on the first day it self.

■ The loading dose of warfarin can vary. Most physicians start with 5 mg or 10 mg for two days, then half the dose for the remaining days. Once the INR>2, overlap with heparin should be maintained for 1–2 days before discontinuing it. Patient can eventually be sent home on warfarin.

■ *Outpatient treatment*: Continue enoxaparin at 1 mg/kg SC bid or 1.5 mg/kg SC daily for 5 days. Start warfarin after the first dose, continue the overlap for 5 days, then recheck INR, and adjust warfarin dose for out patient therapy of DVT.

■ *Thrombolysis*: Rarely done but consider in extensive DVT or massive PE

■ IVC filter placement if anticoagulation is contraindicated. Most new filters are removable.

■ *Duration of warfarin*:

  □ *First event with reversible risk factors*: Continue for 3–6 months

  □ *Second event or cancer and other nonmodifiable risk factor*: Continue treatment for 12 months: life long

■ *Complication*: Postthrombotic syndrome

Consultation

■ Hematology/oncology

TREATMENT OF ELEVATED INR

■ *If INR < 5 but above the therapeutic range and the patient is not actively bleeding*: Hold warfarin and repeat INR in 1–2 days. May need to restart warfarin at a lower dose.

■ *If the INR is between 5 and 9 and the patient is not bleeding*: Hold warfarin, may need to give vitamin K at a dose of 1–2.5 mg orally. Recheck INR in 1–2 days and restart warfarin at a lower dose when INR is in the therapeutic range. If there is bleeding then the treatment would be different.

■ *In case of surgery or dental extraction where a more rapid reversal is needed and INR > 5*: Vitamin K can be given orally in a dose of 2.5–5 mg but with higher INR, a higher dose of vitamin K might be needed. An additional dose of vitamin K 1–2.5 mg can be given if the INR is still elevated after 24 hours. Please note that if the INR is between 1.5 and 3, holding warfarin or FFP prior to procedure might be better. When vitamin K is administered, a certain resistance to warfarin develops and makes it even longer to reach a therapeutic level with warfarin when restarted. Use vitamin K with caution and after careful evaluation of the situation.

■ *If the INR > 9 but clinically significant bleeding has not occurred*: Vitamin K 3–5 mg orally should be administered. INR should be repeated in 6–8 h and vitamin K repeated if necessary.

■ *If INR > 20 or active bleeding occurs*: Vitamin K 5–10 mg slow IV infusion can be given in addition to transfusion of FFP or prothrombin complex concentrate. Extra caution needs to be taken when giving vitamin K intravenously as it has been known to cause anaphylaxis.

■ *In cases of life-threatening bleeding or serious warfarin overdose*: Prothrombin complex concentrate replacement therapy is indicated, supplemented with 10 mg of vitamin K by slow intravenous infusion; this can be repeated, according to the INR.

Source: Ansell J, Hirsh J, Dalen J, et al. Managing oral anticoagulant therapy. *Chest* 2001;119 Suppl:22S–38S.

ENDOCRINE

DIABETIC KETOACIDOSIS (DKA)

Diabetic ketoacidosis (DKA) is an extreme form of hyperglycemia in insulin dependent diabetics where there is an absolute or relative deficiency of insulin. It is accompanied by acidosis, dehydration, and fatigue.

Etiology

- Infection—most common
- Poor compliance with insulin therapy
- Unknown diabetes
- High sugar intake in diet
- Myocardial infarction
- Cerebrovascular accident
- Complicated pregnancy
- Trauma
- Stress
- Cocaine
- Surgery
- Acromegaly
- Idiopathic (20–30%)

History

Classic Symptoms of Hyperglycemia

- Thirst
- Polyuria, polydipsia
- Nocturia

Other Symptoms

- Generalized weakness
- Malaise/lethargy
- Nausea/vomiting
- Decreased perspiration
- Fatigue
- Anorexia or increased appetite
- Confusion

Physical Examination

- *HEENT*: Dry conjunctiva, dry mucous membranes
- *Skin*: Dry skin, decreased skin turgur
- *Neurology*: Decreased reflexes, confusion and even coma
- *Diagnosis*
  - ☐ BMP q2–4h, glucose levels may be as low as 250 mg/dL.
  - ☐ Finger stick could be obtained early if suspecting DKA as the chemistry might take time.
- *Sodium*: The osmotic effect of hyperglycemia drives the extracellular water intravascularly. For each 100 mg/dL of glucose over 100 mg/dL, the serum sodium level is lowered by approximately 1.6 mEq/L. Measure anion gaps CBC: High white blood cell (WBC) counts or marked left shift may suggest underlying infection.
- *CMP*: Glucose is usually in the range of 400–800 with low bicarbonate levels suggesting metabolic acidosis. BUN/creatinine might be elevated due to dehydration. Arterial blood gas (ABG) levels
- *Serum and urine ketones*: It tests for acetone and acetoacetic acid.
- Urinalysis (UA)
- *Osmolality*: Measured as 2 (Na+) (mEq/L) + glucose (mg/dL)/18 + BUN (mg/dL)/2.8.
- *Phosphorus level*: If patient is an alcoholic or malnourished.

Treatment

- Remember "fluids, fluids, fluids, and then insulin" whereas in the hyperosmolar state it is "fluids, fluids, fluids, fluids, and eventually insulin."
- Intravenous insulin needs to be started early in DKA.
- Potassium level needs to be checked every 2 hours during initial treatment.
- BMP inclusive of serum glucose level should be checked every 2 hours during the initial phase of treatment and eventually the frequency could be prolonged.
- Large volume of isotonic saline (1–3 L) should be given in the first hour. Any further therapy would be to maintain hemodynamic status.
- Once the patient is stabilized, IVF can be switched to ½ NS at 200 mL/h or higher. Monitor for CHF. D5 ½ NS should be initiated with or without potassium when the glucose levels are below 250.
- Insulin should be started about ½-1 hour after intravenous fluid replacement is started. Potassium levels need to be checked q2–4h until the patient is stabilized and the anion gap closes. IV insulin should be started after an IV bolus of 10 units and then 0.1 U/kg/h.
- Potassium should be replaced with the initial fluids, as it tends to move back into the cells when the acidosis is corrected and can lead to severe hypokalemia.

It should be replaced even if the values are normal. If the values are high then it needs to be monitored carefully before starting therapy.

■ Add 20–40 mEq/L of KCl to each liter of fluid once K+ is less than 5.5 mEq/L.
■ Bicarbonate is not given unless the pH is <7.1. It is believed that just with fluid and IV insulin the acidosis should be corrected.

Consultation
■ Endocrine

HYPOGLYCEMIA

Hypoglycemia is a syndrome caused by a reduction in plasma glucose concentration to a level that may induce symptoms of low blood sugar.

Etiology

- *Reactive hypoglycemia*: This occurs in patients with a history of previous GI procedures such as (gastrectomy, gastrojejunostomy, vagotomy, pyloroplasty) and allows rapid glucose entry and absorption in the intestine, provoking excessive insulin response to a meal. This may occur within 1–3 hours after a meal.
- Tight glycemic control
- *Exogenous insulin*: Tumors such as islet cell adenoma either isolated or as a part of MEN I, exogenous administration
- *Nonbeta-cell tumors*: Mediastinal tumors.
- *Autoimmune hypoglycemia*: Can be caused by insulin antibodies and insulin receptor antibodies
- Sulfonylurea abuse
- *Hormonal deficiencies*: Hypoadrenalism, glucagon deficiency
- *Acute illnesses*: Sepsis, renal failure, acute MI

History

- Patients commonly present with sweating, tachycardia, tremors, and anxiety. These symptoms are due to sympatho-adrenal activation.
- Neuroglycopenic symptoms are weakness, tiredness, or dizziness, poor concentration, and in severe cases, death.

Physical Examination

- *Heart*: Tachycardia might be present
- *Neuro*: Resting tremors, fatigue, disorientation

Diagnosis

- CBC
- CMP
- Chest x-ray
- *Insulin levels*: Elevated in insulinoma (high C-peptide) and exogenous insulin administration (low C-peptide)
- Sulphonylurea levels
- *C-peptide levels*: Insulinoma is associated with elevated C-peptide concentrations with concurrent hypoglycemia. Exogenous insulin abuse results in low concentrations of C-peptide.

- Oral glucose tolerance test can be done if reactive hypoglycemia is suspected. An oral glucose tolerance test is not the best test for fasting hypoglycemia and provides little benefit.
- A supervised fast is the most reliable test for fasting hypoglycemia.
- ACTH stimulation test or morning cortisol level should be obtained if adrenal insufficiency is suspected.

Imaging Studies

- MRI will be needed to evaluate insulinomas, as they might be too small for CT scans.
- Retroperitoneal tumors that are producing insulin-like growth factor (IGF) can be imaged with a CT scan.

Treatment

- Diet
- Blood glucose in the range of 60–80 mg/dL, dietary therapy can be initiated but if the values are lower than that, then more aggressive IV therapy might be needed.
- Dietary therapy is essential and first-line therapy in treating fasting hypoglycemia. Frequent meals/snacks are recommended especially at night, with complex carbohydrates.
- Consultation with a nutritionist is essential in addition to a diabetic teacher, if the patient is a diabetic.
- If dietary therapy is inadequate, then IV D50 is given and is still not improved the intravenous glucose infusion with D5 half-normal saline or D5 water. Intravenous octreotide can be effective in suppressing endogenous insulin secretion. Reactive hypoglycemia does not require medical care.
- If patient had been on sulphonyl ureas, then the duration of observation should be longer as they remain in the system for a longer duration.

Surgical Care

- Hypoglycemia caused as a result of tumor should be treated surgically. The success rate for benign tumors is very high and is about 50% for malignant tumors.

Consultation

- Endocrine

Types of Insulin

- Rapid-acting insulin, such as insulin lispro or insulin aspart starts to work about 5 minutes after injection, peaks in about 1 hour, and continues to work for 2 to 4 hours.
- Regular or short-acting insulin reaches the bloodstream within 30 minutes after injection, peaks anywhere from 2 to 3 hours after injection, and is effective for approximately 3 to 6 hours.

■ Intermediate-acting insulin reaches the bloodstream about 2 to 4 hours after injection, peaks 4 to 12 hours later and is effective for about 12 to 18 hours.

■ Long-acting insulin (ultralente) can reach the bloodstream 6 to 10 hours after injection and is effective for 20 to 24 hours. Two long-acting analogues of the long-acting insulin exist, namely glargine and detemir. They both tend to lower glucose levels in a similar manner over a 24-hour period with less of a peak of action than ultralente.

SYNDROME OF INAPPROPRIATE ANTIDIURETIC HORMONE SECRETION (SIADH)

The syndrome of inappropriate antidiuretic hormone secretion, as the name suggests is the inappropriate secretion and activity of the antidiuretic hormone that causes hyponatremia by retaining water in excess amounts.

Etiology

■ Some of the causes of SIADH are listed below:

■ *Pulmonary disease*: COPD, pneumonia, malignancy, lung abscess, TB

■ *Neurology*: Tumor, trauma, infection, cerebrovascular accident, subarachnoid hemorrhage, delirium tremens, multiple sclerosis

■ *Carcinoma*: Lung, pancreas, thymoma, ovarian

■ *Drugs*: NSAIDs, nicotine, diuretics, chlorpropamide, carbamazepine, tricyclic antidepressants, SSRIs, vincristine, thioridazine, cyclophosphamide, clofibrate, vasopressin

■ *Surgery*: Postoperative

■ Idiopathic (most common)

History

■ Patients can present with multiple symptoms but initially anorexia, nausea, and malaise are the earliest, followed by headache, irritability, confusion, muscle cramps, weakness, seizures, and possibly coma. These occur due to osmotic fluid shifts that can cause cerebral edema and increased intracranial pressure. History of diet, fluid intake, gastrointestinal losses, amount of urinary output, and medications is important. A detailed history is needed to establish a diagnosis of SIADH. Other potential causes of hyponatremia are CHF, liver failure, adrenal insufficiency, renal failure, and thyroid diseases.

Physical Examination

■ SIADH is characterized by euvolemic hyponatremia.

■ *Extremity*: Edema in a hyponatremic patient could point toward conditions other than SIADH, such as the hypervolemic hyponatremic states (CHF, cirrhosis, and nephrotic syndrome).

■ *Neurology*: Confusion, lethargy, weakness, myoclonus, asterixis, depressed reflexes, generalized seizures, and coma.

Diagnosis

■ CBC

■ *CMP*: Serum electrolytes, BUN, creatinine, and glucose levels

■ Hyponatremia is typical of SIADH

■ If hypokalemia and acidosis are present, then diuretic therapy or vomiting might be the cause.

- Low serum osmolality (<280 mOsm/kg)
- *Urine sodium*: Elevated urinary sodium level (>20 mmol/L)
- *Urine osmolality*: Generally >200 mOsm/L
- *Plasma cortisol level*: To exclude adrenal insufficiency.
- Pseudohyponatremia can occur with severe hyperlipidemia and with hyperproteinemia (levels >10 g/dL, as seen in multiple myeloma).

Imaging Studies

- CXR can discover pneumonias, malignancies, and fibrosis. A more detailed picture can be provided by a CT scan of the chest.
- CT scan of the brain may show evidence of cerebral edema (eg, narrowing of the ventricles) or may identify a CNS disorder responsible for SIADH (eg, brain tumor).

Treatment

- The treatment of hyponatremia should be gradual to prevent central pontine myelinolysis (CPM).
- Free water restriction forms the basis of SIADH treatment.
- The sodium deficit can be calculated by the following formula:
- Na deficit = (Desired Na – Measured Na) $\times$ 0.6 $\times$ (weight in kg)
- The total rate of correction should not exceed 12 mEq/L in the first 24 hours. If risk factors for CPM are present then the rate of correction should be restricted to 10 mEq/L per 24 hours.
- Administration of 3% NaCl should only be required in patients with severely symptomatic hyponatremia (eg, seizures) or potentially in patients with serum sodium level of less than 110 mEq/L.
- The volume of hypertonic saline required to correct the sodium deficit can be calculated by the formula:
  - ☐ Volume of 3% saline = (Na deficit)/513 mEq Na/L
- The rate of correction of chronic hyponatremia should not exceed 0.5 mEq/L/h. Therefore, the amount of time needed to correct a given degree of hyponatremia is as follows:
  - ☐ Time needed for correction = (desired Na : measured Na)/0.5 mEq/L/h
- The rate of infusion of hypertonic saline is as follows:
  - ☐ Rate = (Volume of 3% saline)/(Time needed for correction)
- If hypokalemia is present, it needs to be corrected simultaneously. Monitor serum and urine electrolyte levels every 2 hours, and then at least every 4 hours until the patient's levels are stabilized.
- When the sodium level reaches around 125, reevaluate the therapy. The amount of free water restriction can be reduced or the fluids can be discontinued.
- Furosemide can be used at the dose 1 mg/kg IV as needed to promote extretion of free water in association with isotonic or hypertonic saline.

■ Lithium carbonate and demeclocycline can block the effects of ADH and increase free water excretion but due to the complications associated with its use, it is recommended that appropriate consultations be obtained.

Consultation
■ Nephrology
■ Endocrinology

INFECTIOUS DISEASES

CELLULITIS

The simplest way to define cellulitis is inflammation of the skin. Literally, it means inflammation of the cells. It can involve deeper layers of the skin including the epidermis extending into the dermis and subcutaneous tissues.

Etiology
- Bacterial and fungal infections
- Group A streptococci and *S. aureus*
- Group B streptococci.
- In immunocompromised hosts, gram-negative rods and rarely fungus
- Fresh water wounds: *Aeromonas hydrophila*
- Pneumococcus can cause extensive cellulitis in immunocompromised patients.
- *Cat bite*: *S. aureus*, Group A, B steptococcus, *Pasturella* species
- *Cat scratch*: *Bartonella henselae*
- *Dog bite*: *S. aureus*, Group A, B steptococcus, *Pasturella* species
- Risk factors for developing cellulitis:
  - ☐ Diabetes
  - ☐ Immunodeficiency
  - ☐ Arterial insufficiency or venous stasis
  - ☐ Chronic steroid use
  - ☐ Herpes zoster or simplex

History
- Detailed history should be obtained regarding the mode of entry. Usually a break in the skin is the culprit. Patient with tinea pedis or skin cracks are at higher risk.
- Foreign bodies passing through skin, such as intravenous catheters can be a source of entry.
- Patients with lymphnode dissection following a mastectomy are at risk for recurrent cellulitis.

Physical Examination
- *HEENT*: Lymphadenopathy close to the cellulitis might be present.
- *Skin*: Warmth, erythema, edema, and tenderness of the affected area are present.
- Ascending lymphangitis can be seen as a red streak extending proximally along the lymphatic drainage system.

Diagnosis

- CBC
- CMP with BUN/creatinine
- Blood cultures × 2
- Aspiration of the wound if any evidence of abscess
- Culture and gram stain are of limited use if just the skin is cultured. Yield is positive approximately one-third of the time.
- If an abscess or bullae is present, then a 90% yield could be obtained form the culture and gram stain.
- *Immunofluorescence*: Can be useful in culture negative cellulitis.

Imaging Studies

- Ultrasound of the area could be obtained to evaluate an abscess
- CT scan with IV contrast can also be used to locate and abscess in less dense regions.
- MRI could be more useful for an abscess in dense regions such as the thigh, if the ultrasound was negative and there was high suspicion for an abscess. It could also be useful in the evaluation of osteomyelitis.

Treatment

- If a cut, bite, or a laceration caused the cellulitis, tetanus vaccine should be administered unless received in the last 10 years for a clean wound and less than 5 for a dirty wound.
- Mild cellulitis
- Oral antibiotics like cephalexin 500 mg PO qid for 7–10 days or augmentin 875 mg PO bid for 7–10 days.
- Reevaluate within 24–48 hours. Patients who have failed outpatient treatment should be admitted for intravenous antibiotics.
- *Complicated cellulitis*: Intravenous antibiotics will be needed. First generation cephalosporin or penicillinase-resistant penicillin. Erythromycin or vancomycin can be used if resistant to penicillin. Quinolones are also alternatives.
- Commonly used antibiotics are cepfazolin 500 mg to 1 g IV q6–8h or ceftriaxone 1 g IV q24h or ampicillin-sulbactam 1.5 g to 3 g IV q6h. Vancomycin can be used if MRSA is suspected or if allergic to penicillin.
- In case of cat scratch cellulitis, azithromycin 500 mg IV daily should be administered initially and later switched to PO when patient better for a total of 5–7 days. Doxycycline or ciprofloxacin are other alternatives.
- Keep the affected limb elevated
- If signs of crepitus or necrosis is present, surgery should be consulted immediately.

Consultation

Infectious diseases

DECUBITUS ULCERS (PRESSURE SORES)

Decubitus ulcers commonly occur in dependent area of the body such as the sacral region, ischial tuberosity.

Etiology

- Impaired mobility
- Contractures and spasticity
- Sensory loss also contributes to ulceration
- Malnutrition, hypoproteinemia, and anemia
- Urinary of fecal incontinence resulting in the bacterial contamination of skin

Physical Examination

- There can be varying degrees of pressure ulcers depending on the depth and involvement of various layers of the skin and muscle. Pressure sores can be the greatest at dependent regions and bony prominences and tend to decline at the peripheral sites. Once a small area of skin breakdown has occurred, it is only a matter of time until it develops into a larger lesion

NATIONAL PRESSURE ULCER ADVISORY PANEL STAGING SYSTEM

Stage I: Intact skin, impending ulceration. Erythema, warmth, and induration may be present and may resolve within 24 h of pressure relief.

Stage II: Partial-thickness, loss of epidermis, and some amount of the dermis. Blister, ulceration, or an abrasion may be present.

Stage III: Full-thickness, loss of epidermis, dermis, and extension into the subcutaneous tissue but not the fascia. This lesion presents with or without undermining of adjacent tissue.

Stage IV: Full-thickness, loss of epidermis, dermis, and subcutaneous tissue and extension into muscle, bone, tendon, or joint capsule. Osteomyelitis can be present in association with fractures, bone destruction, and dislocations. Sinus tracts may be present.

Source: Black, J; Baharestani, M et al. National pressure ulcer advisory panel's updated pressure ulcer staging system. *Adv Skin Wound Care.* 2007 May;20(5):269–274.

One should monitor for foul odors, wound drainage, eschar, necrotic material, and soilage from urinary or fecal incontinence. This information can guide us regarding the level of bacterial contamination and the need for debridement.

Anatomic Sites
The most common locations are the hip and buttock areas followed by ischial tuberosity and sacral regions. Less commonly, patellar or the pretibial regions. Very rarely one could discover decubitus ulcers on the nose, chin, elbow, etc.

Diagnosis

- CBC
- CMP

- Wound culture and tissue biopsy
- Blood culture if febrile and systemic involvement suspected.
- MRI of the region if osteomyelitis suspected or bone scan.
- X-ray is not helpful in the initial stages.

Treatment
Medical Therapy

- Air mattress or foam for beds and wheelchairs to decrease the pressure.
- Change the patient position every 2 hours.
- The ulcer and surrounding skin should be clean and free from urine and other contaminants.
- Wound dressings depend on the type of wound. A stage I lesion with signs of breakdown may require no dressing. Stage II ulcers confined to the epidermis or dermis may be treated with a hydrocolloid occlusive dressing (DuoDerm), which maintains a moist environment to facilitate reepithelialization. For more severe ulcers, wet-to-dry dressings, incorporating isotonic sodium chloride solution or dilute Dakins solution (sodium hypochlorite), Silvadene, Sulfamylon, hydrogels (Carrington gel), xerogels (Sorbsan), and vacuum-assisted closure (VAC) sponges. Daily whirlpool use may also be helpful to irrigate and mechanically debride the ulcers.
- Infected ulcers can lead to sepsis, necrotizing fasciitis, and even gangrene if not debrided appropriately. Appropriate antibiotics need to be initiated at that time.
- Nutritional consult should be obtained. Prealbumin and albumin levels should be ordered. Nutritional status should be optimized with enteral, parenteral feeding if patient unable to take po.
- When optimal medical treatment is provided, many stage I and stage II pressure sores heal spontaneously. Surgery might be needed for stage III and stage IV ulcers.

Surgical Therapy

- The postoperative care depends on the surgeon. Mostly a plastic surgeon is given the task of reconstruction.
- Postoperatively, the patient needs to be on a specialized support surface for about 6 weeks.
- After approximately 6 weeks, pressure should be applied gradually to the site but frequent change of position is essential.
- Perform skin care daily.

Consultation

- General surgery
- Plastic surgery

5

ICU Rounds

Manish Mehta, MD

This chapter focuses on the common issues and diseases encountered in the intensive care unit (ICU). The goal is to provide a basic understanding of critical care to make one feel comfortable in that setting.

ADULT RESPIRATORY DISTRESS SYNDROME (ARDS)

In 1994, the American–European Consensus Conference (AECC) on ARDS formulated their definition of ARDS as follows:

- Acute onset of symptoms
- The ratio of the alveolar partial pressure of oxygen (Pao_2) to the fraction of inspired oxygen (FiO_2) of 200 mm Hg or less
- Bilateral infiltrates on chest x-rays
- Pulmonary arterial wedge pressure of 18 mm Hg or less or no clinical signs of left atrial hypertension

ARDS is detected radiographically with leakage of fluid with high protein content into the alveolar spaces suggesting alveolar damage.

Etiology

- *Infection*: Pneumonia of any etiology (especially viral) and systemic sepsis (especially Gram negative)
- *Shock*: Any type, particularly septic and traumatic shock
- *Aspiration*: Gastric contents, toxic inhalation
- *Trauma*: Pulmonary contusion, fat embolization, and multiple trauma
- *Other*: Systemic inflammatory response syndrome, pancreatitis, s/p CABG, massive blood transfusion, drug ingestion (eg, heroin, methadone, barbiturates, salicylates)

History

- ARDS can occur following a variety of pulmonary or nonpulmonary insults. Care must be taken in such patients to prevent development of ARDS
- ARDS can occurs from 4 hr to several days after the injury
- Dyspnea is present in most cases
- Other symptoms, if present, typically are related to the predisposing condition

Physical Examination

Findings on physical examination are not specific for ARDS and can be found in pulmonary edema of any cause.

- *HEENT*: Cyanosis
- *Heart*: Tachycardia, murmurs possible
- *Lungs*: Labored breathing and tachypnea (almost universally present, scattered crackles, increased work of breathing)
- *Neurology*: Agitation, lethargy followed by obtundation

- □ Diffuse pneumonia of any origin (although pneumonia can be a cause of ARDS)
- □ Cardiogenic edema
- □ Pulmonary hemorrhage
- □ Congestive heart failure

Diagnosis

- CBC
- CMP
- EKG
- Blood cultures × 2
- Arterial blood gases (ABG) analysis is the most important laboratory test and allows detection and documentation of hypoxemia.
  - □ Hypocapnia is a typical finding early in ARDS, but hypercapnia is possible at a later stage
  - □ PaO_2 less than 50 mm Hg with an FiO_2 more than 0.6

Imaging Studies

- The chest radiograph reveals characteristic diffuse alveolar-interstitial infiltrates in all lung fields.
- Chest CT may be helpful in advanced cases.
- Echocardiography may be helpful to exclude a cardiogenic etiology for pulmonary edema.

Procedures

- Sputum should be collected for Gram stain and cultures (eg, bacterial, fungal, viral) if a pulmonary infection is present. These are best obtained from the lower respiratory tract shortly after endotracheal (ET) intubation.
- Bronchoscopy with bronchoalveolar lavage may be helpful to identify occult pulmonary infection but is usually performed in the ICU.
- A pulmonary artery catheter may be helpful to exclude cardiogenic causes but usually is placed in the ICU.

Chest X-Ray (Figure 1)

- Symmetrical consolidation with air bronchograms, bilateral infiltrates. Other conditions that could present this way are pneumonias, pulmonary edema, and alveolar hemorrhage. These radiologic features can worsen in a few days or even sooner on occasion.

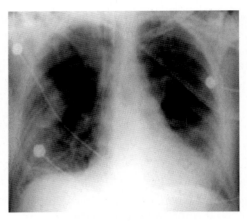

Figure 1

CT Scan

■ Asymmetric, ground-glass opacification is seen for pulmonary causes, whereas for extra-pulmonary causes, symmetric ground-glass opacification is seen.

Treatment

■ ABCs are essential. If this fails then endotracheal intubation will have to be done.

■ Two large-bore IV lines need to be placed if shock is anticipated, otherwise a regular 20-gauge IV should be used at all times.

■ IV fluids if necessary.

■ Mechanical ventilation with positive end-expiratory pressure (PEEP) of 5–10 cm H_2O is effective in reducing intrapulmonary shunting and improving oxygenation.

  ☐ Initiate with an FiO_2 of 100 and decrease only while monitoring pulse oximetry, maintaining the oxygen saturation at 92–94%.

  ☐ Select an initial tidal volume of 8–10 mL/kg and respiratory rate of 10/min.

  ☐ High PEEP is needed to improve the alveolar surface area and avoid collapse.

  ☐ Plateau pressures should be less than 30. This is better managed through pressure-controlled ventilation.

  ☐ Pressure-controlled ventilation is considered better in this setting as the plateau pressures must be kept low.

  ☐ Permissive hypercapnia is allowed in ARDS but only in certain situations. If the pH declines below 7.1, it needs to be corrected.

■ Vitals need to be monitored frequently as the cardiopulmonary status can change based on the ventilator settings.

■ Treat the underlying etiology.

■ Antibiotics based on the condition.

■ Steroids have no benefit in the early phase but may be helpful in the fibroproliferative phase.

Prognosis

■ Mortality rate averages 60%.

■ Patients usually die from sepsis or multiple organ failure.

■ Survivors usually have a good outcome with only minimal pulmonary symptoms but they can persist for a long time.

■ Survivors of severe cases may have some degree of permanent pulmonary fibrosis and symptoms of restrictive lung disease.

Consultation

■ Pulmonary/critical care

SHOCK

■ Shock is a clinically diagnosed syndrome caused by various etiologies. It is characterized by hypotension and in severe cases multisystem organ failure.

Classification of Shock
■ Hypovolemic
■ Distributive
■ Cardiogenic
■ Obstructive
■ Miscellaneous

HYPOVOLEMIC SHOCK

■ Hypovolemic shock is caused as a result of intravascular volume depletion caused by the following conditions. Due to decreased preload, cardiac output is reduced and hence hypotension occurs.

Etiology
■ Intravascular volume loss
  ☐ Diarrhea
  ☐ Burns
  ☐ Diabetes insipidus
  ☐ Heat stroke
■ Hemorrhage
  ☐ Trauma
  ☐ Surgery
  ☐ GI bleeding
■ Other
  ☐ Sepsis
  ☐ Nephrotic syndrome
  ☐ Intestinal obstruction
  ☐ Ascites

DISTRIBUTIVE SHOCK

■ Distributive shock is caused as a result of systemic vasodilation in the setting of sepsis, anaphylaxis, neurological injury and iatrogenic.

Etiology
- Anaphylaxis
  - ☐ Medications (antibiotics, vitamin K, etc.)
  - ☐ Blood products
  - ☐ Foods (shellfish, peanuts)
  - ☐ Latex
- Neurologic causes
  - ☐ Head injury
  - ☐ Spinal shock
- Drugs
- Sepsis

Anaphylaxis causes mast cell degranulation and histamine release with vasodilation. Neurologic injury can interrupt sympathetic input to vasomotor neurons, resulting in vasodilation. Spinal shock may result from cervical cord injuries above T-1, which result in shock from unopposed parasympathetic activity. These patients can present with hypotension and bradycardia. Sepsis results in the release of many vasoactive mediators that may cause vasodilation requiring considerable amount of fluid resuscitation.

CARDIOGENIC SHOCK

- Cardiogenic shock occurs as a result of diminished cardiac output from poor stroke volume. Patients who present in cardiogenic shock are extremely critical. If it occurs following an MI, an urgent catheterization is needed with intra-aortic balloon pump. Many other conditions that can result in cardiogenic shock are:
  - ☐ Acute myocardial infarction
  - ☐ Ventricular wall rupture, papillary muscle rupture
  - ☐ Severe congestive heart failure
  - ☐ Cardiac temponade
  - ☐ Iatrogenic
  - ☐ Sepsis
  - ☐ Dilated cardiomyopathy
  - ☐ Drugs like cocaine
  - ☐ Pulmonary embolism

OBSTRUCTIVE SHOCK

Obstructive shock occurs when:
- Venous return to the heart is obstructed as a result of pressure or mass within the mediastinum such as tension pneumothorax or cardiac temponade.
- The body does not receive adequate oxygen to various parts it begins to fail resulting in multisystem organ failure. This occurs in the later stages of shock and can affect the neurologic status as well. Patients might require aggressive resuscitative efforts.

History
- Patient might complain of fatigue, altered sensorium and some times chest pain. Depending on the type of shock, relevant history should be obtained.

Diagnosis
- CBC
- CMP
- Blood culture $\times$ 2
- Sputum gram stain and culture (if pulmonary source suspected)
- Urine culture
- DIC panel (fibrinogen, D-dimer, PTT, PT)
- Cardiac enzymes
- ACTH stimulation test
- 2-D echocardiogram
- Chest x-ray
- Lactate level

CLINICAL EVALUATION

Acid-Base Status
- Lactic acidosis is present in shock and can be a valuable tool to determine the prognosis.

Mixed Venous Oxygen Saturation
- Sample obtained form the Swan-Ganz catheter is mixed venous blood from the from the right atrium. By comparing the mixed venous oxygen saturation (SvO_2) with the SaO_2, a determination of the arteriovenous oxygen saturation difference can be noted. Normally the SaO_2 is 90–100%, the normal SvO_2 is 70–80%. In a state of shock the oxygen extraction difference is >33%, suggesting that the tissues require more oxygen to meet the demand. If the oxygen extraction difference is <25%, that signifies vasodilation and distributive state.

Central Venous Pressure (CVP) and Pulmonary Capillary Wedge Pressure (PCWP)

- A central venous catheter in the pulmonary vein can detect pressure in that vein as well as the left atrium. It is of tremendous importance to understand the intravascular volume status of a patient.
- A normal CVP in a normal compliant heart is typically 1–3 cm H_2O. Pressures much higher than 10 cm H_2O may reflect volume overload or poor right-sided heart compliance or function. Volume administration is generally thought to be maximal at PCWP measurements of 12–18 cm H_2O in patients with adequate left-sided heart function.

Cardiac Index

- Calculated by $CI = CO/BSA = SV \times HR/BSA$. Normal cardiac index is 3.5–5.5.
- If cardiac index is less than 1.8, patient could be in cardiogenic shock. It is a very useful guide while titrating various pressors and cardiotropic agents.

TREATMENT

- ABCs are extremely essential
- Two large bore IV lines should be placed immediately.
- Airway should be patient, administer 100% oxygen initially. If patient in distress, endotracheal intubation should be considered. (See indication of intubation in the next section).

Septic Shock

- In addition to volume expansion, empiric antibiotics should be initiated early. Commonly used antibiotics are ceftriaxone 1g IV q24h, levofloxacin 750 mg IV q24h. If pseudomonal infection is suspected, then dual coverage with piperacillin/tazobactam, a cephalosporin or quinolones should be initiated. MRSA should be empirically covered with vancomycin.

Volume Expansion

- Intravenous access is extremely necessary in this setting. Two large-bore IVs need to be placed immediately. If vascular access cannot be obtained, then an intraosseous (IO) needle may be placed into the bone marrow.
- Administer 20 mL/kg of an isotonic crystalloid infusion, such as 0.9% isotonic sodium chloride or lactated Ringer solution, over 5 minutes or less. Additional fluid can be administered it needed. Isotonic fluids tend to stay intravascular longer than hypotonic agents.
- If the patient's clinical status does not improve, wide-open infusion should be done.
- In the setting of distributive or hypovolemic shock, aggressive volume expansion is necessary.
- If the patient is actively bleeding and in hypovolemic shock, PRBCs should be transfused immediately and arrangements such as surgery consults, gastroenterology consults should be done simultaneously to treat the source of blood loss.

Vasopressors Used in Shock

The decision on which pressor to use is somewhat complicated but if you understand the physiology behind it, the decision gets easier. Inotropic agents increase myocardial contractility and can have some effects on peripheral vascular resistance. Some of these can be vasoconstrictors such as epinephrine and norepinephrine. Some may be vasodilators such as milrinone. Some vasopressors have beta 1-adrenergic activity resulting in tachycardia thus increasing myocardial oxygen demand causing worsening of myocardial ischemia and others, which are potent vasoconstrictors, can worsen perfusion to peripheral end-organ tissue capillary beds such as the renal or splanchnic vasculature. They are extremely useful in the setting of shock but their side effects have to be understood well before initiating a pressor.

Dopamine

Dopamine is often used either alone or in combination with other inotropic agents. It is recommended for fluid-refractory septic shock. Dopamine is generally useful for its mixed and vasodilatory effect on end-organ perfusion such as renal and splanchnic vasculature at a low dose (ie, 2–5 mcg/kg/min IV). At an intermediate dose (ie, 5–10 mcg/kg/min IV), the beta 1-agonist effect assists by improving myocardial contractility, CO, and enhancing conduction (ie, increasing SA rate) in the heart. At a higher dose (ie, 10–20 mcg/kg/min IV or more), the alpha-agonist effect increases and may increase peripheral vasoconstriction and blood pressure.

Epinephrine

Epinephrine is the pressor of choice for fluid refractory, dopamine resistant non-vasodilatory shock. Epinephrine acts on both alpha- and beta-receptors, resulting in increased myocardial contractility and increased peripheral vasoconstriction. Ventricular dysrhythmias may be precipitated. At high enough doses, it can cause limb ischemia. Usual starting dose is 0.1 mcg/kg/min IV and is titrated upward according to effectiveness and adverse effects. In severe cases, patients may receive doses of 2–3 mcg/kg/min IV or even higher.

Dobutamine

It is a strong inotropic agent with primarily beta 1-agonist effects that increases cardiac contractility. It also has some effect on beta 2-receptors causing peripheral vasodilation that might reduce systemic vascular resistance and afterload. It is very useful in cardiogenic shock or severe systolic congestive heart failure to improve contractility. Dobutamine has fewer side effects than epinephrine. A typical dose begins with 5 mcg/kg/min IV and is gradually increased to 20 mcg/kg/min IV.

Norepinephrine

Norepinephrine is mainly an alpha agonist casuing vasoconstriction and hence increasing the peripheral vascular resistance. It is useful in distributive shock as well as other types of shock. It is a potent pressor and can be initiated early in any type of shock as the first pressor. It can cause some tachycardia and care must be taken in patients with rapid atrial fibrillation or ventricular tachycardias. Typical doses of norepinephrine are similar to epinephrine and begin at 0.1 mcg/kg/min IV, and titrated upward according to effectiveness and adverse effects.

Phosphodiesterase Inhibitors
Inamrinone and milrinone are phosphodiesterase inhibitors produce an increase in intracellular cyclic adenosine monophosphate (cAMP), which raises intracellular calcium levels, improving cardiac inotropy as well as peripheral vasodilation. They can be used in association with other pressors like the catecholamines to improve cardiac contractility and reduce the after load.

Typical doses of inamrinone are a loading dose of 0.75 mg/kg IV over 2–3 min followed by a continuous IV infusion of 5–10 mcg/kg/min. Milrinone may be initiated with a loading dose of 25–50 mcg/kg over 10 min, followed by a continuous IV infusion of 0.375–0.75 mcg/kg/min. Adverse effects of both inamrinone and milrinone may include arrhythmias as well as thrombocytopenia.

Corticosteroids
The use of corticosteroids, particularly in patients with septic shock, is debated. Studies so far have not demonstrated any conclusive benefit in both humans and animals. It might be useful to obtain a random cortisol level and a ACTH stimulation test prior to administration of corticosteroids. Dosage is 1–2 mg/kg hydrocortisone IV every 6 hours to as much as a 50 mg/kg bolus followed by the same amount infused over 24 hours.

Drotrecogin Alfa (Xigris)
■ *Indication*: Xigris is indicated in adult patients with severe sepsis (sepsis associated with acute organ dysfunction) who have a high risk of death (eg, as determined by APACHE II). It is a recombinant form of human activated protein C. It has been proven in studies to improve mortality

■ *Contraindications*: Xigris increases the risk of bleeding. Xigris is contraindicated in patients with high risk of bleeding that could result in increased morbidity and possibly mortality:

☐ Active internal bleeding

☐ Recent (within 3 months) hemorrhagic stroke

☐ Recent (within 2 months) intracranial or intraspinal surgery, or severe head trauma

☐ Trauma with high risk for life threatening bleeding

☐ Presence of an epidural catheter

☐ Intracranial neoplasm or mass lesion or evidence of cerebral herniation

Xigris is contraindicated in patients who have been hypersensitive to drotrecogin alfa (activated) or any of its components.

Dose: 24 mcg/kg/hr IV × 96 hr

When treating shock, the underlying etiology should be identified and treated.

Nutrition
Nutritional assessment has to be done periodically with any critical patient and more so a patient in shock. It is extremely essential to provide adequate nutrition to allow a timely recovery.

VENTILATION

NON-INVASIVE VENTILATION

This is a mode of ventilation that does not require ET tubes and LMA. It plays a very important role when a patient does not want to be resuscitated.

Types
Continuous Positive Airway Pressure (CPAP)
- Delivers a set positive airway pressure more than the atmospheric pressure
- Increases oxygenation by enhancing alveolar recruitment and prevents collapse
- Decreases V/Q mismatch
- Decreases the preload by increasing the intrathoracic pressure on the IVC

Bi-level Positive Airway Pressure (BiPAP)
- Delivers positive pressure in both inspiration and expiration, but more during inspiration, by increasing the tidal volume
- Increases the minute ventilation, hence helps in CO_2 narcosis
- Increases alveolar recruitment and prevents collapse
- Decreases V/Q mismatch

Clinical Conditions
- *COPD*: BiPAP increases the minute ventilation and enhance removal of excess CO_2
- *OSA*: CPAP allows airways to be open and prevents alveolar collapse.
- *Hypoventilation*: BiPAP could be considered
- *Acute hypoxemia*: CPAP can be used.

Contraindications
- Hemodynamic instability
- Respiratory arrest
- Refractory hypoxema
- Aspiration risk
- Copious secretions
- Altered mental status
- Traumatic brain injury

MECHANICAL VENTILATION

One of the first negative-pressure ventilator to be used was the Drinker and Shaw tank-type ventilator in 1929. It included a metal cylinder that surrounded the patient until the neck. It was also termed as the iron lung. The negative pressure was created by a vacuum pump. This helped with the expansion of the lung and in contrast when the vacuum was reduced the negative pressure declined.

Indications for Intubation
■ Conditions causing hypercapnia (Pco_2 >50)
  ☐ Severe COPD
  ☐ Status asthmaticus
  ☐ Hypoventilation
  ☐ Respiratory muscle fatigue with lactic acidosis
■ Conditions causing hypoxia (Po_2 <60)
  ☐ Pulmonary edema
  ☐ Pulmonary embolism
  ☐ Severe pneumonia
  ☐ ARDS/acute lung injury
■ Airway protection
  ☐ Delirium tremens
  ☐ Status epilepticus
  ☐ Aspiration
  ☐ Laryngeal edema
  ☐ Traumatic brain injury
■ Acid base disturbances that require immediate correction
■ Therapeutic hyperventilation to decrease ICP in various intracranial bleeds

Other Indications That Could Help With Judgment
■ Apnea with respiratory arrest
■ Acute lung injury
■ Respiratory rate >30 breaths per min
■ Vital capacity <15 mL/kg
■ Minute ventilation >10 L/min
■ Alveolar-arterial difference in oxygen tension (A-a DO_2) with 100% oxygenation of >450 mm Hg
■ Clinical deterioration
■ Respiratory muscle fatigue
■ Obtundation or coma

- Hypotension
- Tachypnea
- Neuromuscular disease

Clinical judgement to intubate is based on these values. Increasing severity of illness should prompt the clinician to consider starting mechanical ventilation.

PCO$_2$ is dependent on minute ventilation: Tidal volume $\times$ Respiratory rate (Increasing the minute ventilation decreases the PCO$_2$)

PO$_2$ is dependent on FiO$_2$ and PEEP (Increasing the PEEP or FiO$_2$ increases the PO$_2$)

Mode of Ventilation

- Ventilation can either be pressure controlled as is usually done for ARDS or volume cycled as in most cases. It is important to understand each mode of ventilation before using it.

Tidal Volume and Rate

- The 12–12 rule is followed for a patient with preexisting disease. A tidal volume of 12 mL for each kilogram of lean body weight is programmed to be delivered 12 times a minute in the assist-control mode.
- In COPD, the tidal volume is reduced and follows a 10–10 rule. A tidal volume of 10 mL/kg lean body weight is delivered 10 times a minute in the assist-control mode.

Initial FiO$_2$

- When the mechanical ventilation is initiated, oxygenation should be addressed first. Initially the FiO$_2$ should be set at 100% and later titrated to keep the O$_2$ saturation >92%. A short period with an FiO$_2$ of 100% is not dangerous to the patient receiving mechanical ventilation but prolonged use of 100% FiO$_2$ can have serious consequences. Using 100% FiO$_2$ initially prevents hypoxemia and also help us to calculate the shunt fraction.
- The degree of shunt with 100% FiO$_2$ can be estimated by applying this general rule: The measured PaO$_2$ is subtracted from 700 mm Hg. For each difference of 100 mm Hg, the shunt is 5%. A shunt of 25% should remind the clinician to consider the use of positive end-expiratory pressure (PEEP).
- Conditions causing shunts.
  - Major atelectasis
  - Lobar pneumonia
  - ARDS
  - Congestive heart failure
  - Hemorrhage

Initial Settings for Ventilation

- Assist-control mode
- Tidal volume set depending on lung status
  - ☐ Normal = 12 mL/kg ideal body weight
  - ☐ COPD = 10 mL/kg ideal body weight
  - ☐ ARDS = 6–8 mL/kg ideal body weight
- Rate of 10–12 breaths per minute
- FiO_2 of 100%
- Sighs rarely needed
- PEEP only as indicated after first arterial blood gas, started usually at 5 cm of water
- Inability to oxygenate with FiO_2 <60%

PEEP Adjustment

- Generally PEEP is initiated at 5 cm of H_2O but can reduce the systemic blood pressure if a higher level is used. When using a higher setting as in ARDS, proper hemodyamnamic support with volume or cardiac inotropes should be used.
- A PEEP level >10 cm H_2O is generally an indication to monitor cardiac output by using a Swan Ganz catheter.
- Understanding when to wean a patient from the ventilator is extremely important. There are numerous ways to accomplish that and no protocol is 100% effective. The best way is to evaluate each situation separately.
  - ☐ For instance, if the rapid, shallow breathing index (the respiratory rate/tidal volume, or frequency/tidal volume [f/Vt]) is <105, the patient has a good chance to be weaned from the ventilator. For patients >70 yr, a higher value of RSBI could be acceptable.
- Parameters commonly used to assess a patient's readiness to be weaned from mechanical ventilatory support include the following:
  - ☐ Respiratory rate <25 breaths per min
  - ☐ Tidal volume >5 mL/kg
  - ☐ Vital capacity >10 mL/kg
  - ☐ Minute ventilation <10 L/min
  - ☐ PaO_2/FiO_2 >200
  - ☐ f/Vt < 105 or <130 in elderly patients, RSBI

Weaning of Mechanical Ventilation

The weaning modes are synchronized intermittent mandatory ventilation (SIMV), pressure support ventilation (PSV), and a spontaneous breathing trial (SBT).

- In *SIMV*, breaths given are either compulsory ventilator-controlled breath or a spontaneous breath with or without pressure support. This allows the patient to partially breathe on his or her own. It is partial as the patients respiratory muscles rest during the mandatory breaths and work during the spontaneous phase. This is a great mode to begin the weaning process, gradually decreasing the mandatory breaths by 2 breaths every 1–2 hours.

■ *Spontaneous breathing trial* (SBT) is the preferred method of weaning. This is an attempt to gauge how the patient might do if he or she is immediately removed from the ventilator. This method is also referred to as the sink-or-swim trial. The key is to withdraw ventilatory support while oxygenation is continued.

■ The simplest form of SBT is the *T-piece trial*. The patient is disconnected from the ventilator, and the endotracheal or tracheostomy tube is hooked to a flow-by oxygen system, usually from the wall.

Complications of Intubation

■ Upper-airway and nasal trauma

■ Tooth avulsion

■ Oral-pharyngeal laceration

■ Laceration or hematoma of the vocal cords

■ Tracheal laceration

■ Perforation

■ Hypoxemia

■ Esophageal intubation

■ Intubation of the right main stem bronchus is reported in 3–9% of all intubations in adults

■ Aspiration rates are 8–19% in intubations performed in adults without anesthesia

Barotrauma

■ Barotrauma refers to rupture of the alveolus with the development to pneumothorax and pneumomediastinum. Some reports suggest an incidence of 6–25%. Large tidal volumes and elevated peak inspiratory and plateau pressures are risk factors. Monitoring and decreasing the tidal volume when needed and also adjusting the peak and plateau pressures to a safe level can prevent barotrauma.

Oxygen Toxicity

■ Oxygen toxicity occurs as a result of increased FiO_2 and its duration of use. Oxygen toxicity is due to the production of oxygen free radicals, such as superoxide anion, hydroxyl radical, and hydrogen peroxide. When a patient is already on the ventilator, the last thing you need is oxygen toxicity. Try to decrease the FiO_2 as soon as possible to keep the saturation >92%. It can lead to many complications such as tracheobronchitis, hypercarbia due to decrease in the respiratory drive and even ARDS in severe cases.

■ If more oxygenation is needed and the patient has stable hemodyanmics, it might be better to increase the PEEP by a safe amount. Always try to reduce the FiO_2 from 100% to 60% or less within 24 hr.

Ventilator-Associated Pneumonia

This can be a life-threatening condition and can delay the weaning process. The mortality rates reported are 33–50%. VAP can occur in nearly 10–25% of patients on mechanical ventilation.

- VAP can develop within 48 hr after intubation and should be suspected in patients with high fevers, persistant infiltrates on chest x-rays.

- Organisms that cause VAP include *H influenza, Pseudomonas aeruginosa, S pneumonia, Klebsiella,* etc After 7 days of intubation MRSA should be suspected. Broad-spectrum antibiotics should be started when VAP is suspected.

Intrinsic PEEP or Auto-PEEP

- Intrinsic PEEP or auto-PEEP is a complication of mechanical ventilation that most frequently occurs in patients with COPD and/or asthma who require prolonged expiration. When intrinsic PEEP is diagnosed, the patient should temporarily be released from mechanical ventilation to allow for full expiration. The ventilator can then be adjusted to shorten inspiration by decreasing the set tidal volume or by increasing the inspiratory flow rate.

Cardiovascular Effects

- Positive-pressure ventilation can decrease venous return to the heart and in turn reduce preload, stroke volume, and eventually cardiac output.

Consultation

- Pulmonary/critical care

COMMON MEDICAL EQUATIONS

- **A-a O_2 Gradient**

  $[(FiO_2) \times (\text{Atmospheric pressure} - H_2O \text{ pressure}) - (Pa_{CO2}/0.8)] - PaO_2 \text{ from ABG}$

- **Absolute Neutrophil Count**

  $10 \times \text{WBC count in 1000s} \times (\% \text{ PMNs} + \% \text{ Bands})$

- **Anion Gap**

  $Na^+ - (Cl^- + HCO_3^-)$

- **Corrected Calcium**

  $(0.8 \times (\text{Normal albumin} - \text{Patient's albumin})) + \text{Serum } Ca^{2+}$

- **Cockcroft-Gault GFR**

  $(140 - \text{Age}) \times (\text{Weight in kg}) \times (0.85 \text{ if female})/(72 \times Cr)$

- **Fick's Cardiac Output Equation**

  $O_2 \text{ Uptake or consumption}/([\text{Arterial } O_2] - [\text{Venous } O_2])$

- **Fractional Excretion of Sodium (FENa)**

  $(P_{Cr} \times U_{Na})/(P_{Na} \times U_{Cr})\%$

- **Ideal Body Weight (Men)**

  $50 \text{ kg} + 2.3 \text{ kg} \times (\text{Height in inches}) - 60)$

- **Ideal Body Weight (Women)**

  $45.5 \text{ kg} + 2.3 \text{ kg} \times (\text{Height in inches}) - 60)$

- **LDL Cholesterol**

  $\text{Total cholesterol} - \text{HDL} - (TG/5)$

- **Discriminant Function**

  $4.6 \times (\text{Patient's PT} - \text{Control PT}) + TBili$
  (>32 has a poor prognosis and may benefit from steroid therapy)

6

Procedures

Arun Mathews, MD

A*deptness with procedures is one of the defining characteristics of an excellent hospitalist. American Board of Internal Medicine (ABIM) certified residency programs now have stringent competency requirements that include proficiency with a variety of fundamental procedures; the following guide is provided for informational purposes only. If for any reason you feel uncomfortable performing a procedure, the authors strongly advise that you seek the aid of a seasoned proceduralist. Several procedures that are considered essential to the hospitalist's armamentarium will be discussed: central venous catheter placement, lumbar puncture (LP), endotracheal intubation, arthrocentesis, thoracentesis, abdominal paracentesis, arterial blood gas (ABG) sampling, and arterial line placement.*

CENTRAL LINE PLACEMENT

Indications
- To secure IV access for the administration of fluid, blood products, medications, and parenteral nutrition
- IV access in patients without accessible peripheral veins
- Infusion of hypertonic or irritant solutions
- Rapid administration of large volumes of fluid
- Vasopressor administration
- To measure and monitor central venous pressure (CVP)

Contraindications
- Agitated or uncooperative patient
- Prior radiation to the region
- Infection of the area overlying the target vessel
- *Subclavian vein*: Distorted landmarks, trauma to the shoulder girdle, deformity of the chest wall, previous surgery, or fracture of the clavicle
- *Internal jugular vein*: Tracheostomy, excessive pulmonary secretions
- *Femoral vein*: Compromised inferior vena cava due to clot, extrinsic compression, or IVC filter

Complications
Pain, infection, bleeding, arterial or venous laceration, arterial cannulation, pneumothorax, hemothorax, cardiac arrhythmia, and air embolism

Step-by-Step Procedure
1. Explain the procedure, risks, benefits and alternatives to the patient. Obtain written informed consent and verbalized understanding from the patient.
2. Familiarize yourself with the contents of the standard central line or triple lumen catheter (TLC) kit; drape (usually 24 inches × 36 inches with 4-inch fenestration), 5 mL ampule of 1% lidocaine solution, sterile gloves, sterile gown, disinfectant sponge, gauze, tissue dilator, scalpel (usually No. 11 blade), 10% povidone-iodine solution, suture needle, triple lumen catheter with 3 patent ports, 3-way stopcock (for CVP monitoring), adhesive tape, antibiotic ointment, dressing, tuberculin syringe, guidewire in plastic sheath, penetration syringe, dilator, big needle, scalpel, guide syringe and needle, anesthesia syringe and needle, and lidocaine. Ensure the patency of all ports by flushing with saline.

Note: Ask about allergy to iodine-containing solutions. If the patient has an iodine allergy, another topical antiseptic such as rubbing alcohol should be used.

3. Ensure that the patient is optimally positioned and check anatomical landmarks. The authors advise that the patient be hooked up to a cardiac monitor throughout the procedure so that abnormalities such as ectopy or oxygen desaturation can be closely monitored.

4. Perform sterile preparation of at least 2 inches in diameter surrounding the insertion site by applying 10% povodine iodine solution or other antiseptic solution.

5. Using the smallest (25-gauge) needle, anesthetize the area with 1% lidocaine solution by first inserting the needle almost parallel to the skin with the bevel pointing up, forming a small wheal just underneath the skin. Then draw back on the syringe gently while advancing the needle a little deeper in order to anesthetize tissue that is slightly deeper. Continually drawing back on the syringe as you advance the needle and before injection will ensure that you avoid direct administration of lidocaine to the vasculature.

6. While waiting for the lidocaine to take effect, drape the area of planned catheter placement, using sterile fashion.

7. Use the 22-gauge "finder needle" attached to a 10-mL syringe to locate the specific vein by slowly advancing the needle while continuing to draw back on the attached syringe.

8. Upon aspiration of venous blood with the 22-gauge needle, maintain its position and insert the 18-gauge needle, following the same path as the 22-gauge-needle.

9. While holding the 18-gauge (largest bore) needle in place, quickly feed the guidewire into the needle with your dominant hand. Remove the syringe while holding the needle in place and quickly feed the guidewire into the needle while watching for ectopy on the cardiac monitor.

10. Remove the needle over the guidewire while *always* holding onto one section of the guidewire in order to prevent its embolization.

11. Using the scalpel, make a 2-mm nick in the skin at the wire entry site.

12. Pass the dilator approximately 3–4 cm over the guidewire in order to dilate the subcutaneous tissue.

13. Using a twisting motion, pass the catheter over the guidewire while again taking care not to let go of the guidewire. You will eventually see the guidewire exiting from the brown port of the triple lumen catheter.

14. Now you can advance the catheter and remove the guidewire while holding onto the guidewire with one hand.

15. Aspirate blood and flush each port with normal saline.

16. Suture the line in place. A spacer may be necessary in small patients.

17. Depending on the insertion site, it may be necessary to order an x-ray in order to confirm placement and to rule out complications such as pneumothorax.

18. Chart the procedure by writing a brief note detailing the indications for the procedure, relevant labs (eg, INR/PTT, platelet count), technique that was used, sterile prep, amount of anesthetic used, amount of blood loss, and any complications that were encountered during the procedure.

FEMORAL VEIN CANNULATION

Approach

■ Identify the femoral artery by checking for pulsation just below the inguinal ligament. Once you have found the artery, remember that the femoral vein is *medial* to the artery.

■ The insertion site is just medial to the femoral artery and approximately 1 cm inferior to the inguinal ligament.

■ With the bevel up and at a 45- to 60-degree angle above the skin, the needle should be inserted parallel to the vessel. A steeper angle decreases the chance of entering the peritoneum, while a more medial angle decreases the chance of cannulating the femoral artery.

FEMORAL VEIN ANATOMY

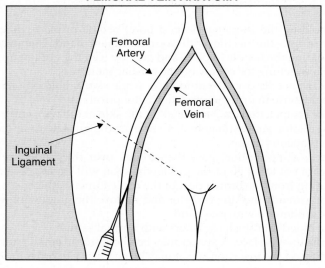

INTERNAL JUGULAR VEIN CANNULATION

Approach

- First approach:
  - ☐ Turn the patient's head approximately 45–60 degrees contralateral to the side of planned catheter insertion. A triangle is formed by the clavicle and the 2 heads of the sternocleidomastoid muscle. At the apex of this triangle and just lateral to the carotid is the optimal point of insertion.
- Second approach:
  - ☐ Turn the patient's head 45 degrees to the contralateral side of insertion. Draw an imaginary line between the sternal notch and the mastoid process on the side of planned catheter insertion. Halfway between these 2 points and just lateral to the carotid artery is the optimal point of insertion.
  - ☐ Insert the needle at a 70-degree angle to the skin and aim toward the ipsilateral nipple. Only insert the needle to a depth of 0.5–1 inches; insertion to a depth greater than 1.5 inches will significantly increase the risk of a pneumothorax. If this direction proves unsuccessful, withdraw the needle and re-insert at a more medial angle. If this again proves unsuccessful, re-assess your landmarks.
  - ☐ Consider using ultrasound guidance if you encounter continued difficulty. Studies have shown that ultrasound guidance works best for cannulation of the internal jugular and femoral veins. Ultrasound reduces the number of complications, the number of failed attempts, and the duration of the procedure.

INTERNAL JUGULAR VEIN ANATOMY

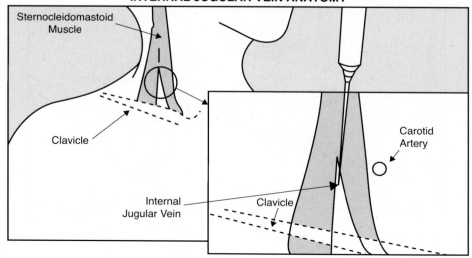

SUBCLAVIAN VEIN CANNULATION

Approach

- Remove the patient's pillow and place a towel roll between the patient's scapulae.
- Place the patient in a 10- to 15-degree Trendelenburg position.
- Turn the patient's head away from the target vessel.
- For catheter insertion in the subclavian vein, the clavicular periosteum should be anesthetized in addition to the skin and fascia. The periosteum is very sensitive.
- Using the nondominant hand to guide placement, place the index finger at the sternal notch and thumb at clavicle.
- Insert the 22-gauge needle right underneath the clavicle, approximately 2-cm inferior to the junction of the lateral 1/3 and medial 2/3 of the clavicle. Pass the needle underneath the clavicle in the direction of the suprasternal notch, parallel to the patient's back. *It is very important to remember to always draw back on the syringe while advancing the needle.*
- Once under the clavicle, continue to advance the needle approximately 4–5 cm. If this proves unsuccessful, withdraw the needle and redirect in a more cephalad direction.

SUBCLAVIAN ANATOMY

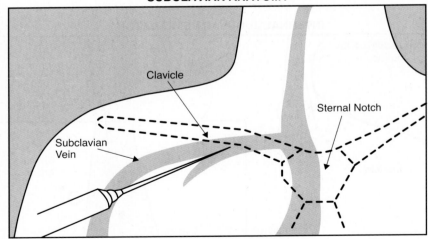

Clavicle

Sternal Notch

Subclavian
Vein

Procedure for Removing Central Lines

■ Ensure that the line is not tunneled; this may require consultation by interventional radiology.

■ Place the patient in the Trendelenburg (reverse Trendenlenburg for femoral lines) position and remove all pillows.

■ Gently remove all dressings along with suture material.

■ Tell the patient to hold his/her breath and quickly but gently pull the catheter out in the same direction that it was placed.

■ Dress the site with sterile gauze and place a Tegaderm or equivalent dressing over the gauze.

ENDOTRACHEAL INTUBATION

Indications

- Insufficient oxygenation measured by decreased arterial Pa_{O_2} that cannot be corrected by supplemental oxygen by mask.
- Insufficient respiratory effort (ventilation), measured by increased arterial Pa_{O_2}.
- Inadequate airway patency such as angioedema or excessively enlarged tonsils
- Need for airway protection due to stroke or seizure in order to prevent aspiration of stomach contents
- Airway protection while under general anesthesia
- Hemodynamic instability

Contraindications

There is no absolute contraindication to tracheal intubation. Relative contraindications to tracheal intubation include:

- Severe airway trauma or obstruction that does not allow safe passage of an endotracheal tube
- Cervical spine injury, in which the need for complete immobilization of the cervical spine makes endotracheal intubation difficult

Equipment

- Self-refilling bag-valve combination or bag-valve unit connector, tubing, and oxygen source. Assemble all items before attempting intubation.
- Laryngoscope with curved (Macintosh type) and straight (Miller type) blades of a size appropriate for the patient.
- Several endotracheal tubes of varying sizes; high-flow, low pressure cuffed balloons are preferred.
- Oral airways (the oral airway is a device that lifts the tongue off the posterior pharynx, often making it easier to mask ventilate a patient).
- Tincture of benzoin and precut tape.
- Introducer (stylets or Magill forceps).
- Suction apparatus (tonsil tip and catheter suction).
- Syringe, 10-mL, to inflate the cuff.
- Mucosal anesthetics (2% lidocaine).
- Water-soluble sterile lubricant.
- Gloves.

Position of the Patient

The patient should be lying on a bed that is adjusted so that the patient's face is at the level of the lower chest of the person performing the procedure. The patient's head should be elevated about 10 cm and in the sniffing position, which serves to align the oral, pharyngeal, and laryngeal axis, so that the passage from the lips to the glottic opening is in a straight line. Obese patients or those with an anticipated "difficult" airway should be positioned with a shoulder roll under their scapulae. This position permits better visualization of the glottis and vocal cords and allows easier passage of the endotracheal tube.

CORRECT POSITION OF PATIENT'S HEAD

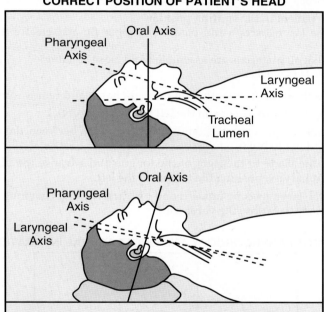

Technique

Mask Ventilation (oxygen delivered with a face mask at a rate of 10–15 L/min)

1. Select the proper-sized mask; it should cover the mouth and nose and fit snugly against the cheeks.
2. Place the patient in the sniffing position.
3. Place the mask over the patient's mouth and nose with the right hand.
4. With the left hand, place the small and ring fingers under the patient's mandible, and lift up to open the airway. Grasp the mask with the thumb and index finger, and press it to the patient's face while lifting the mandible with the ring and small fingers.
5. Compress the bag with the right hand.

6. The chest should rise with each breath, and airflow should be unimpeded. If unable to make the chest rise, one should try the "jaw-thrust" maneuver and "chin lift," or use both hands to hold the mask and ask a second operator to squeeze the bag. Occasionally, insertion of an oral or nasal airway facilitates ventilation by mask. Because of the lack of support for the lips, elderly edentulous patients may be particularly difficult to ventilate using a mask.

Topical Anesthesia
Anesthetize the mucosa of the oropharynx, and upper airway with lidocaine 2%, if time permits and the patient is awake.

Direct Laryngoscopy
1. Place the patient in the sniffing position.
2. Check the laryngoscope and blade for proper fit, and ensure that the light works.
3. Ensure that all materials are assembled and close at hand.
4. *Curved blade technique*:

    a. Open the patient's mouth with the right hand, and remove any dentures.
    b. Grasp the laryngoscope in the left hand (see figure).
    c. Spread the patient's lips, and insert the blade between the teeth, being careful not to break a tooth.
    d. Pass the blade to the right of the tongue and advance the blade into the hypopharynx, pushing the tongue to the left.
    e. Lift the laryngoscope upward and forward without changing the angle of the blade to expose the vocal cords.

DIRECT LARYNGOSCOPY AND OROTRACHEAL INTUBATION

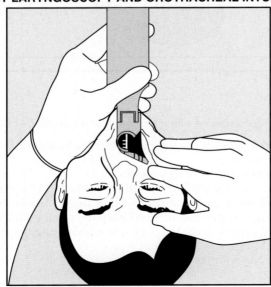

CURVED BLADE PLACEMENT IN OROTRACHEAL INTUBATION

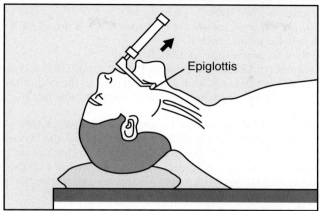

Epiglottis

5. *Straight blade technique*:
   a. Follow the steps outlined for curved blade technique, but advance the blade down the hypopharynx, and lift the epiglottis with the tip of the blade to expose the vocal cords. The tip of the laryngoscope blade fits below the epiglottis, which is no longer visible with the blade in position.

STRAIGHT BLADE PLACEMENT IN OROTRACHEAL INTUBATION

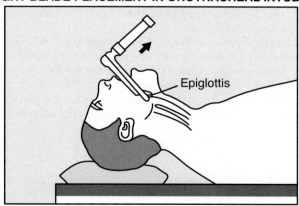

Epiglottis

Orotracheal Intubation

1. Select the proper-sized tube.
2. With the 10-mL syringe, inflate the balloon with 5–8 mL of air. Ensure that the balloon is functional and intact.
3. Lubricate the end of the tube (optional).
4. Insert the stylet, and bend the tube and stylet gently into a crescent shape so that the tip of the stylet is at least 1-cm proximal to the end of the tube.
5. Ventilate the patient with the bag–valve combination for 1–2 minutes with 100% oxygen.
6. Proceed the direct laryngoscopy (as explained above); when visualizing the glottis and vocal cords, gently pass the tube and then the laryngoscope blade through the vocal cords into trachea, far enough so that the balloon is just beyond the cords. Occasionally, gently pressing posteriorly on the anterior neck at the level of the larynx will help to bring an anteriorly placed larynx into view and facilitate intubation.
7. Withdraw the stylet.
8. Connect the bag–valve combination, and begin ventilation with 100% oxygen.
9. Confirm that the tube is properly positioned. First, listen over the stomach with a stethoscope while ventilating the patient. If sounds of airflow are heard or if distension of the stomach occurs, the tube is in the esophagus. If the esophagus has been intubated instead of the trachea, remove the tube and try again.
10. Listen to each side of the chest to be sure that breath sounds are equal in both sides of the thorax. If not, reposition the tube. When breath sounds are equal on both sides and the thorax rises equally on both sides with each inspiration, note the position of the tube (mark the tube at patient's mouth), and inflate the cuff with the 10-mL syringe until there is no air leak around the tube when positive pressure is applied.
11. Apply tincture of benzoin to the cheeks, upper lip, and endotracheal tube.
12. Wrap adhesive tape around the tube where it comes out of the mouth. Then carry the tape over the cheek and around the back of the head onto the other cheek. Fasten the end of the tape around the tube.
13. Obtain a chest x-ray film immediately to check tube placement, and also obtain arterial blood gas measurements to assess the adequacy of ventilation.

ABDOMINAL PARACENTESIS

Indications
Diagnostic:

■ To determine the cause of ascites – new onset ascites or ascites of unknown origin

■ Patients with ascites of known etiology who may have a decompensation clinical state as indicated by fever, painful abdominal distension, peritoneal irritation, hypotension, encephalopathy or sepsis

■ Suspected malignant ascites

■ Peritoneal dialysis patients with fever, abdominal pain or other signs of sepsis (usually the paracentesis fluid may be removed directly from the patient's dialysis catheter)

Therapeutic:

■ To relieve symptoms of ascites.

Contraindications
There are no *absolute* contraindications; below are a few *relative* contraindications.

■ Uncorrected bleeding diathesis, adhesions from prior abdominal surgeries, severe bowel distension, abdominal wall cellulitis at the proposed site of puncture, coagulopathy (INR >1.4), thrombocytopenia (platelets <40), hernia at chosen site, or caput medusae at chosen site.

Equipment
■ Universal precautions materials

■ 1-liter vacuum bottles

■ Blood collection tubing or a secondary IV tubing set

■ 18-gauge needle

■ Skin prep solution

■ Sterile draping

■ 1% or 2% lidocaine with epinephrine for local anesthesia

■ 5-cc syringe with 25 gauge needle for anesthesia infiltration

Step-by-Step Procedure

1. Obtain informed consent and remember to use sterile technique at all times. If ascites is suspected but not evident on physical exam or is small, consider ultrasound to mark the fluid. If an ultrasound machine is available, scan patient to localize fluid collections, and perform the procedure under real-time ultrasound guidance. Ensure the mark is in the most optimal place and have ultrasound quantify the amount of fluid when doing a therapeutic tap.
2. Have the patient urinate or use a Foley catheter to empty the bladder.

3. Place the patient in a semi-recumbent position (45–60 degrees) and percuss the level of dullness; the insertion site should be just inferior to the umbilicus and the level of percussed dullness. The usual insertion site is 2–3 cm below the umbilicus. Midline insertion is the safest and this should be the first choice. Contraindications to midline insertion are midline hernias or umbilical hernias and presence of scar tissue. The second-choice site should be in the right lower quadrant, approximately 2 cm above the inguinal ligament; this site should *only* be used in cases where ascites is particularly large. When using this site, it is important for the patient to be positioned so that he/she is turned slightly to the ipsilateral side of needle insertion.

4. Use skin prep solution to cleanse skin over the proposed puncture site, and drape to define a sterile field.

5. Anesthetize the skin over the proposed puncture site with the lidocaine drawn up in the 5-cc syringe with the attached 25-gauge needle. Anesthetize down to the peritoneum. Aspirate periodically; if ascitic fluid returns, withdraw the needle slightly to re-enter tissue before further anesthetic is infiltrated.

6. Using the Z *technique* retract the skin inferiorly relative to the abdominal wall and use a 20- to 22-gauge needle attached to a 20- to 30-cc syringe to aspirate ascitic fluid. Remember to aspirate continuously.

7. For large volume paracentesis, use the same Z *technique* but always use the Caldwell needle. Once fluid is aspirated, remove the needle from the metal catheter and attach pressurized, noncollapsible tubing. Use the needle just removed and place it on the other end of the tubing and insert the needle into vacutainer bottle(s).

8. To change vacuum bottles as they become full, close the clamp on the tubing. Then remove the needle of the collection tubing from the full bottle, and reinsert into an empty bottle. Reopen clamp to start fluid flowing again.

9. When paracentesis is done, simply remove the needle from abdominal wall. Place a small pressure dressing on the puncture site. Have patient remain supine for 2–4 hours.

10. For each liter removed, consider giving give the patient 50 cc of 25% albumin IV (the studies on this are equivocal but may prevent renal failure).

11. If available, a bedside ultrasound machine is an asset.

Complications
■ Infection (peritonitis), excessive bleeding, renal failure, hypotension, perforated viscous

Diagnostic Studies

■ Send fluid for cell count, differential (lavender top); albumin, total protein (tiger or gold top); Gram stain (black top test tube); culture (culture bottles). Other studies (amylase, cytology, AFB stains, etc.) only if clinically indicated.

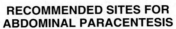

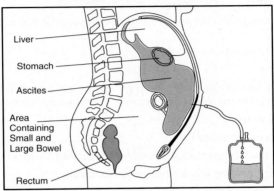

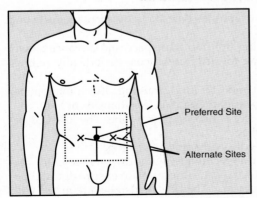
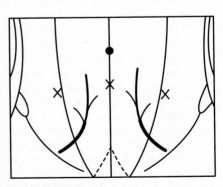

Recommended Sites for Abdominal Paracentesis

LUMBAR PUNCTURE (LP)

Indications

■ Diagnosis of meningitis, subarachnoid hemorrhage, carcinomatosis, multiple sclerosis, measurement of CSF pressure, delivery of medications

Contraindications

■ Increased intracranial pressure; if suspected (papilledema, headache), rule out with head CT

■ Infection near puncture site

■ Coagulopathy

■ If the patient has any of the following criteria, get a head CT prior to performing the LP in order to minimize the risk of brainstem herniation:

☐ Age ≥60 years

☐ Immunocompromised state

☐ History of CNS lesion (mass lesion, stroke, and/or focal CNS infection)

☐ Seizure in the past week prior to presentation

☐ Neurologic findings (altered mental status, inability to answer two questions or follow two commands correctly, and/or any focal neurologic findings such as gaze palsy or arm drift)

Step-by-Step Procedure

1. Place patient on side and have him/her "roll up into a ball" with shoulders and pelvis perpendicular to the bed and chin down. Positioning is key. Locate the vertebral interspace between the posterior iliac crests (should be at L3, L4). Mark site with pen cap.

2. Use sterile technique to prep and drape site. Anesthetize subcutaneously and to vertebrae.

3. Insert spinal needle (bevel pointing up) into interspace and advance slowly with slight cephalad angle, aiming towards umbilicus. Periodically remove stylet fully to check for CSF.

4. Once subarachnoid space reached and CSF fluid draining, attach manometer and measure pressure. Normal opening pressure is less than 20 cm H_2O.

5. Drain CSF into tubes 1–4. Only ~2 cc is necessary per tube. The less CSF removed, the less chance for headache.

6. Re-insert the stylet, remove the needle, and apply a dressing.

7. If difficulty is experienced with this technique, withdraw and re-enter at a different intervertebral space (below L3). It is important to ensure optimal positioning and to ask for help if necessary. The LP can also be attempted with the patient in the upright position. If difficulty persists, consider consulting the neurology or anesthesia services.

8. After the procedure, instruct the patient to remain recumbent for 6–12 hours and encourage fluid intake for postprocedure headache prevention.

Complications

■ Headache, infection, hemorrhage, brainstem herniation

Studies

■ Check your local hospital for specific guidelines on the specific tubes that are necessary for the planned study. Always check a cell count with differential, glucose, total protein, gram stain, and culture. An additional black-top test tube may be used for cytology.

Note: most labs require at least 8–10 cc of CSF for AFB culture.

LUMBAR PUNCTURE POSITIONING

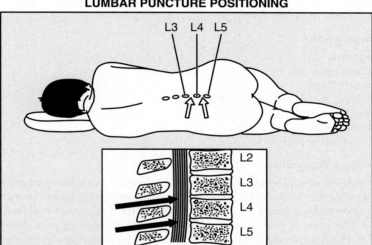

Source: Royal Children's Hospital, Melbourne, Australia.

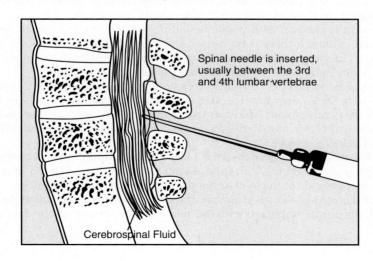

ARTHROCENTESIS

Indications
■ Crystal-induced arthropathy
■ Hemarthrosis
■ Limiting joint damage from an infectious process
■ Symptomatic relief of a large effusion
■ Unexplained joint effusion
■ Unexplained monarthritis

Contraindications
1. Bacteremia
2. Inaccessible joints
3. Joint prosthesis
4. Overlying infection in the soft tissues
5. Severe coagulopathy
6. Severe overlying dermatitis
7. Uncooperative patient

Step-by-Step Procedure
1. The patient is supine on the table with the knee extended (some physicians prefer that the knee be bent to 90 degrees). Some physicians prefer the medial approach for smaller effusions, but the lateral approach will be discussed here. The knee is examined to determine the amount of joint fluid present and to check for overlying cellulitis or coexisting pathology in the joint or surrounding tissues.
2. The superior lateral aspect of the patella is palpated. The skin is marked with a pen, one fingerbreadth above and one fingerbreadth lateral to this site. This location provides the most direct access to the synovium.
3. The skin is washed with povidone-iodine solution. The physician should be gloved, although there is no consensus as to whether sterile gloves must be used. A 21-gauge, 1-inch needle is attached to a 5- to 20-mL syringe, depending on the anticipated amount of fluid present for removal.
4. The needle is inserted through stretched skin. Some physicians administer lidocaine (Xylocaine) into the skin, but stretching the pain fibers in the skin with the nondominant hand can also reduce needle-insertion discomfort. The needle is directed at a 45-degree angle distally and 45 degrees into the knee, tilted below the patella.
5. Once the needle has been inserted 1 to 1.5 inches, aspiration is performed, and the syringe should fill with fluid. Using the nondominant hand to compress the opposite side of the joint or the patella may aid in arthrocentesis.
6. Once the syringe has filled, a hemostat can be placed on the hub of the needle. With the needle stabilized with the hemostat, the syringe can be disconnected

and the fluid sent for studies. Care should be taken not to touch the needle tip against joint surfaces when removing the syringe. A syringe filled with corticosteroid can then be attached to the needle.

7. The skin is cleansed and a bandage is applied over the needle-puncture site. The patient is warned to avoid forceful activity on the joint while it is anesthetized.

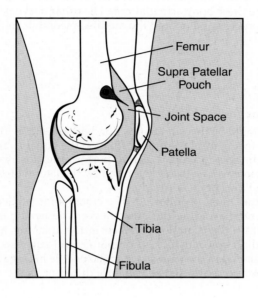

ARTHROCENTESIS OF THE ELBOW JOINT

Anatomy of the Elbow Joint

■   Remember that the elbow joint is formed by three articulations: humerus with radius, humerus with ulna, and radius with ulna. Soft tissues, tendons, and ligaments stabilize these bony articulations. The ulnar nerve passes just medial to the olecranon process and behind the medial epicondyle in the cubital tunnel.

Equipment

■   Syringe 20 mL
■   Needle 18 or 22 gauge, 1.5 inch

Step-by-Step Procedure

1.   The patient should be in a supine position with the elbow flexed to 45 degrees and the hand in a neutral position resting on the patient's thigh.
2.   Essential landmarks to palpate before performing this injection are the soft tissue at the center of the triangle formed by the lateral olecranon, the head of the radius, and the lateral epicondyle.
3.   Sterile technique must be followed. The elbow joint is injected from a lateral approach, thereby avoiding the ulnar nerve. The needle is inserted into the soft tissue within the triangle described in the anatomy, and directed to the opposite (medial) epicondyle. Aspiration of fluid suggests that the needle is properly positioned in the joint space. If the needle hits against bone, it should be pulled back and redirected at a slightly different angle.

ANATOMIC TRIANGLE FOR ASPIRATION

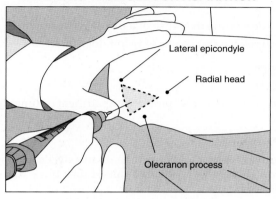

Lateral epicondyle

Radial head

Olecranon process

ELBOW ARTHROCENTESIS

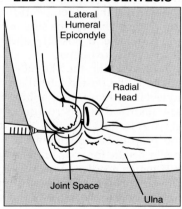

Lateral
Humeral
Epicondyle

Radial
Head

Joint Space

Ulna

THORACENTESIS

Indications
- Diagnostic: to determine the cause of a pleural effusion
- Therapeutic: to relieve symptoms of respiratory distress

Contraindications
- *None are absolute*
- Coagulopathy or any major respiratory impairment or lung disease on the contralateral side

Step-by-Step Procedure
1. Obtain informed consent and remember to use sterile technique at all times.
2. If effusion on chest x-RAY, obtain a lateral decubitus film ipsilateral to the side of the effusion.
3. If the effusion is small (<1 cm on lateral decubitus film) or not free flowing, consider ultrasound to mark the effusion and/or look for loculation. Always go to ultrasound yourself to witness the marking and positioning of the patient! Ensure the mark is in the most optimal place and have ultrasound quantify the amount of fluid when doing a therapeutic tap.
4. Have the patient sit up comfortably on the side of the bed and lean forward slightly on the bedside tray table. If possible, and especially for therapeutic taps, place the patient on a pulse oximeter.
5. Find the optimal site by percussing the patient's chest wall and finding the fluid level. The usual site is the posterolateral aspect of the back, 1–2 interspaces below the fluid level but above the diaphragm. Aim to go just *above* the rib to avoid hitting any neurovascular structures. Mark the spot with a pen cap or something that won't be erased by 10% povodone-iodine solution.
6. Using sterile technique, prep and drape the site.
7. Use a 25-gauge or smaller needle for your initial wheal and subcutaneous anesthesia. Change to a 22-gauge needle (1.5 inch) and infiltrate lidocaine on the rib, marching up until you are just above the rib and into the pleural space. If you obtain fluid at this point, note the depth of the needle.
8. Remember to use the same technique of marching up the rib when using your larger aspiration needle. For a diagnostic tap, use an 18–20 gauge needle attached to a 20–30 cc syringe.
9. If performing a therapeutic tap, use an 18-gauge angiocatheter (or the catheter supplied in your kit) and place a stopcock on the end of the catheter once the needle is removed. Place noncollapsible tubing onto the stopcock and then drain the fluid in your container of choice. The use of vacutainer bottles may place too much negative pressure on the catheter, thereby collapsing the catheter or tubing. Removing more than one liter of pleural fluid increases the chance for re-expansion pulmonary edema.
10. If some fluid comes out and then stops, check your catheter, tubing, etc. Having the patient Valsalva can increase intrathoracic pressure and help the fluid flow.

11. If you aspirate air (see air bubbles in your syringe) or the patient develops hypotension, desaturation, or respiratory distress, stop immediately and obtain a chest x-ray or perform immediate needle decompression for tension pneumothorax. If the patient has recently undergone thoracentesis, however, air bubbles may not indicate a pneumothorax.
12. When removing the needle, have the patient Valsalva to reduce chance of pneumothorax and bandage the site.
13. Obtain a stat chest x-ray postprocedure to rule out pneumothorax.

Complications

■ Pneumothorax, infection, hypotension, hemothorax, re-expansion pulmonary edema, hepatic or splenic puncture

Diagnostic Studies

■ Always send fluid for cell count and differential (lavender top); LDH, total protein (tiger top); Gram stain (black top test tube); culture (culture bottles); pH. Other studies (cytology, glucose, AFB stains, etc.) only if clinically indicated.

EXAMPLE OF THORACENTESIS

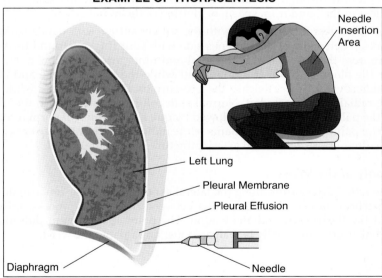

Needle Insertion Area

Left Lung

Pleural Membrane

Pleural Effusion

Diaphragm

Needle

ARTERIAL BLOOD GAS (RADIAL ARTERY PUNCTURE)

■ Radial artery puncture is performed to obtain arterial blood sampling for gas analysis. The partial pressures of oxygen (Pa_{O_2}) and carbon dioxide (Pa_{CO_2}) and the pH of arterial blood are important in assessing pulmonary function, since these data indicate the status of gas exchange between the lungs and the blood.

Contraindications
■ Cellulitis or other infections over the radial artery
■ Absence of palpable radial artery pulse
■ Positive *Allen test* (see below), indicating that only one artery supplies the hand
■ Coagulation defects (relative)

Allen Test
■ It is very important to perform an Allen test to confirm the patency of the ulnar artery, because radial artery puncture is contraindicated in case there is no collateral flow through the ulnar artery, since it can result in a gangrenous finger or loss of the hand from spasm or clotting of the radial artery.

■ The Allen test is performed with the patient sitting with hands supinated on knees. Then stand at the patient's side with your fingers around the wrist and compress the tissue over both radial and ulnar arteries. Allow a few minutes for the blood to drain from the hand while the patient opens and closes the hands several times. Release the pressure on the ulnar artery while keeping the radial artery occluded. Normal skin color should return to the ulnar side of the palm in 1–2 seconds, followed by quick restoration of normal color to the entire palm. A hand that remains white indicates either absence or occlusion of the ulnar artery, and radial artery puncture is contraindicated.

Anatomy of the Wrist
■ The radial artery runs along the lateral aspect of the volar forearm deep to the superficial fascia. The artery runs between the styloid process of the radius and the flexor carpi radialis tendon. The point of maximum pulsation of the radial artery can usually be palpated just proximal to the wrist.

ANATOMY OF THE WRIST

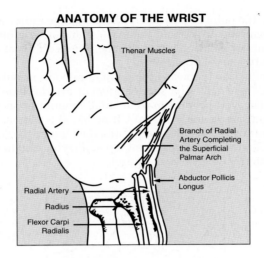

Thenar Muscles

Branch of Radial
Artery Completing
the Superficial
Palmar Arch

Abductor Pollicis
Longus

Radial Artery

Radius

Flexor Carpi
Radialis

Necessary Equipment
1. Alcohol and cotton for skin cleansing
2. Syringe with 3–5 mL of lidocaine 1% and a 23–25-gauge needle
3. Preheparinised 3–5 mL syringe with 23–25 gauge needle
4. Gloves
5. Bag with ice (in which sample will be send to lab)
6. Adhesive bandage and adhesive tape
7. ABG sampling kit (recommended to preserve the integrity of the sample)
8. Collection tubes
9. Appropriate identification labels
10. Appropriate lab requisitions

Step-by-Step Procedure
1. Wash your hands and put on disposable gloves.
2. Locate the approximate position of the artery by slowly rolling your index finger from side to side.

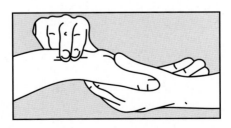

3. Clean the skin over the proposed site of puncture.
4. Anesthetize the skin over the proposed site of puncture with 1% lidocaine 3–5 mL.

5. Identify again the point of maximal pulsation of the radial artery.
6. With your dominant hand hold the syringe and needle puncture (preheparinised) and insert the needle into the anesthetized area at 45 degrees to the skin with needle's bevel uppermost.
7. Guide the needle slowly toward the point of maximum pulsation. When you hit the artery, there will be a sudden gush of arterial blood into the hub of the needle. Then you need to make a small amount of suction to obtain an adequate blood sample (only 1–2 mL). If no blood is obtained with these maneuvers, withdraw the needle to a position just under the skin and try again. Make at least 3 attempts before giving up and trying another site. This can be done with butterfly wings (see in figure).

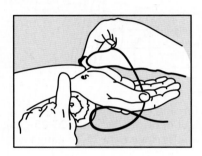

8. Once you have taken blood sample remove the needle from the artery and apply direct pressure over the site for 5 minutes.
9. Expel all air bubbles from the sample holding the syringe upright and allowing the bubbles to collect near the needle hub. Then evacuate it by pushing on the plunger.
10. Carefully cap the needle with a rubber stopper. Don't forget to label the tube with patient's name. Place the sample in the bag containing ice and send it to the lab.
11. It is very important to return about 20 minutes later to check for adequate perfusion of the hand and for possible hematoma formation.

ARTERIAL LINE PLACEMENT

Indications
■ Real time, continuous measurement of arterial blood pressure
■ Arterial lines also facilitate the sampling of arterial blood for blood gases. This is essential in some operative procedures where control of the serum carbon dioxide content (PCO_2) is imperative

Contraindications
■ Severe coagulopathy or platelet count <50,000 (unless confirmed to be corrected)
■ Poor collateral circulation at proposed site (check using Allen test)

Equipment
■ Arterial line insertion kit
  □ General arterial line kits typically consist of an arteriotomy needle (20- or 22-gauge needle), a wire, and an intra-arterial catheter.
■ Chloraprep swabs
■ Disposable chucks
■ Arterial line monitoring equipment
■ Ultrasound with sterile drape kit (if necessary)
■ Pulse doppler (if necessary)

Radial Artery
■ The radial artery is most often used; advantages include ease of placement, relative accuracy, and presence of collateral flow. Note that if a short catheter is used in the radial position, blood pressure may be underestimated on high dose vasopressors in septic patients. Vasopressor effect on the longer catheter normally used is unknown.

Step-by-Step Procedure
1. Obtain informed consent and verbalized understanding from the patient and place consent in chart.
2. The radial pulse is palpated between the distal radius and the flexor carpi-radialis tendon. Prior to line placement, perfusion of the extremity should be checked.
3. An Allen test is recommended before cannulation. The Allen test is performed by compressing both radial and ulnar arteries while the patient tightens his/her fist. Releasing pressure on each respective artery determines the dominant vessel supplying blood to the hand. If both arteries are patent, it is considered safe to place an arterial line. If there is poor collateral flow (from arterial thrombus or peripheral vascular disease), consider using another site for arterial access such as the brachial, femoral, axillary, or dorsalis pedis artery.

4. Position the patient's arm palm-up with the wrist in dorsiflexion; it may also be helpful to place a rolled towel under the patient's wrist. Make sure that the blood pressure cuff is not attached as it will impede blood flow proximal to the site for line placement.
5. The skin is prepped in standard sterile fashion. Subcutaneous infusion of local anesthetic is optional, and if you choose to numb the skin, be aware that excessive amounts of fluid can distort the anatomy and diminish the strength of the pulse.
6. The point of maximal impulse is then identified. It is helpful to find several points to get an idea of the course of the artery. A good point of entry for arteriotomy is just proximal to the flexor retinaculum, though anywhere you can feel a pulse is fair game.
7. Some clinicians like to make a superficial nick in the skin to facilitate passage of the needle and catheter, though this is not necessary. In patients with loose or tough thick skin, this is helpful.
8. Flush the arterial line tubing with normal saline to reduce the risk of air embolism during placement.
9. Hold an 18- or 20-gauge needle like a pencil and puncture skin with needle bevel-up at a 30-degree angle to the patient's wrist. If you are having difficulty palpating the radial artery, use your index and middle finger to locate the artery by starting medially and slowly moving laterally until you feel the pulse. If you are having difficulty finding the radial artery, consider using ultrasound or doppler to visualize the artery.
10. Use your other hand to palpate arterial pulse and then advance the needle until a flash is obtained; once the flash is obtained slowly advance the soft catheter while removing the stylet.
11. There are often 2 catheters in each arterial line kit; make sure to use the longer catheter when possible.
12. Once the wire has been passed, the catheter is passed into the artery over the wire via the Seldinger technique. Arterial lines are placed via guidewire, similar to central line placement.
13. Once the line is placed, hook up the flushed arterial line transducer tubing to the catheter tip. Evaluate your waveform to ensure an accurate reading.
14. Secure your line to the skin with the suture provided.

Helpful Hints

■ Some physicians like to penetrate the back wall of the artery with the needle and then slowly pull the needle back until the tip is in the lumen of the artery.

■ Keep in mind that the artery is typically not very deep (2–3 mm).

■ Use the fingers of your other hand to keep the artery from rolling while performing the stick.

■ When feeling the pulse, most beginners intuitively push down harder when the pulse is weak or difficult to palpate. This actually occludes the artery and you won't feel the pulse at all. Instead, lessen the amount of pressure on the artery and the pulse is usually easier to feel.

Seldinger Technique

■ Advance the needle through the puncture site towards the artery at a shallow angle. As the vessel is punctured, a flashback of arterial blood is seen in the hub. Pass the guide wire through the needle into the artery. Withdraw the needle and pass the cannula over the guide wire. The guide wire is then discarded.

ANATOMY OF WRIST SHOWING RADIAL ARTERY

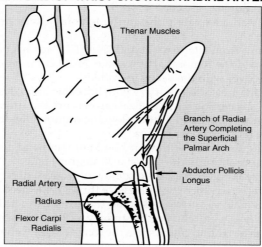

Thenar Muscles

Branch of Radial Artery Completing the Superficial Palmar Arch

Abductor Pollicis Longus

Radial Artery

Radius

Flexor Carpi Radialis

SELDINGER TECHNIQUE

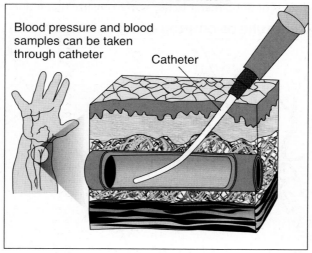

Blood pressure and blood samples can be taken through catheter

Catheter

Femoral Artery

■ The femoral artery is an option that is often employed when radial catheters cannot be placed. It is a relatively easy artery to cannulate, and may be more accurate in sepsis when high dose pressors are used. Disadvantages include an increased risk of infection and it may be problematic when a patient is awake and moving the legs.

Step-by-Step Procedure

1. Ensure there is an adequate pulse in the femoral artery prior to attempting the procedure.
2. Review anatomy, from lateral to medial "NAVL," "venous penis."
3. Prep an area over the femoral artery about 15–20 cm inferior to the inguinal ligament, and cover with the drape provided.
4. Anesthetizing the area over the artery with lidocaine improves comfort and may reduce arterial spasm. Too large a wheal can obscure the artery, so keep it small.
5. Make sure to insert the line 1–2 cm below the inguinal ligament to assure you don't enter the retroperitoneal space.
6. While palpating the artery with your nondominant hand, use the large finder needle to advance through the skin at a 30-degree angle.
7. When the artery is entered, a pulsatile flow of blood will be seen.
8. Once in the artery, advance the guidewire through the needle and remove the needle, always making sure to hold onto the guidewire. If the guidewire will not thread, remove it and the needle, and try a different spot.
9. For a femoral arterial line, always use the long (12-cm) catheter.
10. Place the 12-cm catheter over the guidewire, and advance until the hub is up to the skin.
11. Remove the guidewire, and connect the catheter to a stopcock for measuring. See if an arterial tracing is obtained.
12. Suture the sides of the catheter to the skin to ensure that it doesn't fall out.

PUNCTURE OF COMMON FEMORAL ARTERY (CFA)

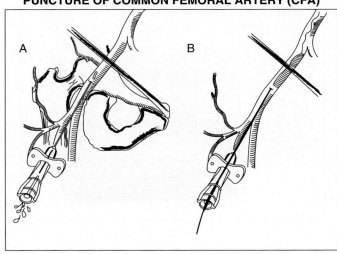

A. The needle enters the CFA.
B. The guidewire is passed through the needle

7

Pre-Op Evaluations

Manish Mehta, MD

Preoperative evaluations are some of the most common consults obtained by hospitalists. Care must be taken to identify the high-risk individuals. It is always a good idea to discuss the type and mode of anesthesia, and the potential complications of the procedure with the surgeon.

FUNCTIONAL STATUS ASSESSMENT

Excellent (>7 METs)	Moderate (4 to 7 METs)	Poor (<4 METs)
Squash	Cycling	Vacuuming
Jogging (10-min mile)	Climbing a flight of stairs	Activities of daily living (eg, eating, dressing, bathing)
Scrubbing floors	Golf (without cart)	Walking 2 mph
Singles tennis	Walking 4 mph	Writing
	Yardwork (eg, raking leaves, weeding, pushing a power mower)	

Source: Reprinted from "Preoperative Cardiac Risk Assessment," *American Family Physician*, Nov. 15, 2002. Copyright © American Academy of Family Physicians. All Rights Reserved.

ACC/AHA PREOPERATIVE CARDIAC RISK ASSESSMENT

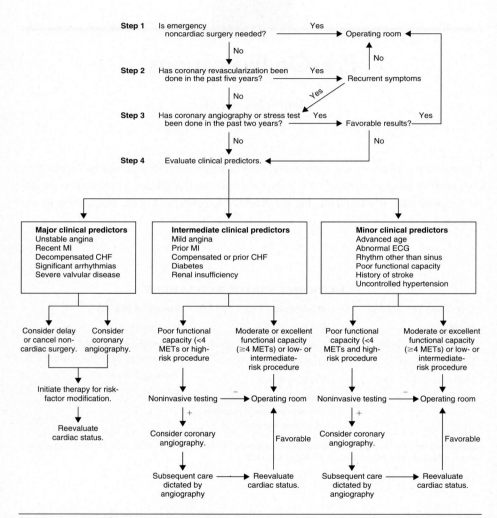

ACP PREOPERATIVE CARDIAC RISK ASSESSMENT

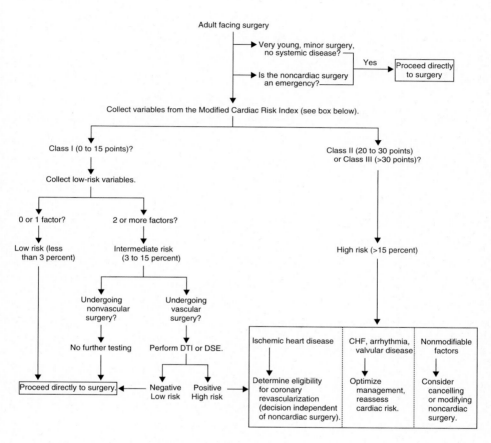

Adult facing surgery

Very young, minor surgery, no systemic disease? ──
Is the noncardiac surgery an emergency?── — Yes → Proceed directly to surgery

Collect variables from the Modified Cardiac Risk Index (see box below).

Class I (0 to 15 points)?

Collect low-risk variables.

0 or 1 factor?   2 or more factors?

Low risk (less than 3 percent)   Intermediate risk (3 to 15 percent)

Undergoing nonvascular surgery?   Undergoing vascular surgery?

No further testing   Perform DTI or DSE.

Proceed directly to surgery.   Negative Low risk   Positive High risk

Class II (20 to 30 points) or Class III (>30 points)?

High risk (>15 percent)

Ischemic heart disease	CHF, arrhythmia, valvular disease	Nonmodifiable factors
Determine eligibility for coronary revascularization (decision independent of noncardiac surgery).	Optimize management, reassess cardiac risk.	Consider cancelling or modifying noncardiac surgery.

Modified Cardiac Risk Index[8]

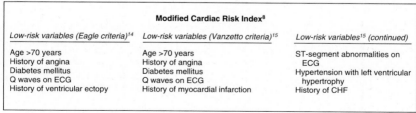

Low-risk variables (Eagle criteria)[14]	Low-risk variables (Vanzetto criteria)[15]	Low-risk variables[15] (continued)
Age >70 years	Age >70 years	ST-segment abnormalities on ECG
History of angina	History of angina	Hypertension with left ventricular hypertrophy
Diabetes mellitus	Diabetes mellitus	History of CHF
Q waves on ECG	Q waves on ECG	
History of ventricular ectopy	History of myocardial infarction	

8

Pacing, Fatigue, and Empathy

Arun Mathews, MD

> *Fatigue makes cowards of us all.*
> —Gen. George S. Patton, Jr.
> Letter of Instruction Number 1, Third Army.
> War As I Knew It, 312

This adage is perhaps truest during the grueling period that is residency training, but can arise in the day to day of a busy acute care physician. From a historical perspective, it was possibly a combination of the primary care physician shortage, coupled by the demands of the traditional call model, that may have resulted in the advent of the shift-work model within hospital medicine. Protected time off and block scheduling aimed to alleviate pressures of continuous medical care. However, fatigue can still rear its head on any given day, largely due to the myriad responsibilities that a hospitalist is beholden to: emergency department admissions, transfers, discharges, consultations, and critical care. In addition, 12-hour shifts leave little time to address "life circumstances" that do not fit neatly into the demands of a block schedule.

It is helpful to recall that fatigue can be deconstructed into physical fatigue and emotional fatigue. Physical fatigue is perhaps easily remedied by adequate sleep, a healthy diet, and regular exercise. A more progressive view suggests, however, that physical and emotional health are inextricably linked and not mutually exclusive. A healthy frame of mind is needed to maintain the discipline needed to make healthy dietary choices and regular exercise. Conversely, exercise physiologists can attest to the milieu of antidepressant endorphins released during rigorous exercise. Simply put, a healthy lifestyle positively affects emotional and physical endurance in the workplace.

The diagram suggests a model for understanding the concept of stress. Simply put, stress tends to occur where there is a mismatch between a demand and one's perceived ability to meet that demand. The insidious nature of stress allows it to build daily with potentially harmful consequences. One strategy for managing stress entails the process of cataloging and chunking each individual demand into manageable tasks. Consider this scenario:

You are on the tail end of a 7-day stretch. It started off easily enough but your service has ballooned, and you are understandably anxious about handing off such a large workload to your oncoming colleague. Furthermore, you have just completed placing a difficult central line, only to find that you've been paged by both the ED as well as the direct admissions operator. Reaching for the phone, you hear an overhead page for you to the OR holding area.

What do you do?

A.   Take a deep breath. Realize that you are in the throes of being overwhelmed; it was with these instances in mind that the term "triage" was born. Call the OR, ED, and Direct Admit operator, explaining to each that you are working as diligently as you can but there may be a patient or two in front of them. Then triage which patient needs to be seen first based on sound clinical judgment. Now exhale.

B.   Begin laughing hysterically.

C.   Fake a seizure.

D.   Do A, but also notify the oncoming physician that it has become quite busy and that you would greatly appreciate a helping hand, in return for coming an hour or two earlier on the next shift or another similarly busy day for him/her.

Granted, a somewhat flippant series of options, but nonetheless, a scenario that is plausible. By taking stock of the various "demands," one is better able to apply strategies to minimize the perception of having lost control—a powerful driver of stress. In this particular scenario, these strategies include knowledge of the triage process as well as an understanding that one is able to call for help. A minute spent cataloging demands as they arise and assessing management or coping strategies can go great lengths in the alleviating the perception of stress.

EMPATHY AS A SKILL

Compassion in medicine can trump even the most stressful circumstances, but like all precious resources, it can be rapidly depleted. The antithesis of compassion or empathy is apathy. The concept of apathy is often a symptom of emotional fatigue, a well-recognized (albeit poorly studied) phenomenon in health care workers. Doebbeling et al reviewed the pitfalls of this phenomenon in health care workers tasked with the care of terminal cancer patients and patients with end-stage AIDS. As hospital medical care also involves palliative care issues, it can be inferred that hospitalists can be subject to similar emotional pressures in caring for chronically ill patients. In fact, despite shift work and block scheduling, we believe that hospitalists are at risk of developing apathy in the midst of their work schedules, given the acuity of the patients that they are caring for and the multiple avenues for admission as detailed in the example above. Like stress, apathy can be insidious in onset and manifest via a host of regrettable behaviors ranging from simple procrastination to unethical decision making and negligence. Hence, it is our opinion that apathy in medical care should be held with the same derision as poor hand-hygiene compliance or incomplete, illegible documentation.

So how does one avoid apathy? Perhaps the solution lies in developing strategies for embracing empathy within our practice by re-defining its role from the peripheral, somewhat vacuous understanding of it to a firm, teachable skill, possibly even a discipline, inhabiting a core directive that drives each and every patient interaction we undertake. Atul Gawande suggests in his book *Better: A Surgeon's Notes on Performance*, that we as practitioners consider asking unscripted questions of our patients. "Ours is a job of talking to strangers," he observes. "Why not learn something about them?" An additional minute spent gathering a detail or two that doesn't necessarily need to be documented in the patient's record ultimately serves to highlight the humanity of the physician/patient interaction. Hence, borrowing shamelessly from the good Dr. Gawande, ask an unscripted question.

Try to make sure that this unscripted question is not asked from the doorway, hand on the doorknob, as if trying to make a quick getaway from the scene. Simply put, make sure that one takes the time to sit and engage with each and every patient, each and every time. Dr. Michael Gregory, chairman and CEO of a nation-wide hospitalist practice, espouses the importance of the bedside chair. Performing a guided physical exam, all the while sharing the results of completed investigations and summing up with an assessment and plan of action, is not only good communication, but in truth, is just good medicine, acknowledging the partnership between patient and practitioner.

Look for instances where one can actually be of service to one's patients. By this, we refer not to the abstract concept of providing the service of medicine to our patients, but to the simpler, more direct *act* of service to our patients. A cup of ice, a piece of paper with a diagram drawn on it by none other than yourself, a sip of water, a warm blanket, a book, a movie review. By practicing the daily act of giving, boundaries are shattered and service truly becomes second nature. Hippocrates would have wept.

PACING AND EFFICIENCY: THE WAY OF THE HOSPITALIST

Acute care physicians thrive on the challenge of building relationships with strangers quickly, managing complex multi-system medical issues, and guiding both patients and their families through the myriad medical decisions that are implicit within modern healthcare. Managing stress and practicing empathic medical care can only be possible if a physician develops efficient workflow habits. The following are some tips garnered from seasoned hospitalists regarding the management of time during the day.

Every minute before 9 A.M. is worth two after mid-day:
In simple terms, the earlier one begins the day, the earlier one completes rounds. The earlier rounds are completed, the earlier one is able to focus on new admissions, follow-up visits, asking unscripted questions, etc. Try to identify in your hospital when the A.M. labs are drawn and become available, in addition to when shift change occurs. It is in the morning that the charts tend to be where they are meant to be and not accompanying the patient to various scheduled tests.

Pick your severances:
It is simply not practical to spend extended amounts of time with each and every patient. Still, patients' (and families') needs can vary from day to day. Recognize this and try to pre-empt the division of your unscripted time, focusing on different groups of patients on different days. Sometimes a brief rundown of care, followed by a "check in" later in the day can be just as effective as a prolonged discourse.

Round with a rounding partner:
Ideally, make attempts to involve nursing as much as possible in the rounding process. Not only is this sound team-based medicine, but also an important safety strategy for bringing up issues of which the physician may not have been aware. If you are unable to round with the nurse, attempt to visit with the nurse following the patient visit, highlighting your plan of care and engaging the nurse to add any additional pertinent information.

Avoid multitasking, but delegate like an octopus:
Multitasking can lead to mistakes. Focus on one task at a time, but utilize the resources available to you. Ask the unit secretary to locate consultants and call them for you, ask nursing assistants about how well the patient ate or ambulated, ask the case managers to arrange the outpatient tests and appointments.

Arrive to work on time and strive to leave on time:
Practicing in a team environment involves being aware of how interdependent our work schedules are. Professionalism and reliability is the glue that holds a team together.

9 A.M. is the unofficial end of written orders and mid-day is the unofficial end of the rounding day:
Having the majority, if not all, of your patients' orders written by 9 A.M. and all documentation (notes) completed by noon translates into additional time to provide follow-up care and to be available for new admissions/consultations.

Manage your consultants:
Insist on verbal consultation requests and return the favor by picking up the phone and discussing targeted problems you wish the consultant to address when you ask for a sub-specialty consultation. Try to learn from each and every consultation, but do not defer disposition control to the consultant. Remember, you are the coordinator of care and are charged with task of constantly evaluating the "big picture" for your patient.

9

Ethical Issues in Hospital Medicine

Arun Mathews, MD

P*racticing physicians are faced with many moral and ethical issues that their years in medical school may not adequately prepare them to face. Medical advances and new technologies have greatly added to medicine's ability to prolong life, sometimes beyond reason.*

With this new-found ability to offer treatments and extend life to patients who years ago would not have survived, there comes a new responsibility to exercise this power judiciously. Today's doctors are called upon to decide when and how these new advances are used, but may often feel ill-equipped to make ethical decisions.

The following is a guide to assist practicing physicians in internal medicine in their basic understanding of some of the common ethical issues that may be faced in caring for their patients. Topics to be addressed are as follows:

- DNR orders
- Withdrawal of treatment
- Informed consent
- Competence and decision-making capacity
- Confidentiality and Health Insurance Portability and Accountability Act (HIPAA)
- Futility and unreasonable patient requests
- The difficult patient
- Pain control and palliative care
- Advance directives
- Ethics consultation

The topics covered are not meant to be all-inclusive, but will provide a basis for an understanding of the issues.

DO NOT RESUSCITATE (DNR) ORDERS

Simply put, do not resuscitate (DNR) orders are orders written by a patient's physician that stipulate that in the event of respiratory or cardiac arrest, no resuscitation is to be attempted. Generally, DNR orders are written when patients who have a life-threatening or inevitably fatal illness wish to have a natural death without painful or invasive medical procedures. Less commonly, patients not in these situations may request DNR status because they hold strong views about what they may perceive as artificial prolongation of life.

Bradley (2005) suggests that there should be a procedure in place to address the withholding of life-sustaining treatment, as follows.

■ *Medical assessment*: There should be a thorough review of the patient's condition, prognosis, and options for treatment outlined clearly in the patient's medical record.

■ *Patient competency assessment*: The patient's attending physician should document clearly his or her evaluation of the patient's competency to make an informed choice regarding withholding of life-sustaining treatment.

   ☐ The patient is deemed competent if he or she is of legal age (over the age of 18) or an emancipated minor who has the ability to comprehend the consequences of a decision to withhold therapy or treatment.

   ☐ The decision should be informed and made only after a consultation with the attending physician regarding condition, prognosis, and options for treatment. If the patient is deemed competent, wishes of an appointed health care agent or family members are not considered of sufficient weight to overrule the patient's decision.

   ☐ The patient is not considered to be competent if he or she is under the legal age of 18 and not an emancipated minor, or if they lack the ability to make informed decisions regarding resuscitation because of impaired mental status. In the case of an incompetent patient, a family member, health care agent, or legally appointed guardian may act as surrogate for the patient.

■ *Documenting DNR orders*: Proper documentation of the DNR order, once decided upon, should be as complete as possible and should include

   ☐ *A summary of the order.* This should include the reason and justification for the order and any staff discussion regarding the patient's condition.

   ☐ *An acknowledgment of competence.* The patient's competence (or incompetence) should be documented.

   ☐ *A description of the circumstances surrounding the patient's consent to the order.* If the patient is deemed not competent, the discussion with family members, health care agent, or legal guardian should be on record.

   ☐ *A statement of the patient's wishes.* This may include comfort measures or the withdrawal of any other care.

■ If at any time a physician feels conflicted regarding DNR status, consultation with an ethics committee may be an option.

Quick Consult:

■ DNR orders are orders written stipulating that the patient does not wish to be resuscitated in the event of respiratory or cardiac arrest.

■ Medical assessment and competency assessment should be carried out on all patients requesting DNR status.

■ Proper documentation is crucial.

WITHDRAWAL OF TREATMENT

Withdrawal of treatment has become an issue because it is now possible to maintain life for long periods of time when there is little or no hope of recovery. Treatment is withdrawn when it is felt that a patient will die despite any treatment given (Cohen & Winter, 1999).

Involvement of the patient's family in the decision-making process regarding withdrawal of treatment is of paramount importance. Families who feel that they have been well informed and involved in the decision to withdraw treatment are more likely to be at peace with the decision. Cohen and Winter point out that it is unwise to withdraw treatment without the family's agreement.

There are three situations that may arise around the issue of withdrawal of care:

- *The family requests withdrawal of treatment inappropriately.* Duty of care is always to the patient, and not to their family members. The astute physician will listen to their concerns and then explain why continuation of treatment is appropriate. Offering a second opinion may appease this situation.

- *The family requests continued treatment when there is no hope of recovery.* Communication with the family is key, remembering that there may be cultural or religious beliefs influencing their request. Again, offering a second opinion may help. If there continues to be conflict with family members, seeking advice from an ethics committee may be called for.

- *The patient requests withdrawal of treatment.* The request may stem from frustration. An honest approach that includes the rationale for continuing treatment is best. In the end, a competent patient has the right to refuse treatment.

There has been much debate about whether there is a distinction between withdrawal of treatment and assisted suicide. Orentlicher (1996) states "Perhaps the most common justification for the distinction is that assisted suicide involves an act of killing, whereas the withdrawal of treatment permits the disease to take its natural course" (p. 663). He also points out that many believe that when patients are fatally ill and there is little benefit to be derived from treatment, it is acceptable to allow patients to die.

Whatever the physician's personal beliefs regarding withdrawal of treatment, this issue is commonly faced and multifaceted. When faced with decision-making regarding the issue of withdrawal of care, it may be prudent to elicit other opinions and, if necessary, the assistance of an ethics committee.

Quick Consult:

■ Withdrawal of treatment decisions are faced when it is believed that a patient will die despite any treatment offered.

■ Involvement of the family in the decision-making process is of paramount importance where possible.

■ Three ethical issues that may be faced in withdrawal of care:

1. The family requests withdrawal of care inappropriately.
2. The family insists on continuing care beyond any hope of recovery.
3. The patient requests withdrawal of treatment ("A competent patient has the right to refuse treatment").

■ When in doubt, obtaining an ethics committee consult is never wrong.

INFORMED CONSENT

Informed consent refers to the ability of a patient to make decisions about their health care on the basis of a full and complete understanding of their treatment options. Informed consent is based on the ethical principles of self-determination and autonomy. Informed consent should be based on discussion between the physician and patient regarding the following elements:

■ *The nature of the decision to be made.* This may include a description of the procedure to be carried out.

■ *Any existing alternatives.* Alternatives to the proposed treatment or procedure should be thoroughly explained.

■ *The known risks and benefits.* Potential for harm should be outlined, as well as any expected positive outcomes of any available treatments.

■ *The patient's understanding.* It should be documented that the patient fully understands the information provided.

■ *The patient's consent.* Whether or not the patient consents to the proposed treatment should be documented.

Two components must be present in order for consent to be considered valid. First, the patient must be considered competent to make any decisions involving the patient's health care. Second, consent must be voluntary.

Voluntary consent refers to the fact that patients may consent to treatment or procedures simply because of the nature of the doctor–patient relationship. Patients may be concerned that refusing treatment options may change this relationship in a negative way. Good, clear communication will go a long way toward mitigating the threat of passive (and unintentional) coercion.

Many states have legislation that sets forth the minimum required standard of care with regard to informed consent. Legislation typically addresses one or more of the following standards:

■ *Reasonable physician standard.* For example, what would a typical physician offer in the way of information about the proposed treatment or procedure in order to make an informed decision?

■ *Reasonable patient standard.* What information would a typical patient need to know about the proposed treatment or procedure in order to make an informed choice?

■ *Subjective standard.* What would this *particular* patient need to know in order to make an informed decision?

Most hospitals or institutions have policies in place regarding which procedures or treatments require a signed consent form, as in operative procedures and blood transfusions. The AMA (2008) states:

> It is important that the communications process itself be documented. Good documentation can serve as evidence in a court of law that the process indeed took place. A timely and thorough documentation in the patient's chart by the physician

providing the treatment and/or performing the procedure can be a strong piece of evidence that the physician engaged the patient in an appropriate discussion (AMA, 2008).

A last important point regarding informed consent is that it should never be presumed, unless the patient is unconscious or incompetent, and there is no surrogate available to make a decision regarding treatment.

Quick Consult:

■ Informed consent is based on the patient's ability to make a decision regarding their health care.

■ Patient must be considered competent, and consent must be voluntary.

■ Should be based on discussion between patient and physician that includes the following elements:

    1. The nature of the decision to be made, or treatment being considered
    2. Alternatives to the proposed treatment or procedure
    3. Known risks and benefits
    4. Patient's understanding of the information presented, and whether or not they give their consent

■ Should be well documented.

COMPETENCY AND DECISION-MAKING CAPACITY

The previous section outlined procedures to be followed in order to obtain informed consent. However, occasions arise in which patients make decisions contrary to what their physician recommends. Appelbaum (2007) states "Hence, the determination of whether patients are competent is critical in striking a proper balance between respecting the autonomy of patients who are capable of making informed decisions and protecting those with cognitive impairment" (p. 1834).

Cognitive impairment may occur in any number of conditions. Psychiatric patients are the most obvious group whose decision-making ability may be affected by their disease. Patients with dementia and Alzheimer's disease are another obvious group. Azar, Gurrera, Karel, and Moye (2006) conducted a study to examine consent capacity among older adults with dementia over a period of 9 months. Their conclusion was as follows: "Some patients with mild-to-moderate dementia develop a clinically relevant impairment of consent capacity within a year. Consent capacity in adults with mild-to-moderate dementia should be reassessed periodically to ensure that it is adequate for each specific informed consent situation" (p. 79).

Legal standards vary considerably from one jurisdiction to the next with regard to decision-making capacity for consent to treatment. There are, however, some basic criteria that should be addressed, as outlined by Appelbaum:

■ *Patients are able to communicate a choice.* Patients should be able to clearly communicate their preferred treatment option; frequently changing their mind may indicate lack of capacity.

■ *Patients are able to understand relevant information.* Patients should have a reasonable grasp of the information given by the physician; information they should understand includes the basic elements of consent, such as the nature of their condition, nature of the proposed treatment, risks and benefits they may reasonably expect, and any alternatives to the treatment offered.

■ *Patients are able to appreciate their situation and its consequences.* Patients should be able to demonstrate knowledge of their condition and consequences of treatment options; lack of insight, delusions, and denial of their situation are the most common causes of impairment.

■ *Patients are able to reason about their treatment options.* The reasoning process focuses on the process by which the patient reaches a decision, not on the decision itself. This distinction is important, as patients are entitled to make "unreasonable" decisions, providing that they are competent to make a decision to begin with.

If, in the physician's opinion, and after taking the above factors into consideration, the patient is deemed incompetent, the physician should seek to remedy the situation when possible. If there is an obvious cause of impairment, such as fever or sedation, attempting to remedy these situations may reverse the situation. Patients who suffer impaired cognition due to psychiatric illness or other disorders should be given every educational opportunity to help them comprehend their situation. For those patients incapacitated by fear or anxiety, enlisting support for the patient in the form of a trusted family member or friend may assist the patient to make a reasoned decision.

When the patient is deemed incompetent to make decisions regarding the patient's medical treatment, efforts should be made to find a surrogate, such as a family member. Patients who have made a prior advance directive may have already decided on a course of action for this type of situation, and their directive may give clear instructions about who may make decisions on their behalf. In an emergency situation, a physician may provide treatment based on the premise that a reasonable person would consent to such treatment.

Physicians should be familiar with the laws in their jurisdictions regarding capacity and decision-making capacity. As mentioned previously, physicians may choose to ask for an ethics consultation if they find their patient's decision at odds with their recommended treatment for them.

Quick Consult:

■ Patients should meet four criteria in order to be judged competent to make decisions regarding their care:

1. Must be able to communicate a choice
2. Must be able to understand relevant information
3. Must be able to appreciate the situation and its consequences
4. Must be able to reason about treatment options

■ Patients may be incompetent as a result of their condition, ie, Alzheimer.

■ If the patient is deemed incompetent, an effort to find a surrogate should be made.

■ Physicians should be aware of the laws in their state regarding competency.

PATIENT CONFIDENTIALITY AND HIPAA REGULATIONS

As long as there have been practicing physicians, doctors have been held to the highest standards of confidentiality. The duty to maintain confidentiality means that a physician may not divulge personal information that a patient provides them, nor can they divulge information they may discover in the course of treating a patient.

The AMA's Council on Ethical and Judicial Affairs states, "The information disclosed to a physician during the course of the patient-physician relationship is confidential to the utmost degree" (AMA, 2007). The Council explains that the purpose of this ethical duty to maintain confidentiality is to allow the patient to feel comfortable making a full disclosure to their physician, knowing that the physician is ethically bound to keep their private information to himself or herself.

Access to new technology, while improving patient care, presents new challenges to securing patient confidentiality. The advent of electronic health records, shared databases, and integrated health care systems allow greater access to patient records, thus increasing the risks of breaches in confidentiality.

The general rule of thumb regarding confidentiality is that information from a patient's medical record may not be disclosed to a third party without the patient's consent. A breach of confidentiality occurs when information is disclosed to a third party without patient consent or a court order. Disclosure may be written or oral, by telephone or fax, or electronically, such as through email (AMA, 2007).

Generally, express authorized permission is required to release medical records in the following situations (AMA, 2007):

- *Patient's lawyer or insurance company.* The patient must give permission for release of medical information even to the patient's own lawyer or insurance company.
- *Patient's employer.* The exception is if a workers' compensation claim is involved.
- *Patient's family.* Medical records can be released to a family member if the family member has durable power of attorney for health care.
- *Government agencies.* Examples might include government welfare agencies, government disability programs, and social services.
- *Other third parties.* Any other parties who request medical records must not be given access without the patient's permission.

State law governs who may grant permission for release of medical records. Generally, the patient is the only one permitted to grant permission if he or she is deemed competent. A legal guardian or parent may grant permission if the patient is a minor or deemed incompetent. If the patient is deceased, an executor or administrator may grant permission (AMA, 2007). Generally, the expected elements of a valid release should include the following:

- *The patient's name and identifying information.* This includes such information as the patient's health care number or date of birth.
- *Address of the sender.* This is the health care professional or institution authorized to release the information.

- *Description of the information to be released.* Examples are lab results, progress notes, and medication lists.
- *The third party.* This identifies the party to whom the information is to be released.
- *Signature.* The signature of the patient (or their surrogate) should be included.
- *Time period.* This refers to the period of time that the release is valid for.

Implied consent refers to special situations in which the patient does not expressly authorize the release of medical records or information. An example of this occurs when a patient is transferred from one hospital to another. In agreeing to be transferred, the patient also agrees to allow their medical information to be shared between the two facilities to provide continuity of care.

HIPAA (Health Insurance Portability and Accountability Act) includes new regulations that provide for the protection of personal identifiers, such as certain health data. Enacted in 1996, HIPAA regulations are enforceable, and address the following areas:

- *Access to medical records.* Patients may ask to see or obtain copies of their health records and request changes or corrections to errors or mistakes.
- *Notice of privacy practices.* Patients must be provided notice of any possible use of their personal health information; patient rights under HIPAA must also be provided.
- *Limits on the use of personal health information.* Basically, HIPAA allows for providers of care to share only that information which is deemed necessary to the care of that patient and does not allow sharing of health care information to parties not immediately involved in the patient's care.
- *Marketing.* HIPAA provides that a patient's permission must be obtained before disclosing personal health care information for the purposes of marketing.
- *Confidential communications.* Health care providers are expected to use their professional judgment when communicating personal health information to interested parties and must ensure communications are confidential, as the situation permits.
- *Authorized representatives.* A surrogate or authorized proxy (ie, an appointed power of attorney) should be treated the same as the patient unless, in the physician's opinion, that person is not acting in the patient's best interest.
- *Reportable conditions.* Conditions that may impact others may be exempt from confidentiality laws, ie, in cases of certain infectious diseases, or driving impairment due to seizures or dementia.
- *Complaints.* Patients are entitled to file complaints for breaches of these privacy practices; however, patients do not have the right to file private lawsuits.

Practitioners should become intimately familiar with HIPAA regulations, but should also bear in mind that physicians using good judgment and acting in good faith should not concern themselves with being found noncompliant with HIPAA regulations.

Quick Consult:

■ General rule of thumb is that information from a patient's medical record may not be disclosed to a third party without patient consent.

■ Third parties may be:
1. A patient's lawyer or insurance company
2. A patient's employer (except in workers' compensation claims)
3. A patient's family (unless family member has legal standing, such as durable power of attorney)
4. Government agencies
5. Other third parties

■ Implied consent refers to special situations in which the patient does not expressly authorize the release of information.

■ HIPAA (1996) regulations are enforceable by law, and expand upon previously existing confidentiality laws.

■ Physicians who are unsure of any element of patient confidentiality should consider seeking advice of hospital legal counsel, if available.

FUTILITY AND UNREASONABLE PATIENT REQUESTS

Arguments concerning futility and/or unreasonable patient requests invariably produce strong feelings among those who debate this issue. The cases that draw the most attention are not common scenarios, and yet they manage to draw national attention when they occur.

Truog (2007) writes that the most infamous cases are "about families insisting on the continued use of life-sustaining treatments that physicians consider medically inappropriate" (p. 1). He goes on to say, "in cases of intractable conflict, the American Medical Association and others have recommended an approach based on due process as a fair method for reaching resolution" (p. 1).

Jecker, Jonsen, and Schneiderman (1996) address several of the common issues surrounding unreasonable patient requests and futility.

Physician-Patient Power Struggle

At the heart of this issue is the notion that physicians wield all the power in decision-making regarding futility, owing to their expert knowledge and control over technology, while the patient (or the patient's surrogate) has none. The authors contend that it is the physician's duty of beneficence to use treatments that provide therapeutic benefits, and that "abuses of power are resolved not by eliminating medical judgment and yielding to unreasonable demands but rather by exercising judgment openly and responsibly according to professional standards" (p. 670). They express the belief that "unreasonable" patient requests are usually misguided attempts by the family to do everything possible for the patient as an expression of how much they care for the individual. They may feel that agreeing with the physician means "giving up" on their loved one.

Consensus on the Definition of Futility

Even physicians disagree about quantifying and qualifying futility. The authors point out that achieving consensus about futility is a gradual process that "begins with public awareness of an issue, proceeds to understanding by working through the issue ... and finally leads to resolution on cognitive, emotional, and moral levels" (p. 670).

They also argue that "every profession declares values and standards" (p. 670), and society rejects or accepts these standards by acting through legal channels.

Physiologic Definition of Futility

The authors have been criticized by some who believe that a physiologic definition of futility is free from moral judgment and is the only ethically defensible option. However, no one has been able to come up with a true working definition of the concept of futility. As stated by the authors, "Contrary to the assertion that physiologic futility is value-free, we argue that it entails a value choice ... it assumes that the goals of medicine are to preserve organ function, body parts, and physiologic activity – an assumption that ... departs dramatically from the patient-centered goals of medicine" (p. 670).

Empirical Treatment Data and Futility

The underlying basis for this argument is that no physician can say for certain that a certain treatment will or will not work. However, most medical treatments are based on evidence that a treatment will be beneficial in a majority of patients, and there is generally empirical evidence that the physician can look to when deciding on a particular treatment. The authors make a valid point: "Thus, the proper question to ask is not whether we can be certain a treatment will not work but how many times we are willing to see a treatment fail before we agree that it does not work" (p. 671).

Futility and Religion

The authors touch on the issue of religious beliefs and futility of care by pointing out that the two can coexist together; they need not be at odds with one another. They argue, "Miracles may be an important goal of prayer for many patients, but they should not be imposed on physicians as a goal of medical practice" (p. 672).

Rationing and Resource Allocation

Monetary considerations should not be a consideration in decisions regarding medical futility. As the authors rightly conclude, "only society has the ethical mandate to decide the relevance of nonmedical criteria in the allocation of scarce resources" (p. 672).

Truog (2007) points out that many of the sensational cases regarding futility of care and unreasonable patient demands "are the product of a severe breakdown of trust in the relationship between the clinicians and the patient's family ... improvement of physician's communication and conflict-resolution skills would no doubt go a long way toward preventing such cases from occurring" (p. 1).

Quick Consult:

■   Points to consder when faced with unreasonable patient requests:

1. Family members may feel that they must prove how much they care by insisting on futile measures and that deciding against futile measures means they are "giving up" on the patient.
2. Physicians and patients may have fundamental differences owing to culture, religion, and class.
3. Communication is key; breakdown in communication may lead to loss of trust in the physician.
4. The AMA recommends an approach to conflict based on due process.
5. An ethics committee consult should be sought if differences between the physician and family are irreconcilable.

THE DIFFICULT PATIENT

Undoubtedly during the course of a physician's career, he or she will encounter patients that they consider to be "problem patients." These patients may engender feelings of frustration, dislike, and anger in their caregivers because of behavioral or emotional aspects that affect their care.

Who are these patients, and why are they problematic to deal with? Steinmetz and Tabenkin (2001) identified the following three categories of patients as considered difficult to deal with in a study of family physicians:

- *Patients with behavioral problems.* These patients may be violent, aggressive, verbally rude, manipulative, lying, and demanding.

- *Patients with repetitive or unsolved complaints.* These patients seek out medical care repetitively for the same complaints, despite numerous negative studies.

- *Patients with psychiatric disorders.* Patients with schizophrenia, bipolar disorder, depression, and anxiety are often noncompliant with care and may have behavioral issues.

There are many underlying reasons why patients may behave as they do. For example, the patient may be suffering from an undiagnosed psychiatric problem. Mood disorders may cause a patient to consult a physician with complaints of insomnia, headache, back pain, or fatigue. Patients suffering from anxiety may present with various physical complaints, or may complain that they feel that not enough is being done to root out the cause of their complaint. Alcoholics or those with borderline personalities may seek care for somatic complaints. Even when the physician becomes aware of or suspects that a psychiatric problem may be the basis for the symptoms, these patients may reject a diagnosis, adding to physician frustration.

Physician factors may also play a part in difficult physician–patient relationships. Studies have shown that physician overwork is correlated with a higher number of patients perceived as being difficult to deal with. In addition, less experienced physicians may be more likely to perceive patients as being difficult (Haas, Leiser, Magill, & Sanyer, 2005). There may be patients who are more apt to raise negative feelings in their physician due to the physician's past experiences. An example of this is a physician who grew up with an alcoholic parent who finds it difficult to deal with alcoholic patients.

The way the health care system is designed does little to mitigate these factors. Managed care has increased patient mistrust in their physicians and in health care in general. Advances in technology, such as the Internet, mean that patients are getting their health information from sources other than their own physicians. Pressure for doctors to treat more patients in less time and using fewer resources has translated to less time spent with patients. All of these changes may lead to greater potential for conflicting expectations of the physician–patient relationship (Haas et al., 2005).

Management of the difficult patient may involve incorporating one or more of the following tips into the treatment plan:

■ *Focus on specific problems.* Ask the patient to focus on their biggest concern at the moment.

■ *Acknowledge and accept the emotional response that some patients bring out.* Acknowledging that the patient brings out negative emotions in the physician allows the physician to focus on the patient's problem, and not the patient's difficult attitude.

■ *Obtain professional support.* Ask other colleagues, who have dealt with similar situations, how they resolved the issue.

■ *Improve listening and understanding skills.* The use of active listening skills, such as repeating back to the patient what the physician heard, will help avoid misunderstandings and make the patient feel as if they have been listened to and understood.

■ *Enlist the patient's help.* Engage the patient in the idea that they are in a partnership with their physician.

■ *Improve skills at expressing negative emotions.* Learning how to discuss negative emotions with the patient may improve communication between patient and physician.

■ *Increase empathy.* Attempting to understand the patient's behavior and reacting to the patient in a nonjudgmental way may improve the physician–patient relationship.

■ *Negotiate with the patient.* Discuss the process of care and agree on a plan for moving forward (Haas et al., 2005).

Ignoring the problem will not likely improve the relationship between the patient and the physician. Referring the patient to another physician will only mean that the new physician will inherit a bigger problem, with a patient who feels angry and rejected. Accusing a patient of being problematic will make for an angry patient, as will attempting to tell the patient there is nothing wrong with him or her.

Dealing with difficult patients may be one of the more frustrating aspects of practicing medicine. Physicians should develop the skills necessary to communicate effectively and should be aware of those patients who "push their buttons" personally. Seeking support or advice from colleagues may be an important tool in dealing with these patients.

Quick Consult:

■ Patients with behavioral problems, repetitive or unsolved complaints, and psychiatric problems are the patients who are most often identified by physicians as being difficult to manage.

■ Physicians' own backgrounds may affect how they view these patients.

■ Good communication skills are important in preventing a bad physician–patient relationship from getting worse.

■ Physicians may find it useful to identify a colleague who may be able to mentor or advise them when dealing with a difficult patient.

PAIN CONTROL AND PALLIATIVE CARE

The World Health Organization provides a good working definition of palliative care:

> The active total care of patients whose disease is not responsive to curative treatment. Control of pain, of other symptoms, and of psychological, social, and spiritual problems is paramount. The goal of palliative care is achievement of the best quality of life for patients and their families (WHO, 1990).

This definition encompasses the principles of palliative care; that is, caring for the whole patient and not just the treatment of symptoms or disease. Fallon and O'Neill (1997) iterate several principles integral to palliative care:

■ *Palliative care affirms life.* The approach to dying is a natural process.

■ *Palliative care accepts death.* Palliative care neither hastens nor postpones death.

■ *Palliative care provides relief from pain.* It also helps to relieve other distressing symptoms.

■ *Palliative care takes a holistic approach.* Palliative care includes psychological and spiritual aspects of care.

■ *Palliative care offers a support system.* Palliative care supports the patient to live as actively as they can until death.

■ *Palliative care offers support to the patient's family.* It assists them in coping with the patient's illness and their own grief.

Pain control is an essential component of palliative care. Achieving adequate pain control allows the dying patient the freedom to address other aspects of the patient's illness comfortably, and provides the opportunity to spend more time at home with family rather than being hospitalized. Many patients can spend most of their time at home with the use of hospice or home care, providing their pain is well controlled. However, it is estimated that "40 percent of patients with advanced cancer experience severe pain at some point, and that 25% of cancer patients die with poorly managed pain" (as cited by Black and Schofield, 2005).

Pain may be caused by the disease itself, as in pain caused by the growth of a tumor, or may be caused as a result of treatment for the disease, as in surgery to remove a tumor. Regardless of the underlying cause of the pain, it must be adequately controlled.

Physicians and patients alike may be hesitant to treat the patient's pain with the full arsenal of medications and treatments available towing to the lack of knowledge or misperceptions regarding pain relief methods. Physicians may not be fully cognizant of new treatments or medications available if palliative care is not their area of expertise. Consulting a pain service or an oncologist may be necessary. Patients may be reluctant to use strong opioids even when appropriate, due to fear of addiction or misinformation about side effects. Concerning the use of morphine, "There is no arbitrary upper limit, but negative attitudes to using morphine still exist; the skilled use of morphine will confer benefit rather than harm, but many patients express fears, which should be discussed" (Fallon & O'Neill, 1997).

The World Health Organization (1996) has recommended a three-step analgesic ladder for pain control management that has been used extensively:

> The analgesic ladder approach is one of regular review of pain and adjustment of analgesia being taken – either by increasing the dose, changing the drug being used, or adding an analgesic with a different action. Drugs are given at regular intervals and orally wherever possible – by the clock and by the mouth. (Black & Schofield, 2005).

Patients should be reassured that side effects with regard to the use of opioids can be managed. The most common side effects are sedation, nausea and vomiting, constipation, and dry mouth. All of these effects can be managed easily with the addition of antiemetics, laxatives, and good mouth care. Sedation generally resolves within a few days of starting opioids.

Perhaps even more important than symptom control in palliative care is establishing a strong, trusting relationship with the dying patient and the patient's family. Honesty at all points, empathy, and an understanding of the patient's fears and concerns will cause the patient to be open and receptive to the physician's advice and will provide comfort to both the patient and family.

Quick Consult:

- Palliative care is the care of the whole patient, including physical, psychological, and spiritual components.
- Adequate pain control is crucial to allowing patients to live their lives as actively as possible until death.
- Both physicians and patients often have misguided or misinformed attitudes toward the use of strong opioids for pain control.
- The WHO advocates a three-step approach to pain control that includes regular assessment of the patient's pain.
- Side effects of opioids can be easily managed and should not be a deterrent in their use.
- There is no upper limit in the use of opioids such as morphine.

ADVANCE DIRECTIVES

Advance directives can be an important tool in guiding a physician's decision-making in regards to end-of-life care. Knowing in advance what the patient's wishes were prior to a critical event helps to avoid treatment that a patient might have refused were they able to speak for themselves (Baranowski-Birkmeier, Johnson, and O'Donnell, 1994).

Advance directives are simply a method by which patients can make their wishes known regarding end-of-life care while they are able to make informed decisions, and ideally before the need to make such decisions arises: "Advance directives (ADs) in the form of living wills or durable powers of attorney represent methods by which individuals can attempt to delineate their wishes about medical care to be applied when decision-making capacity has been lost" (Baranowsk-Birkmeier et al, 1994).

To be deemed valid, an advance directive must comply with state law. Most states have specific forms that patients may complete, and permit any language as long as the document has been appropriately signed and witnessed. The following describes some of the laws of advance directives.

Patient Self-Determination Act

The Patient Self-Determination Act was passed in 1991, and provides that all health care institutions that receive government funds through the Medicaid and Medicare programs provide patients with information about their rights under state law to execute an AD. In addition, written information provided to the patient must clearly state the institution's policies toward end-of-life issues, such as withholding or withdrawing life-sustaining treatment. Institutions found to be in violation of the Act can lose their federal funding.

Durable Power of Attorney for Health Care

In many states, patients can designate an agent to make decisions for them if they become incapacitated or are deemed incompetent to make their own decisions. A DPAHC is drafted to take immediate effect but the agent named is not permitted to make any decisions unless the time comes that the patient is unable to make decisions for himself or herself. Physicians are legally bound to accept the agent's wishes unless the agent is not acting in accordance with the patient's known wishes or in the patient's best interests. A DPAHC can be revoked at any time by a competent patient, either verbally or in writing.

Natural Death Act Declaration

This act directs physicians that the patient does not wish to receive life-sustaining treatments if, in the judgment of two physicians, the patient is certified to be permanently unconscious or is in a terminal situation and is unable to give consent.

The DPAHC takes precedence over a NDAD (patients may have both). However, the presence of a NDAD may reassure physicians that the agent named in the DPAHC is adhering to the patient's wishes, and may be a valuable tool if there are any doubts in this regard.

Physicians should be familiar with the laws of their state regarding ADs. In addition, physicians should feel comfortable raising the issue with their patients, as only a small percentage of the population executes an AD:

> Advance directives have one major goal: to assist in making decisions for patients without decision-making ability that would reflect individual patient preferences. Although multiple concerns have been expressed, many patients and physicians desire a discussion of the issues that would eventually lead to the formation of an AD. This discussion would preferably take place in a physician–patient relationship as part of ongoing health care, without the presence of a crisis situation. (Baranowski-Birkmeier et al, 1995)

Quick Consult:

■ *Advance Directives (ADs)*: Allow patients to voice their wishes for end-of-life care in advance, or before an event that leaves them unable to speak for themselves.

■ *Durable Power of Attorney for Health Care*: Allows a patient to name an agent to make decisions on behalf of the patient in the event that the patient is deemed incompetent or is incapacitated.

■ *Natural Death Act Declaration*: Allows the patient to state that he or she does not wish to receive life-sustaining treatment if deemed to be permanently unconscious or in a terminal situation certified by two physicians.

■ Physicians should be familiar with the laws of their state regarding ADs.

ETHICS CONSULTATION

As stated previously, medical training likely does little to prepare today's physicians for the vast array of ethical issues that they may be faced with. The ability of the medicine to prolong life, and advances in treatments and technology, allows physicians to sustain life beyond what is sometimes appropriate. Savvy consumers of health care may also demand care beyond what should be expected. Laws have often not kept up with new advances. All of these factors may be reason enough for physicians to find themselves in need of an ethics consultation.

Ethics committees involve groups of professionals from diverse backgrounds who provide three main functions: Providing ethics consultations, developing clinical ethics policies, and teaching topical issues in clinical ethics. The goals of an ethics committee are as follows:

- *Promote the rights of patients.* Protecting patient rights is of paramount importance.

- *Promote shared decision-making.* The process should promote the sharing of decision-making between patients (or their surrogates) and physicians.

- *Promote fair policies and procedures.* The end point is to achieve good, client-centered outcomes.

- *Promote education in ethical decision-making.* Another purpose is to enhance the ethical tenor of health care professionals and health care institutions.

- *Promote the resolution of ethical conflicts.* The goal is to answer ethical questions through provision of consultations (University of Washington, 1998).

Members of ethics committees come from a diverse background. The committee may consist of physicians and nurses from the major clinical services, clergy members, legal counsel, and lay public. Ideally, all members receive some training in ethical analysis.

In most cases, anyone involved in the patient's care or who may be involved in decision-making regarding care may request an ethics consultation. The request may come from the physician caring for the patient, a member of the nursing staff, a family member, or anyone else concerned, including patients themselves.

Aulisio, Arnold, and Youngner (2000) make the following recommendations regarding ethics consultations:

- *Open access.* A general policy of open access is important to ensure that the rights and values of all interested parties are respected; exceptions to this policy should be clearly outlined.

- *Notification of interested parties.* Patients or their surrogates should be notified if a consultation is called. The reason for the consultation, the process it will take, and an invitation to attend should be included.

- *Documentation.* Ethics consultation should be clearly documented in the patient's permanent medical record.

- *Case review.* Ethics consultation should have a mechanism for case review.

Aulisio et al. (2000) also caution against the abuse of power and the potential for conflict of interest:

> Ethics consultants have the power to influence clinical care. This power can be abused. For example, ethics consultants have access to privileged information, including highly personal medical, psychological, financial, and legal information. The requirements of confidentiality must be respected. In addition, conflicts of interest can bias consultants' recommendations. If ethics consultants have important personal or professional relationships with one or more parties that could lead to bias, these relationships should be disclosed, and the consultants should perhaps remove themselves from the case. (p. 65)

Ethics consultation can be a powerful tool in assisting physicians who are conflicted regarding a patient's care. When faced with making decisions regarding withdrawal of care, DNR status, informed consent, and competency, the physician may find the advice of an ethics committee invaluable.

Quick Consult:

■ Ethics committees are usually composed of medical, legal, clerical, and lay members.

■ Anyone involved in a patient's care may request a consult, including the patient.

■ Patients and family members should be notified when an ethics consult has been requested, and invited to attend if they desire.

■ Ethics consultations should be documented in the patient's permanent medical record.

■ Ethics consultation can assist the physician faced with difficult decisions, especially if there is conflict surrounding an issue.

Risk Management for Hospitalists

Rosemary Gafner, EdD
Arun Mathews, MD

Hospital medicine is the fastest growing medical specialty in the United States, having gone from a few hundred practitioners in 1996 to about 15,000 by 2006, and hospitalists may already outnumber cardiologists (Lurie et al., 1999). Despite strong initial resistance from primary care physicians and specialists alike, the use and acceptance of hospitalists has expanded dramatically in response to a growing body of evidence that hospitalists improve efficiency by reducing costs and average length of stay without compromising the quality of care (Wachter & Goldman, 2002). Health care facilities also find it beneficial to employ hospitalists because they form a "captive audience" that can be readily trained in new technologies like electronic health records, while office-based physicians benefit by being able to dispense with time-consuming inpatient rounds and concentrate on higher-paying office visits (Pham et al., 2005).

Of particular importance for liability purposes, as discussed in a recent paper by Pham et al. in the Journal of General Internal Medicine, is that different health care systems have evolved different models for employing hospitalists in response to local market forces (Pham et al., 2004). This means that liability issues posing a minor concern for hospitalists practicing in one health care system could pose a major worry for those in another.

ROLE OF THE HOSPITALIST AND UTILIZATION

If you practice in a setting where the primary motivation for establishing a hospitalist program was to control utilization, you are probably at an elevated risk of claims alleging denial of service. In fact, a university medical center recently sued a hospitalist group and the health care insurer that employs them for alleged violations of the Racketeer Influenced and Corrupt Organizations (RICO) Act (Becker, 2007). The suit alleges that the hospitalists, whom the insurer presented as "consultants" tasked with assisting the medical center in managing inpatient care, in fact functioned as utilization reviewers whose primary task was to deny such care. The medical center further alleges that the insurer has used this arrangement to deny the center 20% of the remuneration that it should have received on behalf of patients covered by that insurer.

By contrast, as Pham et al. go on to point out, hospitalist programs initiated primarily with an eye toward relieving PCPs of the burden of inpatient care or to improve patient flow are often faced with pressures to carry large patient loads. The likely consequence is increased liability exposure to claims alleging "failure to monitor" and other risks associated with physicians being spread too thin.

UNDERSTAND YOUR LIMITS AS AN INTERNIST

Another evolutionary change is that, while hospitalists are traditionally responsible for general medicine patients on floors, they are increasingly being called upon to provide care in ICUs, short-stay units associated with EDs, and specialized medical floors. This means that hospitalists, who are usually trained as general internists, are more likely to find themselves in practice situations that require specialty skills. As such, many practitioners have already reported that certain aspects of their training are inadequate relative to their clinical responsibilities (Plauth et al., 2001).

THE CRITICAL ART OF THE HAND-OFF

Whatever the other risks, the single most important liability concern for hospitalists is associated with "hand-offs" between hospitalists and primary care physicians or other follow-up caregivers. Traditionally, the PCP remained the physician of record for hospitalized patients, coordinating the overall plan of care even when multiple specialty consultants became involved. The hospitalist model, however, has developed a hand-off procedure in which the PCP transfers total inpatient care responsibility and does not resume care duties until after discharge. Thus, by design, the hospitalist model interrupts the continuity of care upon the patient's admission to and discharge from the hospital. On both occasions, the hand-off from one physician to another creates situations in which patient information may be lost, mistaken assumptions may be made, and the entire dynamic of patient care may be changed.

THE HAND-OFF GONE AWRY: A TRUE CASE STUDY

An example of how this process can go wrong is shown by the case involving Belle Powell, age 75, who was admitted by infectious disease specialist Morris Allen for the treatment of a methicillin-resistant *Staphylococcus aureus* (MRSA) infection following knee replacement surgery (Kunz v. Little Company of Mary Hospital). Allen prescribed vancomycin, rifampin, and gentamicin. Because of the nephrotoxic potential of gentamicin, Allen gave orders discontinuing it before discharge, but continuing the other two antibiotics. Powell was then discharged to a nursing home. However, the hospital nurse who filled out Powell's patient transfer form wrote instructions to continue IV gentamicin indefinitely.

The nurse then called Allen to confirm the orders before actual discharge. Allen, however, had left on vacation so the call was handled by his partner, Winston Bradley. Bradley had questions about continuing the patient on gentamicin, but the nurse assured him that it was what Allen had ordered. Reasoning that his partner must have had good reason for continuing the drug, Bradley authorized the order.

At the nursing home, Powell was treated by internist David Charles, who continued the gentamicin treatment. Three days later, Powell reported difficulty in urinating. Charles ordered a serum creatinine, which came back elevated. However, he did not discontinue the gentamicin in the belief that Allen and Bradley would not have ordered the drug continued unless they had concluded that the infection posed a greater risk to the patient than the drug. Two days later, with the patient's creatinine continuing to rise, Charles finally decided to discontinue the gentamicin. But by that time, Powell had experienced total and permanent loss of kidney function, and would require dialysis for the rest of her life. Powell sued the hospital, and the nurse admitted responsibility for changing Allen's orders. A jury awarded Powell $3.2 million, upheld on appeal.

THE HAND-OFF GONE AWRY: ANALYSIS

While none of the doctors were sued in this case, all three of them could have been held liable. Allen, knowing that he was about to leave on vacation, should have either filled out the patient transfer form himself or arranged to review it before he left. Bradley breached a duty to perform an independent assessment of the situation, especially given his awareness that continuing a patient on gentamicin would only be indicated under unusual circumstances. As such, he should have reviewed the chart, examined the patient or, at the very least, attempted to contact Allen to confirm the reason behind the orders. Finally, Charles should have conferred with Allen or Bradley at the first indication that the patient was suffering nephrotoxicity. Had any one of the doctors carried out his duties completely, the patient's damages would have been minimal or nonexistent, and the lawsuit avoided.

The failure of succeeding physicians to challenge questionable or even false medical orders is just one of many hand-off errors that can affect the quality of patient care:

- Abnormal test reports requiring immediate follow-up do not arrive until after patients have been discharged.
- Patients languish in the emergency department for hours because it is unclear which physician is supposed to take care of them.
- The hand-off physician receives a battery of reports, but does not understand why the tests were ordered in the first place.
- Patient skips needed follow-up because they do not understand discharge instructions.

These are only a few of the ways that hand-off errors disrupt the continuity of patient care. Because hand-offs are an indispensable part of the hospitalist model, identifying and correcting poor hand-off practices is essential for improving the quality of care you deliver, as well as for reducing your liability exposure.

HAND-OFF AND SIGN-OUT STANDARDS FOR THE HOSPITALIST: SIX BASIC PRINCIPLES

The hand-off process back to the PCP should actually begin the minute you assume control of the patient, and you do this by inviting the primary's input in the care plan. Granted, this can sometimes be difficult because the overlap in expertise between the PCP and the hospitalist can lead to disagreements or tension (Pantilat et al., 1999). Further, not every PCP wants to be fully involved in inpatient care. But in an article in the *American Journal of Medicine*, authors Goldman, Pantilat, and Whitcomb point out that it serves your own best interests to cooperate with the PCP because it is through this doctor that your role as a hospitalist gains legitimacy in the eyes of the patient and family (Goldman, Pantilat, & Whitcomb, 2001). To facilitate the hand-off process, the authors advise hospitalists to follow six basic principles:

1. *Appropriate communication with the PCP is critical*: Primary care physicians report that one of their greatest fears in using hospitalists is that they will be left "out of the loop" and unable to respond appropriately to questions from their patients' families. Neither do they want to be bombarded with more information than they need to know. The solution is to summarize the key information and present it in a manner that meets the PCP's needs. While some PCPs still insist on telephone or fax reports, there is an increasing movement toward email reports. All are acceptable, but whatever method you use, make sure that your reports are focused on the information that will be most useful to the PCP.

2. *Consult the primary care physician*: to make sure that the two of you are in agreement. Such communication is particularly important when dealing with sensitive decisions such as do-not-resuscitate orders, surgical recommendations, and discharge plans. The PCP's input is particularly appreciated by the patient and family in such matters. If you and the PCP have differing opinions about the care plan or other matters, try to resolve them ahead of time and reach a common position such that the patient does not receive conflicting information.

3. *Timeliness is next to godliness*: such that the PCP always receives important news from the hospitalist rather than from the family. Timely communication is particularly critical when important decisions with potentially irreversible consequences are being considered. Discharge information and follow-up instructions must always be provided to the PCP ahead of time, preferably giving key information immediately to be followed later with background and details.

4. *Partner with the patient*: and keep him an active participant in the treatment process. This requires bonding with the patient and making sure that he understands the importance of his own involvement at this critical juncture of his life. The patient – or the family if the patient is not capable – should

understand the diagnosis, treatment, test results, and follow-up plans. The more involved the patient becomes, the more likely he will be to comply with follow-up instructions.

5. *Make clear that you are the patient's advocate*: and that you place his or her interests above those of the hospital or health care plan. In an era of cost-containment, it is easy for the hospitalist to be viewed as part of "the system," whose principal loyalty is to the institution. Beware of any arrangement in which you may be cast in the distasteful role of gatekeeper by denying care being sought by the patient, family, or – especially! – the primary care physician. If you are denying a service because it is not timely or medically indicated, take pains to explain that fact to the patient, lest he or she conclude that you are more concerned with the bottom line than with his or her well-being.

6. *Pass the baton as gracefully as you received it*: or more so. Make sure that appropriate follow-up has been arranged, that the patient knows which doctor to contact and when, and remain available to the patient during the transition. Even if the primary care physician handled his or her responsibilities poorly, or the two of you have a rocky relationship, rise above the situation by placing the patient's interests over every other concern, and hand-off the patient with the same grace, dignity, and professionalism that you wish the other doctor would show toward you.

THE HOSPITALIST DISCHARGE

Hospitalist Discharges to Nursing Facilities

Discharges to skilled nursing facilities and home care require additional consid-erations, according to Goldman et al. Since patients discharged to nursing facili-ties often remain ill and in need of ongoing care, additional information about the hospitalization is often called for. In addition to a concise, detailed, and timely dis-charge summary, the authors suggest providing copies of physician and nursing progress notes, consultant reports, advance directives, and DNR forms and insur-ance information, plus a one-page nursing transfer summary that outlines essen-tial information, including the diagnoses, medications, allergies, diet, status, and code information, along with a contact number if more information is required.

Hospitalist Discharges to Home
Health Agencies

For patients discharged to home care, be prepared to offer interim support until the patient is able to be seen by the PCP. This includes signing short-term orders. Further, if the patient requires care involving potential complications, such as IV antibiotics, you should be prepared to follow the patient after discharge. Alternatively, if the PCP visits the patient in the hospital, it may be best to have him or her review and sign the discharge orders.

HOSPITALIST ADMISSIONS

Admissions Via the ED and the Hospitalist

Possibly the most challenging hand-offs are those involving unassigned patients admitted through the ED. Most admissions from the ED are for medical conditions such as pneumonia or heart failure, which means that hospitalists are frequent recipients of such hand-offs (Government Accounting Office, 2003). Adequate communication is particularly important during this process because poor hand-off practices in the ED have been identified as a key cause of medical error (Croskerry & Wears, 2003). A recent article in *Academic Emergency Medicine* by Apker, Mallak, and Gibson, specifically addressed what the authors called the "gray zone" of communication issues between emergency physicians and hospitalists, and much of this discussion is based on their research and analysis (Apker, Mallak, & Gibson, 2007).

The authors identified three types of information ambiguities that plague EP-hospitalist communications in this gray zone:

- Uncertainty over the diagnosis of patients that present initially to the ED and are assessed and worked up by the ED staff.
- A lack of clarity about patient status when hospital admission is still pending and involves a joint decision between the EP and the hospitalist.
- Uncertainty over which physician is responsible for the care of boarded patients – that is, those who have been admitted to the hospital but physically remain in the ED awaiting an inpatient bed.

An inherent problem with hand-offs in this gray zone is that EPs and hospitalists have different priorities, which often put them at cross purposes. Emergency departments can be busy, hectic places where overcrowding may delay care to even the most urgent cases. As such, the EP's focus is often on stabilizing the patient, then either discharging him or transferring him to another service – any service – as quickly as possible. As a result, the EP may seek to hand-off a patient as soon as the need to admit has been made evident, even though the diagnosis is not clear and test results are still pending.

The hospitalist, on the other hand, is reluctant to accept a patient with an unclear diagnosis, in part because it may well be that the patient would be better served by a different specialty service. This is also true for patients who have multiple conditions and it is not clear which needs attention first. Likewise, there is a reluctance to accept a patient when test results are pending, because a patient who appears to be in stable condition may actually be decompensating, and may become a full-fledged emergency by the time the hospitalist gets to the patient.

THE ED AND THE HOSPITALIST:
A STRUGGLE FOR INFORMATION

Because it serves hospitalists' interests to gather as much up-front information as possible before the hand-off, and because tests ordered through the ED usually get priority over those ordered by other services, hospitalists often press EPs to order additional tests before accepting the transfer. However, delaying the hand-off in order to collect more information can backfire if the delay causes the patient to be kept in the ED through shift changes. That is because many of the communication barriers that impede hand-offs between EPs and hospitalists also bedevil those between fellow EPs. This means that delaying the hand-off until more information can be gathered in the ED may actually have the opposite effect, leaving you trying to pump information from a different emergency physician who knows less about the case than you.

THE ED AND THE HOSPITALIST:
FUNDAMENTAL APPROACHES

The solution begins with the simple recognition of the inherent conflict between your needs as a hospitalist and those of the EP during the hand-off process. You should remain aware of the likely deficits (at least from your perspective) in the information provided by the emergency physician and either negotiate with the EP to fill those gaps or be prepared to get the information yourself. For boarded patients, establish clearly who is responsible for following up on which test results, and who will provide care until the patient is transferred to a floor. Also, be aware of the timing of shift changes in the ED. It may be better to accept the hand-off from the physician who worked up the patient, even with test results and other important information still pending, than to deal with the loss of information created by a hand-off between EPs.

CONCLUSIONS: BE CAREFUL OUT THERE!

Because it would be impossible to outline your likely duty in every conceivable situation, this chapter has aimed at providing you with a general understanding of some of the liability issues confronting hospitalists. Using this knowledge, when you find yourself faced with a situation in which your duty is not immediately clear, you can at least make educated decisions that will maximize the quality of care you deliver while lowering your own risk exposure. When in doubt, however, acting in the best interests of the patient should always be your guide.

A

Abbreviations

ABG	Arterial blood gas
ACLS	Advanced cardiac life support
ACS	Acute coronary syndrome
ADE	Adverse drug event
ARF	Acute renal failures
ARR	Absolute risk reduction
BLS	Basic life support
BMP	Basic metabolic panel
BNP	Brain natriuretic peptide
BSA	Body surface area
CAD	Coronary artery disease
CAP	Community acquired pneumonia
CBC	Complete blood count
CHF	Congestive heart failure
CI	Cardiac index
CMP	Complete metabolic panel
CNS	Central nervous system
CO	Cardiac output
COPD	Chronic obstructive pulmonary disease
CPOE	Computer physician order entry
CSF	Cerebrospinal fluid
CT	Computed tomography
CXR	Chest radiograph
DKA	Diabetic ketoacidosis

DSE	Dipyridamole-thallium imaging and dobutamine stress echocardiography
DSM-IV	Diagnostic and statistical manual of mental disorders (4th ed.)
DVT	Deep vein thrombosis
EBM	Evidence based medicine
EKG	Electrocardiogram
FMEA	Failure mode and effects analysis
GI	Gastrointestinal
HAP	Hospital acquired pneumonia
HHS	Hyperglycemia hyperosmolar state
ICU	Intensive care unit
MRI	Magnetic resonance imaging
NNT	Number needed to treat
NSAIDS	Nonsteroidal anti-inflammatory drugs
NSTEMI	Non-ST-segment elevation myocardial infarction
OTC	Over-the-counter drugs
PBLI	Practice based learning and improvement
PE	Pulmonary embolus
PDI	Pneumonia severity index
PORT	Pneumonia patient outcomes research team
PDSA	Plan do study act
PSI	Pneumonia severity index
QI	Quality improvement
RCA	Root cause analysis
RRR	Relative risk reduction
RVU	Relative value units
SIRS	Systemic inflammatory response syndrome
STEMI	ST-elevation myocardial infarction
SV	Stroke volume
UTI	Urinary tract infection
VTE	Venous thromboembolis

B

Dictation Templates

Manish Mehta, MD
Arun Mathews, MD

Sample history and physical (H&P) examination and discharge summary templates. They could save you a few extra minutes in a busy day.

How to dictate: Most residency programs or hospitals have a dictation system, and chances are that you are already a pro, but if you need a refresher or are new to it, then follow these steps:

INITIAL VISITS (HISTORY AND PHYSICAL) TEMPLATE

Patient Name: **DOB:**
Date of Admit: **Time:**
PCP:

Chief Complaint: Presenting symptom

HPI: Descriptive elements
1. Severity   5. Context
2. Quality   6. Modifying factors
3. Duration   7. Associated signs
4. Timing   8. Location
Pertinent past history:

Allergies:

Medications:

Past Medical History: Pertinent positives and negatives
Past Family History: Pertinent positives and negatives
Past Social History: Pertinent positives and negatives
Review of Systems: Mention each considered system individually including pertinent positives or negatives
1. Integumentary   8. Gastrointestinal
2. Eyes   9. Genitourinary
3. Head, ears, nose, mouth, and throat   10. Musculoskeletal
4. Neck   11. Neurologic
5. Cardiovascular   12. Psychiatric
6. Respiratory   13. Metabolic/Endo
7. Peripheral vascular   14. Hematologic

Physical Exam: Consider examination and document pertinent positives and negatives from these 14 systems
1. Vitals and general   8. Abdomen/Rectal
2. Eyes   9. Genitourinary
3. Ears, nose, mouth, and throat   10. Lymphatics
4. Neck   11. Musculoskeletal
5. Cardiovascular (JVD)   12. Skin
6. Respiratory   13. Neuro
7. Chest/breast   14. Psychiatric

Labs and Image Results: Document all labs and imaging studies considered in evaluating the patient. Document if personally reviewed.

Assessment/Plan: Document a separate assessment and plan for EACH active or considered diagnosis. Documentation should include level of risk and results of therapeutic interventions for each diagnosis.

DISCHARGE SUMMARY TEMPLATE

Admission Date: **Discharge Date:**

Principal Diagnosis at Admission:

Principal Diagnosis at Discharge:

Additional Diagnoses Evaluated and Treated During the Admission:

Consultants: (Include name and specialty)

Procedures: (Name and impression noted)

Hospital Course: (Concise summary of clinical course)

Exam:

Medications at Time of Discharge:

Discharge Plan: (Activities, diet and follow up care)

Issues to be Addressed at Follow Up:

Time Spent on the Day of Discharge:

CC: PCP or other special providers

Death Summary: As above, focusing on events leading to surrounding death: codes, withdrawal of care, date and time of death, who was present.

Bibliography

CARDIOLOGY

Abdon, NJ, Landin, K, Johansson, BW. Athlete's bradycardia as an embolising disorder? Symptomatic arrhythmias in patients aged less than 50 years. Br Heart J 1984;52:660.

Agruss, NS, Rosin, EY, Adolph, RJ, Fowler, NO. Significance of chronic sinus bradycardia in elderly people. Circulation 1972;46:924.

Ahmed, A, Aronow, WS, Fleg, JL. Higher New York Heart Association classes and increased mortality and hospitalization in patients with heart failure and preserved left ventricular function. Am Heart J 2006;151:444.

Ahmed, A, Rich, MW, Fleg, JL, et al. Effects of digoxin on morbidity and mortality in diastolic heart failure: the ancillary digitalis investigation group trial. Circulation 2006;114:397.

Alboni, P, Baggioni, GF, Scarfo, S, et al. Role of sinus node artery disease in sick sinus syndrome in inferior wall acute myocardial infarction. Am J Cardiol 1991;67:1180.

Alexander, KP, Newby, LK, Armstrong, PW, et al. Acute coronary care in the elderly, part II: ST-segment-elevation myocardial infarction: a scientific statement for healthcare professionals from the American Heart Association Council on Clinical Cardiology: in collaboration with the Society of Geriatric Cardiology. Circulation 2007;115:2570.

Alexander, KP, Newby, LK, Cannon, CP, et al. Acute coronary care in the elderly, part I: non-ST-segment-elevation acute coronary syndromes: a scientific statement for healthcare professionals from the American Heart Association Council on Clinical Cardiology: in collaboration with the Society of Geriatric Cardiology. Circulation 2007;115:2549.

Alexander, KP, Roe, MT, Chen, AY, et al. Evolution in cardiovascular care for elderly patients with non-ST-segment elevation acute coronary syndromes: results from the CRUSADE National Quality Improvement Initiative. J Am Coll Cardiol 2005;46:1479.

Al-Faleh, H, Fu, Y, Wagner, G, et al. unraveling the spectrum of left bundle branch block in acute myocardial infarction: insights from the Assessment of the Safety and Efficacy of a New Thrombolytic (ASSENT 2 and 3) trials. Am Heart J 2006;151:10.

Al-Khatib, SM, Pieper, KS, Lee, KL, et al. Atrial fibrillation and mortality among patients with acute coronary syndrome without ST-segment elevation: results from the PURSUIT trial. Am J Cardiol 2001;88:A7.

Alpert, JS. Myocardial infarction with angiographically normal coronary arteries. A personal perspective. Arch Intern Med 1994;154:245.

Alpert, MA, Flaker, GC. Arrhythmias associated with sinus node dysfunction. JAMA 1983;250:2160.

Amat-y-Leon, F, Dhingra, R, Denes, P, et al. The clinical spectrum of chronic His bundle block. Chest 1976;70:747.

Anderson, DC, Kappelle, LJ, Eliasziw, M, et al. Occurrence of hemispheric and retinal isch-emia in atrial fibrillation compared with carotid stenosis. Stroke 2002;33:1963.

Anderson, JL, Karagounis, LA, Califf, RM. Meta-analysis of five reported studies on the relation of early coronary patency grades with mortality and outcomes after acute myo-cardial infarction. Am J Cardiol 1996;78:1.

Andersson, B, Caidahl, K, di Lenarada, A, et al. Changes in early and late diastolic filling patterns induced by long-term adrenergicß-blockade in patients with idiopathic dilated cardiomyopathy. Circulation 1996;94:673.

Angeli, P, Chiesa, M, Caregaro, L, et al. Comparison of sublingual captopril and nifedipine in immediate treatment of hypertensive emergencies. A randomized, single-blind clini-cal trial. Arch Intern Med 1991;151:678.

Antman, EM, Anbe, DT, Armstrong, PW, et al. ACC/AHA guidelines for the management of patients with ST-elevation myocardial infarction.

Antman, EM, Cohen, M, Radley, D, et al. Assessment of the treatment effect of enoxaparin for unstable angina/non-Q-wave myocardial infarction. TIMI 11B-ESSENCE meta-analysis. Circulation 1999 Oct 12;100(15):1602-8.

Antman, EM, Fox, KM. Guidelines for the diagnosis and management of unstable angina and non-Q-wave myocardial infarction: proposed revisions. International Cardiology Forum. Am Heart J 2000 Mar;139(3):461-75.

Antman, EM, Giugliano, RP, Gibson, CM, et al. Abciximab facilitates the rate and extent of thrombolysis: results of the thrombolysis in myocardial infarction (TIMI) 14 trial. The TIMI 14 Investigators. Circulation 1999 Jun 1;99(21):2720-32.

Antman, EM, Hand, M, Armstrong, PW, et al. 2007 Focused update of the ACC/AHA 2004 Guidelines for the Management of Patients With ST-Elevation Myocardial Infarction: A Report of the American College of Cardiology/American Heart Association Task Force on Practice Guidelines

Antman, EM, McCabe, CH, Gurfinkel, EP, et al. Enoxaparin prevents death and cardiac ischemic events in unstable angina/non-Q-wave myocardial infarction. Results of the thrombolysis in myocardial infarction (TIMI) 11B trial. Circulation 1999 Oct 12;100(15):1593-601.

Archer, SL, Huang, JM, Hampl, V, et al. Nitric oxide and cGMP cause vasorelaxation by activation of a charybdotoxin-sensitive K channel by cGMP-dependent protein kinase. Proc Natl Acad Sci U S A 1994;91:7583.

Armstrong, PW, Fu, Y, Chang, WC, et al. Acute coronary syndromes in the GUSTO-IIb trial: prognostic insights and impact of recurrent ischemia. The GUSTO-IIb Investigators. Circulation 1998;98:1860.

Aronow, WS, Kronzon, I. Effect of enalapril on congestive heart failure treated with diuret-ics in elderly patients with prior myocardial infarction and normal left ventricular ejec-tion fraction. Am J Cardiol 1993;71:602.

Atrial fibrillation: current understandings and research imperatives. The National Heart, Lung, and Blood Institute Working Group on Atrial Fibrillation. J Am Coll Cardiol 1993;22:1830.

Aurigemma, GP, Gaasch, WH. Clinical practice. Diastolic heart failure. N Engl J Med 2004;351:1097.

Banerjee, P, Banerjee, T, Khand, A, et al. Diastolic heart failure: neglected or misdiagnosed?. J Am Coll Cardiol 2002;39:138.

Barbash, GI, Birnbaum, Y, Bogaerts, K, et al. Treatment of reinfarction after thrombolytic therapy for acute myocardial infarction: an analysis of outcome and treatment choices in the Global Utilization of Streptokinase and Tissue Plasminogen Activator for Occluded Coronary Arteries (GUSTO I) and Assessment of the Safety of a New Thrombolytic (ASSENT 2) studies. Circulation 2001;103:954.

Bart, BA, Boyle, A, Bank, AJ, et al. Ultrafiltration versus usual care for hospitalized patients with heart failure: the Relief for Acutely Fluid-Overloaded Patients With Decompensated Congestive Heart Failure (RAPID-CHF) trial. J Am Coll Cardiol 2005;46:2043.

Bassan, R, Pimenta, L, Scofano, M, et al. Probability stratification and systematic diagnostic approach for chest pain patients in the emergency department. Crit Pathw Cardiol 2004;3:1.

Bayer, AJ, Chadha, JS, Farag, RR, Pathy, MS. Changing presentation of myocardial infarction with increasing old age. J Am Geriatr Soc 1986;34:263.

Beder, SD, Gillette, PC, Garson, A Jr., et al. Symptomatic sick sinus syndrome in children and adolescents as the only manifestation of cardiac abnormality or associated with unoperated congenital heart disease. Am J Cardiol 1983;51:1133.

Bergstrom, A, Andersson, B, Edner, M, et al. Effect of carvedilol on diastolic function in patients with diastolic heart failure and preserved systolic function. Results of the Swedish Doppler-echocardiographic study (SWEDIC). Eur J Heart Fail 2004;6:453.

Bertrand, ME, Simoons, ML, Fox, KA, et al. Management of acute coronary syndromes: acute coronary syndromes without persistent ST segment elevation; recommendations of the Task Force of the European Society of Cardiology. Eur Heart J 2000;21:1406.

Birchfield, RI, Menefee, EE, Bryant, GD. Disease of the sinoatrial node associated with bradycardia, asystole, syncope, and paroxysmal atrial fibrillation. Circulation 1957;16:20.

Bjerregaard, P. Mean 24 hour heart rate, minimal heart rate, and pauses in healthy subjects 40-79 years of age. Eur Heart J 1983;4:44.

Boahene, KA, Klein, GJ, Yee, R, et al. Termination of acute atrial fibrillation in the Wolff-Parkinson-White syndrome by procainamide and propafenone: importance of atrial fibrillatory cycle length. J Am Coll Cardiol 1990;16:1408.

Boersma, E, Harrington, RA, Moliterno, DJ, et al. Platelet glycoprotein IIb/IIIa inhibitors in acute coronary syndromes: a meta-analysis of all major randomised clinical trials. Lancet 2002;359:189.

Bogaty, P, Dumont, S, O'Hara, GE, et al. Randomized trial of a noninvasive strategy to reduce hospital stay for patients with low-risk myocardial infarction. J Am Coll Cardiol 2001;37:1289.

Bolognese, L, Falsini, G, Liistro, F, et al. Randomized comparison of upstream tirofiban versus downstream high bolus dose tirofiban or abciximab on tissue-level perfusion and troponin release in high-risk acute coronary syndromes treated with percutaneous coronary interventions: the EVEREST trial. J Am Coll Cardiol 2006;47:522.

Borzak, S, Cannon, CP, Kraft, PL, et al. Effects of prior aspirin and anti-ischemic therapy on outcome of patients with unstable angina. TIMI 7 Investigators. Thrombin Inhibition in Myocardial Ischemia. Am J Cardiol 1998;81:678.

Boura, JA, Grines, CL, Keeley, EC. Primary angioplasty versus intravenous thrombolytic therapy for acute myocardial infarction: a quantitative review of 23 randomised trials. Lancet 2003;361:13.

Braunwald, E, Domanski, MJ, Fowler, SE, et al. Angiotensin-converting-enzyme inhibition in stable coronary artery disease. N Engl J Med 2004;351:2058.

Braunwald, E, Mark, DB, et al. Unstable angina: diagnosis and management. Rockville, MD: Agency for Healthcare Policy and Research and National Heart, Lung and

Blood Institute, US Public Health Service. US Department of Health and Human Services;1994:1. AHCPR Publication no. 94-0602.

Brodie, BR, Stuckey, TD, Wall, TC, et al. Importance of time to reperfusion for 30-day and late survival and recovery of left ventricular function after primary angioplasty for acute myocardial infarction. J Am Coll Cardiol 1998 Nov;32(5):1312-9.

Brodsky, M, Wu, D, Denes, P, et al. Arrhythmias documented by 24 hour continuous electro-cardiographic monitoring in 50 male medical students without apparent heart disease. Am J Cardiol 1977;39:390.

Brodsky, MA, Hwang, C, Hunter, D, et al. Life-threatening alterations in heart rate after the use of adenosine in atrial flutter. Am Heart J 1995;130:564.

Brown, H, Goldberg, PA, Selter, JG, et al. Hemorrhagic pheochromocytoma associated with systemic corticosteroid therapy and presenting as myocardial infarction with severe hypertension. J Clin Endocrinol Metab 2005;90:563.

Burkart, F, Pfisterer, M, Kiowski, W. Effect of antiarrhythmic therapy on mortality in survivors of MI with asymptomatic complex ventricular arrhythmias. Basel Antiarrhythmic Study of Infarct Survival (BASIS). J Am Coll Cardiol 1990;16:1711.

Burns, RJ, Gibbons, RJ, Yi, Q, et al. The relationships of left ventricular ejection fraction, end-systolic volume index and infarct size to 6-month mortality after hospital discharge following myocardial infarction treated by thrombolysis. J Am Coll Cardiol 2002;39:30.

Buxton, AE, Lee, KL, Fisher, JD, et al, for the Multicenter Unsustained Tachycardia Trial Investigators. A randomized study of the prevention of sudden death in patients with coronary artery disease. N Engl J Med 1999;341:1882.

Buxton, AE. Patients with nonsustained ventricular tachycardia. In: Sudden Cardiac Death: Prevalence, Mechanisms, and Approach to Diagnosis and Management, Akhtar, M, Myerburg, R, Ruskin, J (Eds), Williams & Wilkins, Baltimore 1994.

Buxton, AE. Prevention of sudden death in patients with coronary artery disease: the Multicenter Unsustained Tachycardia Trial (MUSTT). Prog Cardiovasc Dis 1993; 36:215.

Cairns, JA, Connolly, SJ, Roberts, R, et al. Randomised trial of outcome after myocardial infarction in patients with frequent or repetitive ventricular premature depolarisations: CAMIAT. Lancet 1997;349:675.

Camm, AJ, Garratt, CJ. Adenosine and supraventricular tachycardia. N Engl J Med 1991;325:1621.

Cannon, CP, Braunwald, E, McCabe, CH, et al. Intensive versus moderate lipid lowering with statins after acute coronary syndromes. N Engl J Med 2004;350:1495.

Cannon, CP, Hand, MH, Bahr, R, et al. Critical pathways for management of patients with acute coronary syndromes: an assessment by the National Heart Attack Alert Program. Am Heart J 2002;143:777.

Cannon, CP, Weintraub, WS, Demopoulos, LA, et al. Comparison of early invasive and conservative strategies in patients with unstable coronary syndromes treated with the glycoprotein IIb/IIIa inhibitor tirofiban. N Engl J Med 2001;344:1879.

Chobanian, AV, Bakris, GL, Black, HR, Cushman, WC. The seventh report of the joint national committee on prevention, detection, evaluation, and treatment of high blood pressure: the JNC 7 report. JAMA 2003;289:2560.

Chobanian, AV, Bakris, GL, Black, HR, et al. The seventh report of the Joint National Committee on Prevention, Detection, Evaluation, and Treatment of High Blood Pressure: the JNC 7 report. JAMA 2003;289:2560.

Clarke, M, Sutton, R, Ward, D, et al. Recommendations for pacemaker prescription for symptomatic bradycardia. Report of a Working Party of the British Pacing and Electrophysiology Group. Br Heart J 1991;66:185.

Cleland, JG, Tendera, M, Adamus, J, et al. The perindopril in elderly people with chronic heart failure (PEP-CHF) study. Eur Heart J 2006;27:2338.

Collins, LJ, Silverman, DI, Douglas, PS, Manning, WJ. Cardioversion of nonrheumatic atrial fibrillation: reduced thromboembolic complications with 4 weeks of pre-cardioversion anticoagulation are related to atrial thrombus resolution. Circulation 1995;92:160.

Compton, S. Ventricular tachycardia; eMedicine journal [serial online], October 2008. Available from http://emedicine.medscape.com/article/159075-overview.

Corley, SD, Epstein, AE, DiMarco, JP, et al. Relationships between sinus rhythm, treatment, and survival in the Atrial Fibrillation Follow-Up Investigation of Rhythm Management (AFFIRM) Study. Circulation 2004;109:1509.

Costanzo, MR, Guglin, ME, Saltzberg, MT, et al. Ultrafiltration versus intravenous diuretics for patients hospitalized for acute decompensated heart failure. J Am Coll Cardiol 2007;49:675.

Cotter, G, Metzkor, E, Faigenberg, Z, et al. Randomised trial of high-dose isosorbide dinitrate plus low-dose furosemide versus high-dose furosemide plus low-dose isosorbide dinitrate in severe pulmonary oedema. Lancet 1998;351:389.

Da Costa, A, Isaaz, K, Faure, E, et al. Clinical characteristics, aetiological factors and long-term prognosis of myocardial infarction with an absolutely normal coronary angiogram. A 3-year follow-up study of 91 patients. Eur Heart J 2001;22:1459.

Dargie, HJ. Effect of carvedilol on outcome after myocardial infarction in patients with left-ventricular dysfunction: the CAPRICORN randomised trial. Lancet 2001;357:1385.

Davies, AB, Stephens, MR, Davies, AG. Carotid sinus hypersensitivity in patients presenting with syncope. Br Heart J 1979;42:583.

Dhingra, RC, Denes, P, Wu, D, et al. The significance of second degree atrioventricular block and bundle branch block: observations regarding site and type of block. Circulation 1974;49:638.

Dhingra, RC, Palileo, E, Strasberg, B, et al. Significance of the HV interval in 517 patients with chronic bifascicular block. Circulation 1981;64:1265.

Dickstein, K, Kjekshus, J. Effects of losartan and captopril on mortality and morbidity in high-risk patients after acute myocardial infarction: the OPTIMAAL randomised trial. Optimal Trial in Myocardial Infarction with Angiotensin II Antagonist Losartan. Lancet 2002;360:752.

Dikshit, K, Vyden, JK, Forrester, JS, et al. Renal and extrarenal hemodynamic effects of furosemide in congestive heart failure after acute myocardial infarction. N Engl J Med 1973;288:1087.

Disch, DL, Greenberg, ML, Holzberger, PT, et al. Managing chronic atrial fibrillation: a Markov decision analysis comparing warfarin, quinidine and low-dose amiodarone. Ann Intern Med 1994;120:449.

Dittrich, HC, Erickson, JS, Schneiderman, T, et al. Echocardiographic and clinical predictors for outcome of elective cardioversion of atrial fibrillation. Am J Cardiol 1989;63:193.

Diver, DJ, Bier, JD, Ferreira, PE, et al. Clinical and arteriographic characterization of patients with unstable angina without critical coronary arterial narrowing (from the TIMI-IIIA trial). Am J Cardiol 1994;74:531.

Donges, K, Schiele, R, Gitt, A, et al. Incidence, determinants, and clinical course of reinfarction in-hospital after index acute myocardial infarction (results from the pooled data of the maximal individual therapy in acute myocardial infarction. Am J Cardiol 2001;87:1039.

Donoso, E, Adler, LN, Ffriedberg, CK. Unusual forms of second-degree atrioventricular block, including mobitz type-II block, associated with the morgagni-adams-stokes syndrome. Am Heart J 1964;67:150.

Donovan, KD, Powers, BM, Hockings, BE, et al. Intravenous flecainide versus amiodarone for recent onset atrial fibrillation. Am J Cardiol 1995;75:693.

Eagle, KA, Goodman, SG, Avezum, A, et al. Practice variation and missed opportunities for reperfusion in ST-segment-elevation myocardial infarction: findings from the Global Registry of Acute Coronary Events (GRACE). Lancet 2002;359:373.

Early effects of tissue-type plasminogen activator added to conventional therapy on the culprit coronary lesion in patients presenting with ischemic cardiac pain at rest. Results of the Thrombolysis in Myocardial Ischemia (TIMI IIIA) Trial. Circulation 1993;87:38.

Eberli, FR, Apstein, CS, Ngoy, S, et al. Exacerbation of left ventricular ischemic diastolic dysfunction by pressure-overload hypertrophy: modification by specific inhibition of cardiac angiotensin converting enzyme. Circ Res 1992;70:931.

Echt, DS, Liebson, PR, Mitchell, LB, et al. Mortality and morbidity in patients receiving encainide, flecainide or placebo. The Cardiac Arrhythmia Suppression Trial. N Engl J Med 1991;324:781.

Effect of the antiarrhythmic agent moricizine on survival after myocardial infarction. The Cardiac Arrhythmia Suppression Trial II Investigators. N Engl J Med 1992;327:227.

Effectiveness of spironolactone added to an angiotensin-converting enzyme inhibitor and a loop diuretic for severe chronic congestive heart failure (the Randomized Aldactone Evaluation Study [RALES]). Am J Cardiol 1996;78:902.

Effects of tissue plasminogen activator and a comparison of early invasive and conservative strategies in unstable angina and non-Q-wave myocardial infarction. Results of the TIMI IIIB Trial. Thrombolysis in Myocardial Ischemia. Circulation 1994;89:1545.

Ellenbogen, KA, Dias, VC, Cardello, FP, et al. Safety and efficacy of intravenous diltiazem in atrial fibrillation or atrial flutter. Am J Cardiol 1995;75:45.

Epstein, AE, DiMarco, JP, Ellenbogen, KA, et al. ACC/AHA/HRS 2008 guidelines for device-based therapy of cardiac rhythm abnormalities: a report of the American College of Cardiology/American Heart Association Task Force on Practice Guidelines (Writing Committee to Revise the ACC/AHA/NASPE 2002 Guideline Update for Implantation of Cardiac Pacemakers and Antiarrhythmia Devices) developed in collaboration with the American Association for Thoracic Surgery and Society of Thoracic Surgeons. J Am Coll Cardiol 2008;51:e1.

Evans, R, Shaw, DB. Pathological studies in sinoatrial disorder (sick sinus syndrome). Br Heart J 1977;39:778.

Every, NR, Hlatky, MA, McDonald, KM, et al. Estimating the proportion of post-myocardial infarction patients who may benefit from prophylactic implantable defibrillator placement from analysis of the CAST registry. Am J Cardiol 1998;82:683.

Farshi, R, Kistner, D, Sarma, JSM, et al. Ventricular rate control in chronic atrial fibrillation during daily activity and programmed exercise: a crossover open-label study of five drug regimens. J Am Coll Cardiol 1999;33:304.

Felker, GM, Allen, LA, Pocock, SJ, et al. Red cell distribution width as a novel prognostic marker in heart failure: data from the CHARM Program and the Duke Databank. J Am Coll Cardiol 2007;50:40.

Ferrer, MI. The sick sinus syndrome in atrial disease. JAMA 1968;206:645.

Ferrer, MI. The Sick Sinus Syndrome. New York, Futura Press, 1974.

Ferrer, MI. The etiology and natural history of sinus node disorders. Arch Intern Med 1982;142:371.

Fonarow, GC, Ballantyne, CM. In-hospital initiation of lipid-lowering therapy for patients with coronary heart disease: the time is now. Circulation 2001;103:2768.

Franzosi, MG, Santoro, E, De Vita, C, et al. Ten-year follow-up of the first megatrial testing thrombolytic therapy in patients with acute myocardial infarction: results of the Gruppo Italiano per lo Studio della Sopravvivenza nell'Infarto-1 study. The GISSI Investigators. Circulation 1998;98:2659.

Friedman, LM. Effect of propranolol in patients with myocardial infarction and ventricular arrhythmia. J Am Coll Cardiol 1986;7:1.

Friedrich, SP, Lorell, BH, Rousseau, MF, et al. Intracardiac angiotensin-converting enzyme inhibition improves diastolic function in patients with left ventricular hypertrophy due to aortic stenosis. Circulation 1994;90:2761.

Frost, L, Engholm, G, Johnsen, S, et al. Incident stroke after discharge from the hospital with a diagnosis of atrial fibrillation. Am J Med 2000;108:36.

Fu, Y, Goodman, S, Chang, WC, et al. Time to treatment influences the impact of ST-segment resolution on one-year prognosis: insights from the assessment of the safety and efficacy of a new thrombolytic (ASSENT-2) trial. Circulation 2001;104:2653.

Fuster, V, Ryden, LE, Cannom, DS, et al. ACC/AHA/ESC 2006 guidelines for the management of patients with atrial fibrillation – a report of the American College of Cardiology/American Heart Association Task Force on Practice Guidelines and the European Society of Cardiology Committee for Practice Guidelines (Writing Committee to Revise the 2001 Guidelines for the Management of Patients With Atrial Fibrillation). J Am Coll Cardiol 2006;48:e149.

Gage, J, Rutman, H, Lucido, D, et al. Additive effects of dobutamine and amrinone on myocardial contractility and ventricular performance in patients with severe heart failure. Circulation 1986;74:367.

Garratt, CJ, Griffith, MJ, O'Nunain, S, et al. Effects of intravenous adenosine on antegrade refractoriness of accessory atrioventricular connections. Circulation 1991;84:1962.

Ghali, JK, Pina, IL, Gottlieb, SS, et al. Metoprolol CR/XL in female patients with heart failure: analysis of the experience in Metoprolol Extended-Release Randomized Intervention Trial in Heart Failure (MERIT-HF). Circulation 2002;105:1585.

Gheorghiade, M, Zannad, F, Sopko, G, et al. Acute heart failure syndromes: current state and framework for future research. Circulation 2005;112:3958.

Giardina, EG, Heissenbuttel, RH, Bigger, JT Jr. Intermittent intravenous procaine amide to treat ventricular arrhythmias. Correlation of plasma concentration with effect on arrhythmia, electrocardiogram, and blood pressure. Ann Intern Med 1973;78:183.

Gibler, WB. Evaluation of chest pain in the emergency department. Ann Intern Med 1995;123:315.

Gibson, CM, de Lemos, JA, Murphy, SA, et al. Combination therapy with abciximab reduces angiographically evident thrombus in acute myocardial infarction: a TIMI 14 substudy. Circulation 2001 May 29;103(21):2550-4.

Gibson, CM, Karha, J, Murphy, SA, et al. Early and long-term clinical outcomes associated with reinfarction following fibrinolytic administration in the Thrombolysis in Myocardial Infarction trials. J Am Coll Cardiol 2003;42:7.

Gilard, M, Arnaud, B, Cornily, JC, et al. Influence of omeprazole on the antiplatelet action of clopidogrel associated with aspirin: the randomized, double-blind OCLA (Omeprazole CLopidogrel Aspirin) study. J Am Coll Cardiol 2008;51:256.

Go, AS, Hylek, EM, Chang, Y, et al. Anticoagulation therapy for stroke prevention in atrial fibrillation: how well do randomized trials translate into clinical practice?. JAMA 2003;290:2685.

Go, AS, Hylek, EM, Phillips, KA, et al. Prevalence of diagnosed atrial fibrillation in adults: national implications for rhythm management and stroke prevention: the AnTicoagulation and Risk Factors in Atrial Fibrillation (ATRIA) Study. JAMA 2001;285:2370.

Goldberg, RJ, McCormick, D, Gurwitz, JH, et al. Age-related trends in short- and long-term survival after acute myocardial infarction: a 20-year population-based perspective (1975-1995). Am J Cardiol 1998;82:1311.

Goldstein, S, Fagerberg, B, Hjalmarson, A, et al. Metoprolol controlled release/extended release in patients with severe heart failure. Analysis of the experience in the MERIT-HF study. J Am Coll Cardiol 2001;38:932.

Gomes, JA, Cain, ME, Buxton, AE, et al. Prediction of long-term outcomes by signal-averaged electrocardiography in patients with unsustained ventricular tachycardia, coronary artery disease, and left ventricular dysfunction. Circulation 2001;104:436.

Gomes, JA, Kang, PS, Matheson, M, et al. Coexistence of sick sinus rhythm and atrial flutter-fibrillation. Circulation 1981;63:80.

Goodfriend, MA, Barold, SS. Tachycardia-dependent and bradycardia-dependent Mobitz type II atrioventricular block within the bundle of His. Am J Cardiol 1974;33:908.

Granger, CB, McMurray, JJ, Yusuf, S, et al. Effects of candesartan in patients with chronic heart failure and reduced left-ventricular systolic function intolerant to angiotensin-converting-enzyme inhibitors: the CHARM-Alternative trial. Lancet 2003;362:772.

Greenwood, RD, Rosenthal, A, Sloss, LJ, et al. Sick sinus syndrome after surgery for congenital heart disease. Circulation 1975;52:208.

Gregoratos, G, Abrams, J, Epstein, AE, et al. ACC/AHA/NASPE 2002 guideline update for implantation of cardiac pacemakers and antiarrhythmia devices: summary article. A report of the American College of Cardiology/American Heart Association task force on practice guidelines (ACC/AHA/NASPE committee to update the 1998 pacemaker guidelines). Circulation 2002;106:2145.

Gregoratos, G, Cheitlin, MD, Conill, A, et al. ACC/AHA guidelines for implantation of cardiac pacemakers and antiarrhythmia devices: executive summary. A report of the American College of Cardiology/American Heart Association Task Force on Practice Guidelines (Committee on Pacemaker Implantation). Circulation 1998;97:1325.

Griffith, MJ, Linker, NJ, Garratt, CJ, et al. Relative efficacy and safety of intravenous drugs for termination of sustained ventricular tachycardia. Lancet 1990;336:670.

Grigioni, F, Enriquez-Sarano, M, Zehr, KJ, et al. Ischemic mitral regurgitation: long-term outcome and prognostic implications with quantitative doppler assessment. Circulation 2001;103:1759.

Grossman, E, Messerli, FH, Grodzicki, T, et al. Should a moratorium be placed on sublingual nifedipine capsules for hypertensive emergencies or psuedoemergencies? JAMA 1996;276:1328.

Grzybowski, M, Clements, EA, Parsons, L, et al. Mortality benefit of immediate revascularization of acute ST-segment elevation myocardial infarction in patients with contraindications to thrombolytic therapy: a propensity analysis. JAMA 2003;290:1891.

Guidelines 2000 for Cardiopulmonary Resuscitation and Emergency Cardiovascular Care. Part 6: advanced cardiovascular life support: 7D: the tachycardiaalgorithms. The American Heart Association in collaboration with the International Liaison Committee on Resuscitation. Circulation 2000;102:I158.

Gupta, PK, Lichstein, E, Chadda, KD. Chronic His bundle block. Clinical, electrocardiographic, electrophysiological, and followup studies on 16 patients. Br Heart J 1976;38:1343.

Haas, DC, Streeten, DHP, Kim, RC, et al. Death from cerebral hypoperfusion during nitroprusside treatment of acute angiotensin-dependent hypertension. Am J Med 1983;75:1071.

Harrington, RA, Becker, RC, Ezekowitz, M, et al. Antithrombotic therapy for coronary artery disease: the Seventh ACCP Conference on Antithrombotic and Thrombolytic Therapy. Chest 2004;126:513S.

Harrison, MJ, Marshall, J. Atrial fibrillation, TIAs and completed strokes. Stroke 1984;15:441.

Hart, RG, Pearce, LA, Rothbart, RM, et al. Stroke with intermittent atrial fibrillation: incidence and predictors during aspirin therapy. Stroke Prevention in Atrial Fibrillation Investigators. J Am Coll Cardiol 2000;35:183.

Hatle, L, Bathen, J, Rokseth, R. Sinoatrial disease in acute myocardial infarction. Long-term prognosis. Br Heart J 1976;38:410.

Hayashi, M, Tsutamoto, T, Wada, A, et al. Immediate administration of mineralocorticoid receptor antagonist spironolactone prevents post-infarct left ventricular remodeling associated with suppression of a marker of myocardial collagen synthesis in patients with first anterior acute myocardial infarction. Circulation 2003;107:2559.

Hayashida, W, Van Eyll, C, Rousseau, MF, Pouleur, H. Regional remodeling and nonuniform changes in diastolic function in patients with left ventricular dysfunction: modification by long-term enalapril treatment. The SOLVD Investigators. J Am Coll Cardiol 1993;22:1403.

Hayes, CJ, Gersony, WM. Arrhythmias after the Mustard operation for transposition of the great arteries: a long-term study. J Am Coll Cardiol 1986;7:133.

Heart Failure Society of America. Evaluation and management of patients with acute decompensated heart failure. J Card Fail 2006;12:e86.

Hebert, PC, Fergusson, DA. Do transfusions get to the heart of the matter?. JAMA 2004;292:1610.

Hebert, PC, Yetisir, E, Martin, C, et al. Is a low transfusion threshold safe in critically ill patients with cardiovascular diseases? Crit Care Med 2001;29:227.

Heeschen, C, Hamm, CW, Goldmann, B, et al. Troponin concentrations for stratification of patients with acute coronary syndromes in relation to therapeutic efficacy of tirofiban. PRISM Study Investigators. Platelet Receptor Inhibition in Ischemic Syndrome Management. Lancet 1999;354:1757.

Hellestrand, KJ. Intravenous flecainide acetate for supraventricular tachycardias. Am J Cardiol 1988;62:16D.

Herzog, E, Saint-Jacques, H, Rozanski, A. The PAIN pathway as a tool to bridge the gap between evidence and management of acute coronary syndrome. Crit Pathw Cardiol 2004;3:20.

Hilgard, J, Ezri, MD, Denes, P. Significance of ventricular pauses of three seconds or more detected on twenty-four hour Holter recordings. Am J Cardiol 1985;55:1005.

Hirschl, MM, Binder, M, Bur, A, et al. Clinical evaluation of different doses of intravenous enalaprilat in patients with hypertensive crises. Arch Intern Med 1995;155:2217.

Hiss, RG, Lamb, LE, Allen MF. Electrocardiographic findings in 67,375 asymptomatic subjects. X. Normal Values. Am J Cardiol 1960;6:200.

Ho, DS, Zecchin, RP, Richards, DA, et al. Double-blind trial of lignocaine versus sotalol for acute termination of spontaneous sustained ventricular tachycardia [see comments]. Lancet 1994;344:18.

Ho, PM, Spertus, JA, Masoudi, FA, et al. Impact of medication therapy discontinuation on mortality after myocardial infarction. Arch Intern Med 2006;166:1842.

Hochman, JS, Tamis, JE, Thompson, TD, et al, for the Global Use of Strategies to Open Occluded Coronary Arteries in Acute Coronary Syndromes IIb Investigators. Sex, clinical presentation, and outcomes in patients with acute coronary syndromes. N Engl J Med 1999;341:226.

Hsu, HO, Hickey, RF, Forbes, AR, et al. Morphine decreases peripheral vascular resistance and increases capacitance in man. Anesthesiology 1979;50:98.

Hudson, MP, Granger, CB, Topol, EJ, et al. Early reinfarction after fibrinolysis: experience from the Global Utilization of Streptokinase and Tissue plasminogen activator (alteplase) for Occluded coronary arteries (GUSTO I) and global use of strategies to open occluded coronary arteries (GUSTO III) trials. Circulation 2001;104:1229.

Hudson, RE. The human pacemaker and its pathology. Br Heart J 1960;22:153.

International Liaison Committee on Resuscitation. 2005 International consensus on cardiopulmonary resuscitation and emergency cardiovascular care science with treatment recommendations. Circulation 2005;112:III.

Invasive compared with non-invasive treatment in unstable coronary-artery disease: FRISC II prospective randomised multicentre study. FRagmin and Fast Revascularisation during InStability in Coronary artery disease Investigators. Lancet 1999;354:708.

Israel, CW, Gronefeld, G, Ehrlich, JR, et al. Long-term risk of recurrent atrial fibrillation as documented by an implantable monitoring device. Implications for optimal patient care. J Am Coll Cardiol 2004;43:47.

James, TN. The sinus node. Am J Cardiol 1977;40:965.

James, TN, Birk, RE. Pathology of the cardiac conduction system in polyarteritis nodosa. Arch Intern Med 1966;117:561.

James, TN, Rupe, CE, Monto, RW. Pathology of the cardiac conduction system in systemic lupus erythematosus. Ann Intern Med 1965;63:402.

Jordaens, L, Gorgels, A, Stroobandt, R, Temmerman, J. Efficacy and safety of intravenous sotalol for termination of paroxysmal supraventricular tachycardia. The Sotalol versus Placebo Multicenter Study Group. Am J Cardiol 1991;68:35.

Kaplan, BM, Langendorf, R, Lev, M, Pick, A. Tachycardia-bradycardia syndrome (so-called "sick sinus syndrome"). Pathology, mechanisms and treatment. Am J Cardiol 1973;31:497.

Kaplan, NM. Management of hypertensive emergencies. Lancet 1994;344:1335.

Kaplan, NM. Hypertensive crises in clinical hypertension, 9th ed. Lippincott; Williams & Wilkins, Philadelphia, 2006, p. 390.

Kastor, JA. Multifocal atrial tachycardia. N Engl J Med 1990;322:1713.

Keeley, EC, Boura, JA, Grines, CL. Primary angioplasty versus intravenous thrombolytic therapy for acute myocardial infarction: a quantitative review of 23 randomised trials. Lancet 2003;361:13.

Kerensky, RA, Wade, M, Deedwania, P, et al. Revisiting the culprit lesion in non-Q-wave myocardial infarction. Results from the VANQWISH trial angiographic core laboratory. J Am Coll Cardiol 2002;39:1456.

Kouvaras, G, Cokkinos, DV, Halal, G, et al. The effective treatment of multifocal atrial tachycardia with amiodarone. Jpn Heart J 1989;30:301.

Krahn, AD, Klein, GJ, Kerr, CR. How useful is thyroid function testing in patients with recent-onset atrial fibrillation? Arch Intern Med 1996;156:2221.

Krum, H, Mohacsi, P, Katus, HA, et al. Are beta-blockers needed in patients receiving spironolactone for severe chronic heart failure? An analysis of the COPERNICUS study. Am Heart J 2006;151:55.

Lagerqvist, B, Safstrom, K, Stahle, E, et al. Is early invasive treatment of unstable coronary artery disease equally effective for both women and men? FRISC II Study Group Investigators. J Am Coll Cardiol 2001;38:41.

Lamas, GA, Lee, KL, Sweeney, MO, et al. Ventricular pacing or dual-chamber pacing for sinus-node dysfunction. N Engl J Med 2002;346:1854.

Langendorf, R, Cohen, H, Gozo, EG Jr. Observations on second degree atrioventricular block, including new criteria for the differential diagnosis between type I and type II block. Am J Cardiol 1972;29:111.

Langer, A, Krucoff, MW, Klootwijk, P, et al, for the GUSTO-I ECG Monitoring Substudy Group. Prognostic significance of ST segment shift early after resolution of ST elevation in patients with myocardial infarction treated with thrombolytic therapy: the GUSTO-I ST segment monitoring substudy. J Am Coll Cardiol 1998;31:783.

Larson, DM, Menssen, KM, Sharkey, SW, et al. "False-positive" cardiac catheterization laboratory activation among patients with suspected ST-segment elevation myocardial infarction. JAMA 2007;298:2754.

Latini, R, Masson, S, Anand, I, et al. Effects of valsartan on circulating brain natriuretic peptide and norepinephrine in symptomatic chronic heart failure: the Valsartan Heart Failure Trial (Val-HeFT). Circulation 2002;106:2454.

Lau, J, Antman, EM, Jimenez-Silva, J, Kupelnick, B. Cumulative meta-analysis of therapeutic trials for myocardial infarction. N Engl J Med 1992;327:248.

Ledingham, JG, Rajagopalan, B. Cerebral complications in the treatment of accelerated hypertension. Q J Med 1979;48:25.

Lemos, PA. Hidden drugs, hidden risks – is cocaine use a new risk factor for stent thrombosis?. Catheter Cardiovasc Interv 2007;69:959.

Liebson, PR, Klein, LW. The non-Q wave myocardial infarction revisited: 10 years later. Prog Cardiovasc Dis 1997;39:399.

Linde, C, Leclercq, C, Rex, S, et al. Long-term benefits of biventricular pacing in congestive heart failure: results from the MUltisite STimulation in cardiomyopathy (MUSTIC) study. J Am Coll Cardiol 2002;40:111.

Lip, GY, Beevers, M, Beevers, DG. Does renal function improve after diagnosis of malignant phase hypertension? J Hypertens 1997;15:1309.

Lip, GY, Metcalfe, MJ, Rae, AP. Management of paroxysmal atrial fibrillation. Q J Med 1993;86:467.

Lown, B. Electrical reversion of cardiac arrhythmias. Br Heart J 1967;29:469.

Lundstrom, T, Ryden, L. Ventricular rate control and exercise performance in chronic atrial fibrillation: effects of diltiazem and verapamil. J Am Coll Cardiol 1990;16:86.

MacCarthy, PA, Kearney, MT, Nolan, J, et al. Prognosis in heart failure with preserved left ventricular systolic function: prospective cohort study. BMJ 2003;327:78.

Macdonald, PS, Keogh, AM, Aboyoun, CL, et al. Tolerability and efficacy of carvedilol in patients with New York Heart Association class IV heart failure. J Am Coll Cardiol 1999;33:924.

Mager, G, Klocke, RK, Kux, A, et al. Phosphodiesterase III inhibition or adrenoreceptor stimulation: milrinone as an alternative to dobutamine in the treatment of severe heart failure. Am Heart J 1991;121:1974.

Maintenance of sinus rhythm in patients with atrial fibrillation: an AFFIRM substudy of the first antiarrhythmic drug. J Am Coll Cardiol 2003;42:20.

Malmberg, K. Prospective randomised study of intensive insulin treatment on long term survival after acute myocardial infarction in patients with diabetes mellitus. DIGAMI (Diabetes Mellitus, Insulin Glucose Infusion in Acute Myocardial Infarction) Study Group. BMJ 1997;314:1512.

Mandel, WJ, Laks, MM, Obayashi, K, et al. The Wolff-Parkinson-White syndrome: pharmacologic effects of procaine amide. Am Heart J 1975;90:744.

Mark, DB, Nelson, CL, Anstrom, KJ, et al. Cost-effectiveness of defibrillator therapy or amiodarone in chronic stable heart failure: results from the Sudden Cardiac Death in Heart Failure Trial (SCD-HeFT). Circulation 2006;114:135.

Mark, DB, Sigmon, K, Topol, EJ, et al. Identification of acute myocardial infarction patients suitable for early hospital discharge after aggressive interventional therapy. Results from the Thrombolysis and Angioplasty in Acute Myocardial Infarction Registry. Circulation 1991;83:1186.

Maron, BJ, McKenna, WJ, Danielson, GK, et al. American College of Cardiology/European Society of Cardiology Clinical Expert Consensus Document on Hypertrophic Cardiomyopathy. A Report of the American College of Cardiology Foundation Task Force on Clinical Expert Consensus Documents and the European Society of Cardiology Committee for Practice Guidelines. J Am Coll Cardiol 2003;42:1687.

Masip, J, Roque, M, Sanchez, B, et al. Noninvasive ventilation in acute cardiogenic pulmonary edema: systematic review and meta-analysis. JAMA 2005;294:3124.

McCord, J, Jneid, H, Hollander, JE, et al. Management of cocaine-associated chest pain and myocardial infarction: a scientific statement from the American Heart Association Acute Cardiac Care Committee of the Council on Clinical Cardiology. Circulation 2008;117:1897.

McGinn, AP, Rosamond, WD, Goff, DC Jr, et al. Trends in prehospital delay and use of emergency medical services for acute myocardial infarction: experience in 4 US communities from 1987-2000. Am Heart J 2005;150:392.

McKee, SA, Applegate, RJ, Hoyle, JR, et al. Cocaine use is associated with an increased risk of stent thrombosis after percutaneous coronary intervention. Am Heart J 2007;154:159.

McKelvie, RS, Yusuf, S, Pericak, D, et al. Comparison of candesartan, enalapril, and their combination in congestive heart failure: Randomized Evaluation of Strategies for Left Ventricular Dysfunction (RESOLVD) Pilot Study: the RESOLVD Pilot Study Investigators. Circulation 1999;100:1056.

McMurray, J, Solomon, S, Pieper, K, et al. The effect of valsartan, captopril, or both on atherosclerotic events after acute myocardial infarction an analysis of the Valsartan in Acute Myocardial Infarction Trial (VALIANT). J Am Coll Cardiol 2006;47:726.

McMurray, JJ, Ostergren, J, Swedberg, K, et al. Effects of candesartan in patients with chronic heart failure and reduced left-ventricular systolic function taking angiotensin-converting-enzyme inhibitors: the CHARM-Added trial. Lancet 2003;362:767.

Mehta, RH, Montoye, CK, Gallogly, M, et al. Improving quality of care for acute myocardial infarction: the Guidelines Applied in Practice (GAP) Initiative. JAMA 2002;287:1269.

Mehta, RH, Rathore, SS, Radford, MJ, et al. Acute myocardial infarction in the elderly: differences by age. J Am Coll Cardiol 2001;38:736.

Mehta, SR, Cannon, CP, Fox, KA, et al. Routine vs selective invasive strategies in patients with acute coronary syndromes: a collaborative meta-analysis of randomized trials. JAMA 2005;293:2908.

Mehta, SR, Yusuf, S, Peters, RJG, et al, for the Clopidogrel in Unstable angina to prevent Recurrent Events trial (CURE) Investigators. Effects of pretreatment with clopidogrel and aspirin followed by long-term therapy in patients undergoing percutaneous coronary intervention: the PCI-CURE study. Lancet 2001;358:527.

Meine, TJ, Patel, MR, Washam, JB, et al. Safety and effectiveness of transdermal nicotine patch in smokers admitted with acute coronary syndromes. Am J Cardiol 2005;95:976.

Menon, V, Harrington, RA, Hochman, JS, et al. Thrombolysis and adjunctive therapy in acute myocardial infarction: the Seventh ACCP Conference on Antithrombotic and Thrombolytic Therapy. Chest 2004;126:549S.

Metra, M, Nodari, S, D'Aloia, A, et al. Beta-blocker therapy influences the hemodynamic response to inotropic agents in patients with heart failure: a randomized comparison of dobutamine and enoximone before and after chronic treatment with metoprolol or carvedilol. J Am Coll Cardiol 2002;40:1248.

Meylaerts, L, Ooms, V, Lyra, S, et al. Hypertensive brain stem encephalopathy in a patient with chronic renal failure. Clin Nephrol 2006;65:138.

Milanesi, R, Baruscotti, M, Gnecchi-Ruscone, T, DiFrancesco, D. Familial sinus bradycardia associated with a mutation in the cardiac pacemaker channel. N Engl J Med 2006;354:151.

Mobitz, W. Über die unvollständige Störung der Erregungsüberleitung zwischen Vorhof und Kammer des menschlichen Herzens. Z Gesamte Exp Med 1924;41:180.

Mobitz, W. Über den partriellen Harzblock. Ztschr klin Med 1928;107:449.

Moller, JE, Hillis, GS, Oh, JK, et al. Left atrial volume: a powerful predictor of survival after acute myocardial infarction. Circulation 2003;107:2207.

Moller, JE, Sondergaard, E, Poulsen, SH, Egstrup, K. Pseudonormal and restrictive filling patterns predict left ventricular dilation and cardiac death after a first myocardial infarction: a serial color M-mode Doppler echocardiographic study. J Am Coll Cardiol 2000;36:1841.

Morrow, DA, Antman, EM, Parsons, L, et al. Application of the TIMI risk score for ST-elevation MI in the National Registry of Myocardial Infarction 3. JAMA 2001;286:1356.

Morrow, DA, Antman, EM, Snapinn, SM, et al. An integrated clinical approach to predicting the benefit of tirofiban in non-ST elevation acute coronary syndromes. Application of the TIMI risk score for UA/NSTEMI in PRISM-PLUS. Eur Heart J 2002;23:223.

Moss, AJ, Fadl, Y, Zareba, W, et al, for the Multicenter Defibrillator Implantation Trial Research Group. Survival benefit with an implanted defibrillator in relation to mortality risk in chronic coronary heart disease. Am J Cardiol 2001;88:516.

Moss, AJ, Hall, WJ, Cannom, DS, et al. Improved survival with an implanted defibrillator in patients with coronary disease at high risk for ventricular arrhythmia. N Engl J Med 1996;335:1933.

Murphy, MB, Murray, C, Shorten, GD. Drug therapy: Fenoldopam – a selective peripheral dopamine-receptor agonist for the treatment of severe hypertension. N Engl J Med 2001;345:1548.

Murphy, MB, Murray, C, Shorten, GD. Fenoldopam: a selective peripheral dopamine-receptor agonist for the treatment of severe hypertension. N Engl J Med 2001;345:1548.

Naccarelli, GV, Jalal, S. Intravenous amiodarone, another option in the acute management of sustained ventricular tachyarrhythmias. Circulation 1995;92:3154.

Narula, OS. Atrioventricular conduction defects in patients with sinus bradycardia. Analysis by His bundle recordings. Circulation 1971;44:1096.

Narula, OS. Conduction disorders in the AV transmission system. In: Cardiac Arrhythmias, Dreifus, L, Likoff, W (Eds), Grune and Stratton, New York, 1973, p. 259.

Narula, OS, Narula, JT. Junctional pacemakers in man. Response to overdrive suppression with and without parasympathetic blockade. Circulation 1978;57:880.

Narula, OS. Atrioventricular block. In: Cardiac Arrhythmias: Electrophysiology, Diagnosis and Management, Narula, OS (Ed), Williams & Wilkins, Baltimore, 1979, p. 85.

National Cholesterol Education Program: Executive Summary of the Third Report of the National Cholesterol Education Program (NCEP) Expert Panel on Detection, Evaluation, and Treatment of High Blood Cholesterol In Adults (Adult Treatment Panel III). JAMA 2001 May 16;285(19):2486-97.

Neutel, JM, Smith, DH, Wallin, D, et al. A comparison of intravenous nicardipine and sodium nitroprusside in the immediate treatment of severe hypertension. Am J Hypertens 1994;7:623.

Newby, KH, Thompson, T, Stebbins, A, et al, for the GUSTO Investigators. Sustained ventricular arrhythmias in patients receiving thrombolytic therapy: incidence and outcomes. Circulation 1998;98:2567.

Newby, LK, Eisenstein, EL, Califf, RM, et al. Cost effectiveness of early discharge after uncomplicated acute myocardial infarction. N Engl J Med 2000;342:749.

Ng, FH, Wong, SY, Lam, KF, et al. Gastrointestinal bleeding in patients receiving a combination of aspirin, clopidogrel, and enoxaparin in acute coronary syndrome. Am J Gastroenterol 2008;103:865.

Nieminen, MS, Bohm, M, Cowie, MR, et al. Executive summary of the guidelines on the diagnosis and treatment of acute heart failure: the Task Force on Acute Heart Failure of the European Society of Cardiology. Eur Heart J 2005;26:384.

Nijland, F, Kamp, O, Karreman, AJP, et al. Prognostic implications of restrictive left ventricularfilling in myocardial infarction: serial Doppler echocardiographic study. J Am Coll Cardiol 1997;30:1618.

Nissen, SE. High-dose statins in acute coronary syndromes: not just lipid levels. JAMA 2004;292:1365.

O'Nunain, S, Garratt, CJ, Linker, NJ, et al. A comparison of intravenous propafenone and flecainide in the treatment of tachycardias associated with the Wolff-Parkinson-White syndrome. Pacing Clin Electrophysiol 1991;14:2028.

Ohman, EM, Califf, RM, Topol, EJ, et al. Consequences of reocclusion after successful reperfusion therapy in acute myocardial infarction. Circulation 1990;82:781.

Ornato, JP. Chest pain emergency centers: improving acute myocardial infarction care. Clin Cardiol 1999;22:IV3.

Packard, JM, Graettinger, JS et al. Analysis of the electrocardiograms obtained from 1000 young healthy aviators: ten year follow-up. Circulation 1954;10:384.

Page, RL, Wilkinson, WE, Clair, WK, et al. Asymptomatic arrhythmias in patients with symptomatic paroxysmal atrial fibrillation and paroxysmal supraventricular tachycardia. Circulation 1994;89:224.

Paul, SD, O'Gara, PT, Mahjoub, ZA, et al. Geriatric patients with acute myocardial infarction: cardiac risk factor profiles, presentation, thrombolysis, coronary interventions, and prognosis. Am Heart J 1996;131:710.

Pedersen, TR. Statin trials and goals of cholesterol-lowering therapy after AMI. Am Heart J 1999 Aug;138(2 Pt 2):S177-82.

Persson, H, Lonn, E, Edner, M, et al. Diastolic dysfunction in heart failure with preserved systolic function: need for objective evidence: results from the CHARM Echocardiographic Substudy-CHARMES. J Am Coll Cardiol 2007;49:687.

Peterson, ED, Roe, MT, Mulgund, J, et al. Association between hospital process performance and outcomes among patients with acute coronary syndromes. JAMA 2006;295:1912.

Peuch, P. The value in intracardiac recordings. In: Cardiac Arrhythmias, Krikler, D, Gododwin, JF (Eds), Saunders, Philadelphia, 1975, p. 81.

Pfeffer, MA, McMurray, JJ, Velazquez, EJ, et al. Valsartan, captopril, or both in myocardial infarction complicated by heart failure, left ventricular dysfunction, or both. N Engl J Med 2003;349:1893.

Pfisterer, M, Kiowski, W, Burckhardt, D, et al. Beneficial effect of amiodarone on cardiac mortality in patients with asymptomatic complex ventricular arrhythmias after acute MI but not impaired left ventricular function. Am J Cardiol htt1992;69:1399.

Pitt, B, Krum, H, Nicolau, JC, et al. The EPHESUS Trial: effect of eplerenone in patients with a baseline history of hypertension. Abstracts from Scientific Sessions 2003, November 9-12, Orlando, Florida. Circulation, 2003;106 Suppl 17:IV-599. Abstract 2727.

Pitt, B, Loscalzo, J, Ycas, J, Raichlen, JS. Lipid levels after acute coronary syndromes. J Am Coll Cardiol 2008;51:1440.

Pitt, B, Poole-Wilson, PA, Segal, R, et al. Effect of losartan compared with captopril on mortality in patients with symptomatic heart failure: randomised trial – the Losartan Heart Failure Survival Study ELITE II. Lancet 2000;355:1582.

Pitt, B, Remme, W, Zannad, F, Neaton, J. Eplerenone, a selective aldosterone blocker, in patients with left ventricular dysfunction after myocardial infarction. N Engl J Med 2003;348:1309.

Pitt, B, Segal, R, Martinez, FA, et al. Randomised trial of losartan versus captopril in patients over 65 with heart failure(Evaluation of Losartan in the Elderly Study, ELITE). Lancet 1997;349:747.

Pitt, B, White, H, Nicolau, J, et al. Eplerenone reduces mortality 30 days after randomization following acute myocardial infarction in patients with left ventricular systolic dysfunction and heart failure. J Am Coll Cardiol 2005;46:425.

Platia, EV, Michelson, EL, Porterfield, JK, Das, G. Esmolol versus verapamil in the acute treatment of atrial fibrillation or atrial flutter. Am J Cardiol 1989;63:925.

Poulsen, SH, Jensen, SE, Egstrup, K. Effects of long-term adrenergic beta-blockade on left ventricular diastolic filling in patients with acute myocardial infarction. Am Heart J 1999;138:710.

Pretre, R, Von Segesser, LK. Aortic dissection. Lancet 1997;349:1461.

Prichard, BN, Ross, EJ. Use of propranolol in conjunction with alpha receptor blocking drugs in pheochromocytoma. Am J Cardiol 1966;18:394.

Pritchett, EL. Management of atrial fibrillation. N Engl J Med 1992;326:1264.

Puech, P, Wainwright, RJ. Clinical electrophysiology of atrioventricular block. Cardiol Clin 1983;1:209.

Pur-Shahriari, AA, Mills, RA, Hoppin, FG Jr, Dexter, L. Comparison of chronic and acute effects of morphine sulfate on cardiovascular function. Am J Cardiol 1967;20:654.

Randomised trial of intravenous streptokinase, oral aspirin, both, or neither among 17,187 cases of suspected acute myocardial infarction: ISIS-2. ISIS-2 (Second International Study Infarct Survival) Collaborative Group. Lancet 1988;2:349.

Raymond, R, Lynch, J, Underwood, D, et al. Myocardial infarction and normal coronary arteriography: a 10 year clinical and risk analysis of 74 patients. J Am Coll Cardiol 1988;11:471.

Risk factors for stroke and efficacy of antithrombotic therapy in atrial fibrillation. Analysis of pooled data from five randomized controlled trials. Arch Intern Med 1994;154:1449.

Roe, MT, Harrington, RA, Prosper, DM, et al. Clinical and therapeutic profile of patients presenting with acute coronary syndromes who do not have significant coronary artery disease. The Platelet Glycoprotein IIb/IIIa in Unstable Angina: Receptor Suppression Using Integrilin Therapy (PURSUIT) Trial Investigators. Circulation 2000;102:1101.

Roger, VL, Jacobsen, SJ, Weston, SA, et al. Trends in the incidence and survival of patients with hospitalized myocardial infarction, Olmsted County, Minnesota, 1979 to 1994. Ann Intern Med 2002;136:341.

Rogers, WJ, Bowlby, LJ, Chandra, NC, et al. Treatment of myocardial infarction in the United States (1990 to 1993). Observations from the National Registry of Myocardial Infarction. Circulation 1994;90:2103.

Rokseth, R, Hatle, L. Sinus arrest in acute myocardial infarction. Br Heart J 1971;33:639.

Rosei, EA, Salvetti, M, Farsang, C. European Society of Hypertension Scientific Newsletter: treatment of hypertensive urgencies and emergencies. J Hypertens 2006;24:2482.

Rosen, KM, Dhingra, RC, Loeb, HS, Rahimtoola, SH. Chronic heart block in adults. Clinical and electrophysiological observations. Arch Intern Med 1973;131:663.

Rosen, KM, Loeb, HS, Sinno, MZ, et al. Cardiac conduction in patients with symptomatic sinus node disease. Circulation 1971;43:836.

Rosenthal, L, et al. Atrial fibrillation; eMedicine journal [serial online]; July 2009. Available from http://emedicine.medscape.com/article/151066-overview

Roy, D, Talajic, M, Dorian, P, et al. Amiodarone to prevent recurrence of atrial fibrillation. Canadian Trial of Atrial Fibrillation Investigators. N Engl J Med 2000;342:913.

Rubenstein, JJ, Schulman, CL, Yurchak, PM, DeSanctis, RW. Clinical spectrum of the sick sinus syndrome. Circulation 1972;46:5.

Sabatine, M: Clopidogrel Shines in STEMI Reperfusion: CLARITY-TIMI 28. Paper presented at: American College of Cardiology Annual Scientific Session Late-Breaking Clinical Trials. March 9, 2005; Orlando, FL.

Sabatine, M, et al. Pocket Medicine, 2nd ed, Lippincott Williams & Wilkins, Philadelphia, PA, 2001.

Salerno, DM, Dias, VC, Kleiger, RE, et al. Efficacy and safety of intravenous diltiazem for treatment of atrial fibrillation and atrial flutter. Am J Cardiol 1989;63:1046.

Salvador, D, Rey, N, Ramos, G, Punzalan, F. Continuous infusion versus bolus injection of loop diuretics in congestive heart failure. Cochrane Database Syst Rev 2004;1:CD003178.

Sanders, GD, Hlatky, MA, Owens, DK. Cost-effectiveness of implantable cardioverter-defibrillators. N Engl J Med 2005;353:1471.

Saxon, LA, Bristow, MR, Boehmer, J, et al. Predictors of sudden cardiac death and appropriate shock in the Comparison of Medical Therapy, Pacing, and Defibrillation in Heart Failure (COMPANION) Trial. Circulation 2006;114:2766.

Schomig, A, Kastrati, A, Dirschinger, J, et al. Coronary stenting plus platelet glycoprotein IIb/IIIa blockade compared with tissue plasminogen activator in acute myocardial infarction. Stent versus Thrombolysis for Occluded Coronary Arteries in Patients with Acute Myocardial Infarction Study Investig. N Engl J Med 2000 Aug 10;343(6):385-91.

Schulz, V. Clinical pharmacokinetics of nitroprusside, cyanide, thiosulphate and thiocyanate. Clin Pharmacokinet 1984;9:239.

Schutzenberger, W, Leisch, F, Kerschner, K, et al. Clinical efficacy of intravenous amiodarone in the short term treatment of recurrent sustained ventricular tachycardia and ventricular fibrillation. Br Heart J 1989;62:367.

Schwartz, GG, Olsson, AG, Ezekowitz, MD, et al. Effects of atorvastatin on early recurrent ischemic events in acute coronary syndromes: the MIRACL study: a randomized controlled trial. JAMA 2001 Apr 4;285(13):1711-8.

Scott, O, Williams, GJ, Fiddler, GI. Results of 24 hour ambulatory monitoring of electrocardiogram in 131 healthy boys aged 10 to 13 years. Br Heart J 1980;44:304.

Senges, JC, Becker, R, Schreiner, KD, et al. Variability of Holter electrocardiographic findings in patients fulfilling the noninvasive MADIT criteria. Multicenter Automatic Defibrillator Implantation Trial. Pacing Clin Electrophysiol 2002;25:183.

Setaro, JF, Zaret, BL, Schulman, DS, et al. Usefulness of verapamil for congestive heart failure associated with abnormal left ventricular diastolic filling and normal left ventricular systolic performance. Am J Cardiol 1990;66:981.

Shakar, SF, Abraham, WT, Gilbert, EM, et al. Combined oral positive inotropic and beta-blocker therapy for treatment of refractory class IV heart failure. J Am Coll Cardiol 1998;31:1336.

Sharma, AD, Klein, GJ, Yee, R. Intravenous adenosine triphosphate during wide QRS complex tachycardia: safety, therapeutic efficacy, and diagnostic utility. Am J Med 1990; 88:337.

Sharon, A, Shpirer, I, Kaluski, E, et al. High-dose intravenous isosorbide-dinitrate is safer and better than Bi-PAP ventilation combined with conventional treatment for severe pulmonary edema. J Am Coll Cardiol 2000;36:832.

Sheehan, FH, Doerr, R, Schmidt, WG, et al. Early recovery of left ventricular function after thrombolytic therapy for acute myocardial infarction: an important determinant of survival. J Am Coll Cardiol 1988;12:289.

Short, DS. The syndrome of alternating bradycardia and tachycardia. Br Heart J 1954; 16:208.

Sigurdsson, A, Swedberg, K. Left ventricular remodelling, neurohormonal activation and early treatment with enalapril (CONSENSUS II) following myocardial infarction. Eur Heart J 1994;15 Suppl B:14.

Silber, S, Albertsson, P, Aviles, FF, et al. Guidelines for percutaneous coronary interventions. The Task Force for Percutaneous Coronary Interventions of the European Society of Cardiology. Eur Heart J 2005;26:804.

Simonsen, E, Nielsen, BL, Nielsen, JS. Sinus node dysfunction in acute myocardial infarction. Acta Med Scand 1980;208:463.

Simonsen, E, Nielsen, JS, Nielsen, BL. Sinus node dysfunction in 128 patients. A retrospective study with follow-up. Acta Med Scand 1980;208:343.

Simoons, ML. Effect of glycoprotein IIb/IIIa receptor blocker abciximab on outcome in patients with acute coronary syndromes without early coronary revascularisation: the GUSTO IV-ACS randomised trial. Lancet 2001;357:1915.

Singer, DE, Albers, GW, Dalen, JE, et al. Antithrombotic therapy in atrial fibrillation: the Seventh ACCP Conference on Antithrombotic and Thrombolytic Therapy. Chest 2004;126:429S.

Singh, BN, Singh, SN, Reda, DJ, et al. Amiodarone versus sotalol for atrial fibrillation. N Engl J Med 2005;352:1861.

Singh, SN, Fisher, SG, Carson, PE, et al and the Department of Veteran Affairs CHF-STAT Investigators. Prevalence and significance of nonsustained ventricular tachycardia in patients with premature ventricular contractions and heart failure treated with vasodilator therapy. J Am Coll Cardiol 1998;32:942.

Smith, SC Jr, Allen, J, Blair, SN, et al. AHA/ACC guidelines for secondary prevention for patients with coronary and other atherosclerotic vascular disease: 2006 update endorsed by the National Heart, Lung, and Blood Institute. J Am Coll Cardiol 2006;47:2130.

Snow, V, Weiss, KB, LeFevre, M, et al. Management of newly detected atrial fibrillation: a clinical practice guideline from the American Academy of Family Physicians and the American College of Physicians. Ann Intern Med 2003;139:1009.

Solomon, SD, Glynn, RJ, Greaves, S, et al. Recovery of ventricular function after myocardial infarction in the reperfusion era: the Healing and Early Afterload Reducing Therapy study. Ann Intern Med 2001;134:451.

Solomon, SD, Janardhanan, R, Verma, A, et al. Effect of angiotensin receptor blockade and antihypertensive drugs on diastolic function in patients with hypertension and diastolic dysfunction: a randomised trial. Lancet 2007;369:2079.

Soumerai, SB, McLaughlin, TJ, Spiegelman, D, et al. Adverse outcomes of underuse of beta-blockers in elderly survivors of acute myocardial infarction. JAMA 1997;277:115.

Spencer, FA, Lessard, D, Gore, JM, et al. Declining length of hospital stay for acute myocardial infarction and postdischarge outcomes: a community-wide perspective. Arch Intern Med 2004;164:733.

Spodick, DH. Normal sinus heart rate: sinus tachycardia and sinus bradycardia redefined. Am Heart J 1992;124:1119.

Spodick, DH, Raju, P, Bishop, RL, Rifkin, RD. Operational definition of normal sinus heart rate. Am J Cardiol 1992;69:1245.

Stampfer, M, Epstein, SE, Beiser, GD, Braunwald, E. Hemodynamic effects of diuresis at rest and during intense upright exercise in patients with impaired cardiac function. Circulation 1968;37:900.

Steinhubl, SR, Berger, PB, Mann, JT III, et al. Early and sustained dual oral antiplatelet therapy following percutaneous coronary intervention: a randomized controlled trial. JAMA 2002;288:2411.

Stone, PH, Thompson, B, Anderson, HV, et al. Influence of race, sex, and age on management of unstable angina and non-Q-wave myocardial infarction: the TIMI III registry. JAMA 1996;275:1104.

Strasberg, B, Amat-Y-Leon, F, Dhingra, RC, et al. Natural history of chronic second degree atrioventricular nodal block. Circulation 1981;63:1043.

Sutton, MG, Plappert, T, Hilpisch, KE, et al. Sustained reverse left ventricular structural remodeling with cardiac resynchronization at one year is a function of etiology: quantitative Doppler echocardiographic evidence from the Multicenter InSync Randomized Clinical Evaluation (MIRACLE). Circulation 2006;113:266.

Swedberg, K, Held, P, Kjekshus, J, et al, for the CONSENSUS II Study Group. Effects of the early administration of enalapril on mortality in patients with acute myocardial infarction. N Engl J Med 1992;327:678.

Talan, DA, Bauernfeind, RA, Ashley, WW, et al. Twenty-four hour continuous ECG recordings in long-distance runners. Chest 1982;82:19.

Tatum, JL, Jesse, RL, Kontos, MC, et al. Comprehensive strategy for the evaluation and triage of the chest pain patient. Ann Emerg Med 1997;29:116.

Tavazzi, L. Clinical epidemiology of acute myocardial infarction. Am Heart J 1999 Aug;138(2 Pt 2):S48-54.

The Digitalis Investigation Group. The effect of digoxin on mortality and morbidity in patients with heart failure. N Engl J Med 1997;336:525.

The effect of low-dose warfarin on the risk of stroke in patients with nonrheumatic atrial fibrillation. The Boston Area Anticoagulation Trial for Atrial Fibrillation Investigators. N Engl J Med 1990;323:1505.

The GUSTO Angiographic Investigators. The effects of tissue plasminogen activator, streptokinase, or both on coronary artery patency, ventricular function, and survival after acute myocardial infarction. N Engl J Med 1993;329:1615.

Topol, EJ, Burek, K, O'Neill, WW, et al. A randomized controlled trial of hospital discharge three days after myocardial infarction in the era of reperfusion. N Engl J Med 1988;318:1083.

Topol, EJ, Califf, RM, George, BS, et al. A randomized trial of immediate versus delayed elective angioplasty after intravenous tissue plasminogen activator in acute myocardial infarction. N Engl J Med 1987;317:581.

Totterman, KJ, Turto, H, Pellinen, T. Overdrive pacing as treatment of sotalol-induced ventricular tachyarrhythmias (torsade de pointes). Acta Med Scand Suppl 1982;668:28.

Touboul, P, Atallah, G, Kirkorian, G, et al. Effects of intravenous sotalol in patients with atrioventricular accessory pathways. Am Heart J 1987;114:545.

Tresch, DD, Fleg, JL. Unexplained sinus bradycardia: clinical significance and long term prognosis in apparently healthy persons older than 40 years. Am J Cardiol 1986;58:1009.

Tzivoni, D, Banai, S, Schuger, C. Treatment of torsades de pointes with magnesium sulfate. Circulation 1988;77:392.

Tzivoni, D, Keren, A, Cohen, AM, et al. Magnesium therapy for torsades de pointes. Am J Cardiol 1984;53:528.

Unverferth, DV, Magorien, RD, Altschuld, R, et al. The hemodynamic and metabolic advantages gained by a three-day infusion of dobutamine in patients with congestive cardiomyopathy. Am Heart J 1980;100:622.

van den, Born, BJ, Honnebier, UP, Koopmans, RP, van Montfrans, GA. Microangiopathic hemolysis and renal failure in malignant hypertension. Hypertension 2005;45:246.

Van Gelder, IC, Hagens, VE, Bosker, HA, et al. A comparison of rate control and rhythm control in patients with recurrent persistent atrial fibrillation. N Engl J Med 2002;347:1834.

Vaughan, CJ, Delanty N. Hypertensive emergencies. Lancet 2000;356:411.

Vermes, E, Tardif, JC, Bourassa, MG, et al. Enalapril decreases the incidence of atrial fibrillation in patients with left ventricular dysfunction: insight from the Studies Of Left Ventricular Dysfunction (SOLVD) trials. Circulation 2003;107:2926.

Wachtell, K, Bella, JN, Rokkedal, J, et al. Change in diastolic left ventricular filling after one year of antihypertensive treatment: the Losartan Intervention for Endpoint Reduction in Hypertension (LIFE) Study. Circulation 2002;105:1071.

Wallentin, L, Lagerqvist, V, Husted, S, et al, for the FRISC II Investigators. Outcome at 1 year after an invasive compared with a non-invasive strategy in unstable coronary-artery disease: the FRISC II invasive randomised trial. Lancet 2000;356:9.

Walter, PF, Crawley, IS, Dorney, ER. Carotid sinus hypersensitivity and syncope. Am J Cardiol 1978;42:396.

Ware, LB, Matthay, MA. Clinical practice. Acute pulmonary edema. N Engl J Med 2005; 353:2788.

Wilhelmsson, C, Vedin, JA, Elmfeldt, D, et al. Smoking and myocardial infarction. Lancet 1975;1:415.

Wolf, PA, Kannel, WB, McGee, DL, et al. Duration of atrial fibrillation and imminence of stroke: the Framingham study. Stroke 1983;14:664.

Wong, GC, Morrow, DA, Murphy, S, et al. Elevations in troponin T and I are associated with abnormal tissue level perfusion: a TACTICS-TIMI 18 substudy. Treat Angina with Aggrastat and Determine Cost of Therapy with an Invasive or Conservative Strategy-Thrombolysis in Myocardial Infarction. Circulation 2002;106:202.

Wong, M, Staszewsky, L, Latini, R, et al. Severity of left ventricular remodeling defines outcomes and response to therapy in heart failure: Valsartan Heart Failure Trial (Val-HeFT) echocardiographic data. J Am Coll Cardiol 2004;43:2022.

Woods, JW, Blythe, WB. Management of malignant hypertension complicated by renal insufficiency. N Engl J Med 1967;277:57.

Wu, AH, Parsons, L, Every, NR, Bates, ER. Hospital outcomes in patients presenting with congestive heart failure complicating acute myocardial infarction. A report from the Second National Registry of Myocardial Infarction (NRMI-2). J Am Coll Cardiol 2002;40:1389.

Wu, WC, Rathore, SS, Wang, Y, et al. Blood transfusion in elderly patients with acute myocardial infarction. N Engl J Med 2001;345:1230.

Wyse, DG, Talajic, M, Hafley, GE, et al. Antiarrhythmic drug therapy in the Multicenter UnSustained Tachycardia Trial (MUSTT): drug testing and as-treated analysis. J Am Coll Cardiol 2001;38:344.

Wyse, DG, Waldo, AL, DiMarco, JP, et al. A comparison of rate control and rhythm control in patients with atrial fibrillation. The atrial fibrillation follow-up investigation of rhythm management (AFFIRM) investigators. N Engl J Med 2002;347:1825.

Yabek, SM, Jarmakani, JM. Sinus node dysfunction in children, adolescents, and young adults. Pediatrics 1978;61:593.

Yancy, CW, Lopatin, M, Stevenson, LW, et al. Clinical presentation, management, and in-hospital outcomes of patients admitted with acute decompensated heart failure with preserved systolic function: a report from the Acute Decompensated Heart Failure National Registry (ADHERE) Database. J Am Coll Cardiol 2006;47:76.

Yusuf, S, Pfeffer, MA, Swedberg, K, et al. Effects of candesartan in patients with chronic heart failure and preserved left-ventricular ejection fraction: the CHARM-Preserved trial. Lancet 2003;362:777.

Yusuf, S, Zhao, F, Mehta, SR, et al. Effects of clopidogrel in addition to aspirin in patients with acute coronary syndromes without ST-segment elevation. N Engl J Med 2001;345:494.

Zafari, AM, Taylor, WR. Antiplatelet agents in coronary heart disease: case studies. Hosp Physician 2000;5:1-10.

Zaret, BL, Wackers, FJ, Terrin, ML, et al. Value of radionuclide rest and exercise left ventricular ejection fraction in assessing survival of patients after thrombolytic therapy for acute MI: results of Thrombolysis in Myocardial Infarction (TIMI) Phase II Study. The TIMI Study Group. J Am Coll Cardiol 1995;26:73.

Zile, MR, Brutsaert, DL. New concepts in diastolic dysfunction and diastolic heart failure: part I: diagnosis, prognosis, and measurements of diastolic function. Circulation 2002;105:1387.

Zipes, DP, Camm, AJ, Borggrefe, M, et al. ACC/AHA/ESC 2006 guidelines for management of patients with ventricular arrhythmias and the prevention of sudden cardiac death: executive summary. A Report of the American College of Cardiology/American Heart Association Task Force and the European Society of Cardiology Committee for Practice Guidelines (Writing Committee to Develop Guidelines for Management of Patients With Ventricular Arrhythmias and the Prevention of Sudden Cardiac Death). J Am Coll Cardiol 2006;48:1064.

Zornoff, LA, Skali, H, Pfeffer, MA, et al. Right ventricular dysfunction and risk of heart failure and mortality after myocardial infarction. J Am Coll Cardiol 2002;39:1450.

Zuanetti, G, Latini, R, Maggioni, AP, et al, for the GISSI-3 Investigators. Effect of the ACE inhibitor lisinopril on mortaltiy in diabetic patients with acute myocardial infarction: data from the GISSI-3 study. Circulation 1997;96:4239.

Zwanziger, J, Hall, WJ, Dick, AW, et al. The cost effectiveness of implantable cardioverter-defibrillators: results from the Multicenter Automatic Defibrillator Implantation Trial (MADIT)-II. J Am Coll Cardiol 2006;47:2310.

EKG REVIEW

Feldman, H, et al. A guide to reading and understanding EKG, 1999, Available from http://www.scribd.com/doc/6454322/Easy-ECG-Guide

PULMONARY DISEASES

Aaron, SD, Vandemheen, KL, Fergusson, D, et al. Tiotropium in combination with placebo, salmeterol, or fluticasone-salmeterol for treatment of chronic obstructive pulmonary disease: a randomized trial. Ann Intern Med 2007;146:545.

Aklog, L, Williams, CS, Byrne, JG, et al. Acute pulmonary embolectomy: a contemporary approach. Circulation 2002;105:1416.

Alkhayer, M, Jenkins, PF, Harrison, BD. The outcome of community acquired pneumonia treated on the intensive care unit. Respir Med 1990;84:13.

Almirall, J, Bolibar, I, Balanzo, X, Gonzalez, CA. Risk factors for community-acquired pneumonia in adults: a population-based case-control study. Eur Respir J 1999;13:349.

Almirall, J, Bolibar, I, Vidal, J, et al. Epidemiology of community-acquired pneumonia in adults: a population-based study. Eur Respir J 2000;15:757.

Almirall, J, Mesalles, E, Klamburg, J, et al. Prognostic factors of pneumonia requiring admission to the intensive care unit. Chest 1995;107:511.

Almirall, J, Morato, I, Riera, F, et al. Incidence of community-acquired pneumonia and Chlamydia pneumoniae infection: a prospective multicentre study. Eur Respir J 1993;6:14.

American Thoracic Society. A statement by the Committee on Diagnostic Standards for Nontuberculous Respiratory Diseases. Chronic bronchitis, asthma, and pulmonary emphysema. Am Rev Respir Dis 1962;85:762.

Anderson, FA, Wheeler, HB, Goldberg, RJ, et al. A population-based perspective of the hospital incidence and case-fatality rates of deep vein thrombosis and pulmonary embolism. Arch Intern Med 1991;151:933.

Anzueto, A, Tashkin, D, Menjoge, S, Kesten, S. One-year analysis of longitudinal changes in spirometry in patients with COPD receiving tiotropium. Pulm Pharmacol Ther 2005;18:75.

Aoshiba, K, Nagai, A. Differences in airway remodeling between asthma and chronic obstructive pulmonary disease. Clin Rev Allergy Immunol 2004;27:35.

Arancibia, F, Bauer, TT, Ewig, S, et al. Community-acquired pneumonia due to gram-negative bacteria and Pseudomonas aeruginosa: incidence, risk, and prognosis. Arch Intern Med 2002;162:1849.

Arancibia, F, Ewig, S, Martinez, JA, et al. Antimicrobial treatment failures in patients with community-acquired pneumonia: causes and prognostic implications. Am J Respir Crit Care Med 2000;162:154.

Arnold, FW, Summersgill, JT, Lajoie, AS, et al. A worldwide perspective of atypical pathogens in community-acquired pneumonia. Am J Respir Crit Care Med 2007; 175:1086.

Aubertin, J, Dabis, F, Fleurette, J, et al. Prevalence of legionellosis among adults: a study of community-acquired pneumonia in France. Infection 1987;15:328.

Baddour, LM, Yu, VL, Klugman, KP, et al. Combination antibiotic therapy lowers mortality among severely ill patients with pneumococcal bacteremia. Am J Respir Crit Care Med 2004;170:440.

Badgett, RG, Tanaka, DJ, Hunt, DK, et al. Can moderate chronic obstructive pulmonary disease be diagnosed by historical and physical findings alone?. Am J Med 1993;94:188.

Baraldo, S, Turato, G, Badin, C, et al. Neutrophilic infiltration within the airway smooth muscle in patients with COPD. Thorax 2004;59:308.

Barritt, DW, Jordan, SC. Anticoagulant drugs in the treatment of pulmonary embolism. A controlled trial. Lancet 1960;1:1309.

Bartlett, JG, Dowell, SF, Mandell, LA, et al. Practice guidelines for the management of community-acquired pneumonia in adults. Infectious Diseases Society of America. Clin Infect Dis 2000;31:347.

Bartlett, JG, Mundy, LM. Community-acquired pneumonia. N Engl J Med 1995;333:1618.

Bastien, N, Anderson, K, Hart, L, et al. Human coronavirus NL63 infection in Canada. J Infect Dis 2005;191:503.

Bateman, ED, Bousquet, J, Keech, ML, et al. The correlation between asthma control and health status: the GOAL study. Eur Respir J 2007;29:56.

Bates, JH, Campbell, GD, Barron, AL, et al. Microbial etiology of acute pneumonia in hospitalized patients. Chest 1992;101:1005.

Battleman, DS, Callahan, M, Thaler, HT. Rapid antibiotic delivery and appropriate antibiotic selection reduce length of hospital stay of patients with community-acquired pneumonia: link between quality of care and resource utilization. Arch Intern Med 2002;162:682.

Berntsson, E, Lagergard, T, Strannegard, O, Trollfors, B. Etiology of community-acquired pneumonia in out-patients. Eur J Clin Microbiol 1986;5:446.

Bijl-Hofland, ID, Cloosterman, SG, van Schayck, CP, et al. Perception of respiratory sensation assessed by means of histamine challenge and threshold loading tests. Chest 2000;117:954.

Blanquer, J, Blanquer, R, Borras, R, et al. Aetiology of community acquired pneumonia in Valencia, Spain: a multicentre prospective study.Thorax 1991;46:508.

Bloomfield, P, Boon, NA, DeBono, DP. Indications for pulmonary embolectomy. Lancet 1988;2:329.

Bochud, PY, Moser, F, Erard, P, et al. Community-acquired pneumonia. A prospective outpatient study. Medicine (Baltimore) 2001;80:75.

Bohte, R, van Furth, R, van den, Broek PJ. Aetiology of community-acquired pneumonia: a prospective study among adults requiring admission to hospital. Thorax 1995;50:543.

Boulain, T, Lanotte, R, Legras, A, Perrotin, D. Efficacy of epinephrine therapy in shock complicating acute PE. Chest 1993;104:300.

Boulet, LP, Boulet, V, Milot, J. How should we quantify asthma control? A proposal. Chest 2002;122:2217.

Brady, AJB, Crake, T, Oakley, CM. Percutaneous catheter fragmentation and distal dispersion of proximal pulmonary embolus. Lancet 1991;338:1186.

Brandjes, DPM, Heijboer, H, Buller, HR, et al. Acenocoumarol and heparin compared with acenocoumarol alone in the initial treatment of proximal-vein thrombosis. N Engl J Med 1992;327:1485.

Brender, E. Use of emboli-blocking filters increases, but rigorous data are lacking. JAMA 2006;295:989.

British Thoracic Society Standards of Care Committee. BTS guidelines for the management of community acquired pneumonia in adults. Thorax 2001;56 Suppl 4:IV1.

Bruns, AH, Oosterheert, JJ, Prokop, M, et al. Patterns of resolution of chest radiograph abnormalities in adults hospitalized with severe community-acquired pneumonia. Clin Infect Dis 2007;45:983.

BTS guidelines for the management of chronic obstructive pulmonary disease. The COPD Guidelines Group of the Standards of Care Committee of the BTS. Thorax 1997;52 Suppl 5:S1.

BTS Guidelines for the Management of Community Acquired Pneumonia in Adults-2004. Available from www.Brit-thoracic.org/guideline.

BTS guidelines for the management of community acquired pneumonia in adults. Thorax 2001;56 Suppl 4:IV1.

Buist, AS, McBurnie, MA, Vollmer, WM, et al. International variation in the prevalence of COPD (the BOLD Study): a population-based prevalence study. Lancet 2007; 370:741.

Buller, HR, Agnelli, G, Hull, RD, et al. Antithrombotic therapy for venous thromboembolic disease: the Seventh ACCP Conference on Antithrombotic and Thrombolytic Therapy. Chest 2004;126:401S.

Burge, PS, Calverley, PM, Jones, PW, et al. Randomised, double blind, placebo controlled study of fluticasone propionate in patients with moderate to severe chronic obstructive pulmonary disease: the ISOLDE trial. BMJ 2000;320:1297.

Burman, LA, Trollfors, B, Andersson, B, et al. Diagnosis of pneumonia by cultures, bacterial and viral antigen detection tests, and serology with special reference to antibodies against pneumococcal antigens. J Infect Dis 1991;163:1087.

Calverley, PM, Anderson, JA, Celli, B, et al. Salmeterol and fluticasone propionate and survival in chronic obstructive pulmonary disease. N Engl J Med 2007;356:775.

Carson, JL, Kelley, MA, Duff, A, et al. The clinical course of pulmonary embolism. N Engl J Med 1992;326:1240.

Casaburi, R, Briggs, DD Jr, Donohue, JF, et al. The spirometric efficacy of once-daily dosing with tiotropium in stable COPD: a 13-week multicenter trial. The US Tiotropium Study Group. Chest 2000;118:1294.

Casaburi, R, Mahler, DA, Jones, PW, et al. A long-term evaluation of once-daily inhaled tiotropium in chronic obstructive pulmonary disease. Eur Respir J 2002;19:217.

Castro, M, Zimmermann, NA, Crocker, S, et al. Asthma intervention program prevents readmissions in high healthcare users. Am J Respir Crit Care Med 2003;168:1095.

Celli, BR. Change in the BODE index reflects disease modification in COPD: lessons from lung volume reduction surgery. Chest 2006;129:835.

Celli, BR, Cote, CG, Marin, JM, et al. The body-mass index, airflow obstruction, dyspnea, and exercise capacity index in chronic obstructive pulmonary disease. N Engl J Med 2004;350:1005.

Celli, BR, MacNee, W. Standards for the diagnosis and treatment of patients with COPD: a summary of the ATS/ERS position paper. Eur Respir J 2004;23:932.

Chen, KY, Ko, SC, Hsueh, PR, et al. Pulmonary fungal infection: emphasis on microbiological spectra, patient outcome, and prognostic factors. Chest 2001;120:177.

Clarke, DB. Pulmonary embolectomy re-evaluated. Ann R Coll Surg Engl 1981;63:18.

Clarke, DB, Abrams, LD. Pulmonary embolectomy: a 25-year eperience. J Thorac Cardiovasc Surg 1986;92:442.

Community-acquired pneumonia in adults in British hospitals in 1982-1983: a survey of aetiology, mortality, prognostic factors and outcome. The British Thoracic Society and the Public Health Laboratory Service. Q J Med 1987;62:195.

Crapo, RO. Pulmonary function testing. N Engl J Med 1994;331:25.

Crum, NF, Russell, KL, Kaplan, EL, et al. Pneumonia outbreak associated with group a Streptococcus species at a military training facility. Clin Infect Dis 2005;40:511.

Cunha, B. Community acquired pneumonia; eMedicine journal [serial online], 2009. Available from http://emedicine.medscape.com/article/234240-overview

Dagan, E, Novack, V, Porath, A. Adverse outcomes in patients with community acquired pneumonia discharged with clinical instability from Internal Medicine Department. Scand J Infect Dis 2006;38:860.

Dalen, JE, Alpert, JS. Natural history of pulmonary embolism. Prog Cardiovasc Dis 1975;17:257.

Dalhoff, K, Maass, M. Chlamydia pneumoniae pneumonia in hospitalized patients. Clinical characteristics and diagnostic value of polymerase chain reaction detection in BAL. Chest 1996;110:351.

Dauphine, C, Omari, B. Pulmonary embolectomy for acute massive pulmonary embolism. Ann Thorac Surg 2005;79:1240.

de Roux, A, Marcos, MA, Garcia, E, et al. Viral community-acquired pneumonia in nonimmunocompromised adults. Chest 2004;125:1343.

Decousus, H, Leizorovicz, A, Parent, F, et al. A clinical trial of vena caval filters in the prevention of pulmonary embolism in patients with proximal deep-vein thrombosis. N Engl J Med 1998;338:409.

Decramer, M, Celli, B, Tashkin, DP, et al. Clinical trial design considerations in assessing long-term functional impacts of tiotropium in COPD: the UPLIFT trial. COPD 2004;1:303.

Demir, T, Ikitimur, HD, Koc, N, Yildirim, N. The role of FEV6 in the detection of airway obstruction. Respir Med 2005;99:103.

Dennis, DT, Inglesby, TV, Henderson, DA, et al. Tularemia as a biological weapon: medical and public health management. JAMA 2001;285:2763.

Dismuke, SE, Wagner, EH. Pulmonary embolism as a cause of death. The changing mortality in hospitalized patients. JAMA 1986;255:2039.

Donaldson, GA, Williams, C, Schnnel, JG, Shaw, RS. A reappraisal of the application of the Trendelenburg operation to massive fatal embolism. Report of a successful pulmonary-artery thrombectomy using a cardiopulmonary bypass. N Engl J Med 1963;268:171.

Donohue, JF, van Noord, JA, Bateman, ED, et al. A 6-month, placebo-controlled study comparing lung function and health status changes in COPD patients treated with tiotropium or salmeterol. Chest 2002;122:47.

Dooley, KE, Golub, J, Goes, FS, et al. Empiric treatment of community-acquired pneumonia with fluoroquinolones, and delays in the treatment of tuberculosis. Clin Infect Dis 2002;34:1607.

Dufour, P, Gillet, Y, Bes, M, et al. Community-acquired methicillin-resistant Staphylococcus aureus infections in France: emergence of a single clone that produces Panton-Valentine leukocidin. Clin Infect Dis 2002;35:819.

Dunn, AS, Peterson, KL, Schechter, CB, et al. The utility of an in-hospital observation period after discontinuing intravenous antibiotics. Am J Med 1999;106:6.

Dusser, D, Bravo, ML, Iacono, P. The effect of tiotropium on exacerbations and airflow in patients with COPD. Eur Respir J 2006;27:547.

Dutoit, JI, Salome, CM, Woolcock, AJ. Inhaled corticosteroids reduce the severity of bronchial hyperresponsiveness in asthma but oral theophylline does not. Am Rev Respir Dis 1987;136:1174.

Eight-year follow-up of patients with permanent vena cava filters in the prevention of pulmonary embolism: the PREPIC (Prevention du Risque d'Embolie Pulmonaire par Interruption Cave) randomized study. Circulation 2005;112:416.

El Solh, AA, Aquilina, AT, Gunen, H, Ramadan, F. Radiographic resolution of community-acquired bacterial pneumonia in the elderly. J Am Geriatr Soc 2004;52:224.

Enright, PL, Lebowitz, MD, Cockcroft, DW. Physiologic measures: pulmonary function test. Am J Respir Crit Care Med 1994;149:S9.

Ewig, S, de Roux, A, Bauer, T, et al. Validation of predictive rules and indices of severity for community acquired pneumonia. Thorax 2004;59:421.

Falco, V, Fernandez de, Sevilla, T, Alegre, J, et al. Legionella pneumophila. A cause of severe community-acquired pneumonia. Chest 1991;100:1007.

Falguera, M, Sacristan, O, Nogues, A, et al. Nonsevere community-acquired pneumonia: correlation between cause and severity or comorbidity. Arch Intern Med 2001;161:1866.

Fee, C, Weber, EJ. Identification of 90% of patients ultimately diagnosed with community-acquired pneumonia within four hours of emergency department arrival may not be feasible. Ann Emerg Med 2007;49:553.

File, TM. Community-acquired pneumonia. Lancet 2003;362:1991.

File, TM Jr, Gross, PA. Performance measurement in community-acquired pneumonia: consequences intended and unintended. Clin Infect Dis 2007;44:942.

File, TM Jr, Niederman, MS. Antimicrobial therapy of community-acquired pneumonia. Infect Dis Clin North Am 2004;18:993.

Fine, MJ, Stone, RA, Singer, DE, et al. Processes and outcomes of care for patients with community-acquired pneumonia: results from the Pneumonia Patient Outcomes Research Team (PORT) cohort study. Arch Intern Med 1999;159:970.

Flamaing, J, Engelmann, I, Joosten, E, et al. Viral lower respiratory tract infection in the elderly: a prospective in-hospital study. Eur J Clin Microbiol Infect Dis 2003;22:720.

Francis, JS, Doherty, MC, Lopatin, U, et al. Severe community-onset pneumonia in healthy adults caused by methicillin-resistant Staphylococcus aureus carrying the Panton-Valentine leukocidin genes. Clin Infect Dis 2005;40:100.

Genne, D, Sommer, R, Kaiser, L, et al. Analysis of factors that contribute to treatment failure in patients with community-acquired pneumonia. Eur J Clin Microbiol Infect Dis 2006;25:159.

Ghignone, M, Girling, L, Prewitt, RM. Volume expansion versus norepinephrine in treatment of a low cardiac output complicating an acute increase in right ventricular afterload in dogs. Anesthesiology 1984;60:132.

Gibson, PG, Coughlan, J, Wilson, AJ, et al. Self-management education and regular practitioner review for adults with asthma. Cochrane Database Syst Rev 2000;CD001117.

Gillet, Y, Issartel, B, Vanhems, P, et al. Association between Staphylococcus aureus strains carrying gene for Panton-Valentine leukocidin and highly lethal necrotizing pneumonia in young immunocompetent persons. Lancet 2002;359:753.

Gillet, Y, Vanhems, P, Lina, G, et al. Factors predicting mortality in necrotizing community-acquired pneumonia caused by Staphylococcus aureus containing Panton-Valentine leukocidin. Clin Infect Dis 2007;45:315.

GINA report, global strategy for asthma management and prevention 2006. Global Initiative for Asthma (GINA). Available from http://www.ginasthma.com. (Accessed August 31, 2007).

Global Initiative for Chronic Obstructive Lung Disease, Executive Summary: Global Strategy for the Diagnosis, Management, and Prevention of COPD, 2006, www.goldcopd.com (Accessed January 30, 2008).

Global strategy for the diagnosis, management, and prevention of chronic obstructive pulmonary disease: executive summary 2006. Global Initiative for Chronic Obstructive Lung Disease (GOLD). Available from http://www.goldcopd.org. (Accessed August 31, 2007).

Goldhaber, SZ. Pulmonary embolism. N Engl J Med 1998;339:93.

Goldhaber, SZ, Haire, WD, Feldstein, ML, et al. Alteplase versus heparin in acute pulmonary embolism: randomized trial assessing right ventricular function and pulmonary perfusion. Lancet 1993;341:507.

Goldhaber, SZ, Visani, L, De Rosa, M. Acute pulmonary embolism: clinical outcomes in the International Cooperative Pulmonary Embolism Registry (ICOPER). Lancet 1999;353:1386.

Greenfield, LJ. Evolution of venous interruption for pulmonary thromboembolism. Arch Surg 1992;127:622.

Greenfield, LJ, Kimmell, GO, McCurdy, WC III. Transvenous removal of pulmonary emboli by vacuum-cup catheter technique. J Surg Res 1969;9:347.

Guidelines on diagnosis and management of acute pulmonary embolism. Task Force on Pulmonary Embolism, European Society of Cardiology. Eur Heart J 2000;21:1301.

Gutierrez, F, Masia, M, Rodriguez, JC, et al. Community-acquired pneumonia of mixed etiology: prevalence, clinical characteristics, and outcome. Eur J Clin Microbiol Infect Dis 2005;24:377.

Haahtela, T, Jarvinen, M, Kava, T, et al. Comparison of a beta 2-agonist, terbutaline, with an inhaled corticosteroid, budesonide, in newly detected asthma. N Engl J Med 1991;325:388.

Hageman, JC. Severe community-acquired pneumonia due to Staphylococcus aureus, 2003-04 influenza season. Emerg Infect Dis 2006;12:894.

Halbert, RJ, Natoli, JL, Gano, A, et al. Global burden of COPD: systematic review and meta-analysis. Eur Respir J 2006;28:523.

Halm, EA, Fine, MJ, Marrie, TJ, et al. Time to clinical stability in patients hospitalized with community-acquired pneumonia: implications for practice guidelines. JAMA 1998;279:1452.

Harding, SM. Recent clinical investigations examining the association of asthma and gastroesophageal reflux. Am J Med 2003;115 Suppl 3A:39S.

Hasegawa, M, Nasuhara, Y, Onodera, Y, et al. Airflow limitation and airway dimensions in chronic obstructive pulmonary disease. Am J Respir Crit Care Med 2006;173:1309.

Hirani, NA, Macfarlane, JT. Impact of management guidelines on the outcome of severe community acquired pneumonia. Thorax 1997;52:17.

Hogg, JC. Pathophysiology of airflow limitation in chronic obstructive pulmonary disease. Lancet 2004;364:709.

Hogg, JC, Chu, F, Utokaparch, S, et al. The nature of small-airway obstruction in chronic obstructive pulmonary disease. N Engl J Med 2004;350:2645.

Holmberg, H. Aetiology of community-acquired pneumonia in hospital treated patients. Scand J Infect Dis 1987;19:491.

Hone, R, Haugh, C, O'Connor, B, Hollingsworth, J. Legionella: an infrequent cause of adult community acquired pneumonia in Dublin. Ir J Med Sci 1989;158:230.

Hooi, LN, Looi, I, Ng, AJ. A study on community acquired pneumonia in adults requiring hospital admission in Penang. Med J Malaysia 2001;56:275.

Horlander, KT, Mannino, DM, Leeper, KV. Pulmonary embolism mortality in the United States, 1979-1998: an analysis using multiple-cause mortality data. Arch Intern Med 2003;163:1711.

Houck, PM, Bratzler, DW, Nsa, W, et al. Timing of antibiotic administration and outcomes for Medicare patients hospitalized with community-acquired pneumonia. Arch Intern Med 2004;164:637.

http://www.qualitynet.org/dcs/ContentServer?cid=1192804535739 & pagename=QnetPubli c%2FPage%2FQnetTier3 & c=Page (Accessed April 15, 2008).

Hull, RD, Raskob, GE, Hirsh, J, et al. Continuous intravenous heparin compared with intermittent subcutaneous heparin in the initial treatment of proximal-vein thrombosis. N Engl J Med 1986;315:1109.

Inglesby, TV, Henderson, DA, Bartlett, JG et al. Anthrax as a biological weapon. Medical and public health management. JAMA 1999;281:1735.

Irvin, CG, Eidelman, D. Airways mechanics in asthma. In: Rhinitis and Asthma, Holgate, S, Busse, W (Eds), Blackwell Scientific Publications, Boston, 1995.

Ishida, T, Hashimoto, T, Arita, M, et al. Etiology of community-acquired pneumonia in hospitalized patients. Chest 1998;114:1588.

Jardin, F, Genevray, B, Brun-Ney, D, Margairaz, A. Dobutamine: a hemodynamic evaluation in pulmonary embolism shock. Crit Care Med 1985;13:1009.

Jeffery, PK. Comparison of the structural and inflammatory features of COPD and asthma. Giles F. Filley Lecture. Chest 2000;117:251S.

Jokinen, C, Heiskanen, L, Helvi, J, et al. Microbial etiology of community-acquired pneumonia in the adult population of 4 municipalities in eastern Finland. Clin Infect Dis 2001;32:1141.

Jones, PW, Bosh, TK. Quality of life changes in COPD patients treated with salmeterol. Am J Respir Crit Care Med 1997;155:1283.

Juniper, EF, Kline, PA, Vanzieleghem, MA, et al. Effect of long-term treatment with an inhaled corticosteroid (budesonide) on airway hyperresponsiveness and clinical asthma in nonsteroid-dependent asthmatics. Am Rev Respir Dis 1990;142:832.

Juniper, EF, O'Byrne, PM, Guyatt, GH, et al. Development and validation of a questionnaire to measure asthma control. Eur Respir J 1999;14:902.

Kanwar, M, Brar, N, Khatib, R, Fakih, MG. Misdiagnosis of community-acquired pneumonia and inappropriate utilization of antibiotics: side effects of the 4-h antibiotic administration rule. Chest 2007;131:1865.

Karalus, NC, Cursons, RT, Leng, RA, et al. Community acquired pneumonia: aetiology and prognostic index evaluation. Thorax 1991;46:413.

Karwa, M, Currie, B, Kvetan, V. Bioterrorism: preparing for the impossible or the improbable. Crit Care Med 2005;33:S75.

Kawai, S, Ochi, M, Nakagawa, T, Goto, H. Antimicrobial therapy in community-acquired pneumonia among emergency patients in a university hospital in Japan. J Infect Chemother 2004;10:352.

Kikuchi, Y, Okabe, S, Tamura, G, et al. Chemosensitivity and perception of dyspnea in patients with a history of near-fatal asthma. N Engl J Med 1994;330:1329.

Klein, JS, Gamsu, G, Webb, WR, et al. High-resolution CT diagnosis of emphysema in symptomatic patients with normal chest radiographs and isolated low diffusing capacity. Radiology 1992;182:817.

Koning, R, Cribier, A, Gerber, L, et al. A new treatment for severe pulmonary embolism: percutaneous rheolytic thrombectomy. Circulation 1997;96:2498.

Konstantinides, S, Geibel, A, Heusel, G, et al. Heparin plus alteplase compared with heparin alone in patients with submassive pulmonary embolism. N Engl J Med 2002;347:1143.

Kucher, N, Goldhaber, SZ. Management of massive pulmonary embolism. Circulation 2005;112:e28.

Kucher, N, Rossi, E, De Rosa, M, Goldhaber, SZ. Massive pulmonary embolism. Circulation 2006;113:577.

Labandeira-Rey, M, Couzon, F, Boisset, S, et al. Staphylococcus aureus Panton-Valentine leukocidin causes necrotizing pneumonia. Science 2007;315:1130.

Laheij, RJF, Sturkenboom, MCJM. Risk of community-acquired pneumonia and use of gastric acid-suppressive drugs. JAMA 2004;292:1955.

Leroy, O, Santre, C, Beuscart, C, et al. A five-year study of severe community-acquired pneumonia with emphasis on prognosis in patients admitted to an intensive care unit. Intensive Care Med 1995;21:24.

Levine, MN, Raskob, G, Beyth, RJ, et al. Hemorrhagic complications of anticoagulant treatment: the Seventh ACCP Conference on Antithrombotic and Thrombolytic Therapy. Chest 2004;126:287S.

Li, JZ, Winston, LG, Moore, DH, Bent, S. Efficacy of short-course antibiotic regimens for community-acquired pneumonia: a meta-analysis. Am J Med 2007;120:783.

Lim, WS, Macfarlane, JT, Boswell, TC, et al. Study of community acquired pneumonia aetiology (SCAPA) in adults admitted to hospital: implications for management guidelines. Thorax 2001;56:296.

Lin, K, Watkins, B, Johnson, T, et al. Screening for chronic obstructive pulmonary disease using spirometry: summary of the evidence for the U.S. Preventive Services Task Force. Ann Intern Med 2008;148:535.

Lode, H, File, TM Jr, Mandell, L, et al. Oral gemifloxacin versus sequential therapy with intravenous ceftriaxone/oral cefuroxime with or without a macrolide in the treatment of patients hospitalized with community-acquired pneumonia: a randomized, open-label, multicenter study of clinical efficacy and tolerability. Clin Ther 2002; 24:1915.

Lopez, AD, Shibuya, K, Rao, C, et al. Chronic obstructive pulmonary disease: current burden and future projections. Eur Respir J 2006;27:397.

Luna, CM, Famiglietti, A, Absi, R, et al. Community-acquired pneumonia: etiology, epidemiology, and outcome at a teaching hospital in Argentina. Chest 2000;118:1344.

Lung function testing: selection of reference values and interpretative strategies. American Thoracic Society. Am Rev Respir Dis 1991;144:1202.

MacFarlane, JT, Finch, RG, Ward, MJ, Macrae, AD. Hospital study of adult community-acquired pneumonia. Lancet1982;2:255.

Mandell, LA, Marrie, TJ, Grossman, RF, et al. Canadian guidelines for the initial management of community-acquired pneumonia: an evidence-based update by the Canadian Infectious Diseases Society and the Canadian Thoracic Society. Clin Infect Dis 2000;31:383.

Mandell, LA, Wunderink, RG, Anzueto, A, et al. Infectious Diseases Society of America/ American Thoracic Society consensus guidelines on the management of community-acquired pneumonia in adults. Clin Infect Dis 2007;44 Suppl 2:S27.

Mannino, DM, Buist, AS, Petty, TL, et al. Lung function and mortality in the United States: data from the First National Health and Nutrition Examination Survey follow up study. Thorax 2003;58:388.

Mannino, DM, Gagnon, RC, Petty, TL, Lydick, E. Obstructive lung disease and low lung function in adults in the United States: data from the National Health and Nutrition Examination Survey, 1988-1994. Arch Intern Med 2000;160:1683.

Marik, PE. The clinical features of severe community-acquired pneumonia presenting as septic shock. Norasept II Study Investigators. J Crit Care 2000;15:85.

Marrie, TJ, Poulin-Costello, M, Beecroft, MD, Herman-Gnjidic, Z. Etiology of community-acquired pneumonia treated in an ambulatory setting. Respir Med 2005;99:60.

Marrie, TJ, Shariatzadeh, MR.Community-acquired pneumonia requiring admission to an intensive care unit: a descriptive study. Medicine (Baltimore) 2007;86:103.

Marston, BJ, Plouffe, JF, File, TM Jr, et al. Incidence of community-acquired pneumonia requiring hospitalization. Results of a population-based active surveillance Study in Ohio. The Community-Based Pneumonia Incidence Study Group. Arch Intern Med 1997;157:1709.

Martin, RJ, Pak, J. Overnight theophylline concentrations and effects on sleep and lung function in chronic obstructive pulmonary disease. Am Rev Respir Dis 1992;145:540.

Mason, CM, Nelson, S. Pulmonary host defenses and factors predisposing to lung infection. Clin Chest Med 2005;26:11.

Mathru, M, Venus, B, Smith, RA, et al. Treatment of low cardiac output complicating acute pulmonary hypertension in normovolemic goats. Crit Care Med 1986;14:120.

Matthay, RA, Niederman, MS, Wiedemann, HP. Cardiovascular-pulmonary interaction in chronic obstructive pulmonary disease with special reference to the pathogenesis and management of cor pulmonale. Med Clin North Am 1990;74:571.

Melbye, H, Berdal, BP, Straume, B, et al. Pneumonia – a clinical or radiographic diagnosis? Etiology and clinical features of lower respiratory tract infection in adults in general practice. Scand J Infect Dis 1992;24:647.

Menendez, R, Cordoba, J, de La, Cuadra, P, et al. Value of the polymerase chain reaction assay in noninvasive respiratory samples for diagnosis of community-acquired pneumonia. Am J Respir Crit Care Med 1999;159:1868.

Menendez, R, Torres, A, Rodriquez de Castro, F, et al. Reaching stability in community-acquired pneumonia: the effects of the severity of disease, treatment, and the characteristics of patients. Clin Infect Dis 2004;39:1783.

Menendez, R, Torres, A, Zalacain, R, et al. Risk factors of treatment failure in community acquired pneumonia: implications for disease outcome. Thorax 2004;59:960.

Meneveau, N, Seronde, MF, Blonde, MC, et al. Management of unsuccessful thrombolysis in acute massive pulmonary embolism. Chest 2006;129:1043.

Metersky, ML, Sweeney, TA, Getzow, MB, et al. Antibiotic timing and diagnostic uncertainty in Medicare patients with pneumonia: is it reasonable to expect all patients to receive antibiotics within 4 hours?. Chest 2006;130:16.

Michetti, G, Pugliese, C, Bamberga, M, et al. Community-acquired pneumonia: is there difference in etiology between hospitalized and out-patients?. Minerva Med 1995;86:341.

Miller, MR, Hankinson, J, Brusasco, V, et al. Standardisation of spirometry. Eur Respir J 2005;26:319.

Mitka, M. JCAHO tweaks emergency departments' pneumonia treatment standards. JAMA 2007;297:1758.

Mittl, RJ Jr, Schwab, RJ, Duchin, JS, et al. Radiographic resolution of community-acquired pneumonia. Am J Respir Crit Care Med 1994;149:630.

Moine, P, Vercken, JB, Chevret, S, et al. Severe community-acquired pneumonia. Etiology, epidemiology, and prognosis factors. French Study Group for Community-Acquired Pneumonia in the Intensive Care Unit. Chest 1994;105:1487.

Molloy, WD, Lee, KY, Girling, L, et al. Treatment of shock in a canine model of pulmonary embolism. Am Rev Respir Dis 1984;130:870.

Mortensen, EM, Coley, CM, Singer, DE, et al. Causes of death for patients with community-acquired pneumonia: results from the Pneumonia Patient Outcomes Research Team cohort study. Arch Intern Med 2002;162:1059.

Moser, KM. Venous thromboembolism. Am Rev Respir Dis 1990;141:235.

Muller, MP, Low, DE, Green, KA, et al. Clinical and epidemiologic features of group A streptococcal pneumonia in Ontario, Canada. Arch Intern Med 2003;163:467.

Murciano, D, Auclair, MH, Pariente, R, Aubier, M. A randomized, controlled trial of theophylline in patients with severe chronic obstructive pulmonary disease. N Engl J Med 1989;320:1521.

Nathan, RA, Sorkness, CA, Kosinski, M, et al. Development of the asthma control test: a survey for assessing asthma control. J Allergy Clin Immunol 2004;113:59.

Nathan, RV, Rhew, DC, Murray, C, et al. In-hospital observation after antibiotic switch in pneumonia: a national evaluation. Am J Med 2006;119:512.

National Asthma Education and Prevention Program: Expert panel report III: Guidelines for the diagnosis and management of asthma. Bethesda, MD: National Heart, Lung, and Blood Institute, 2007. (NIH publication no. 08-4051).

National Asthma Education Program. Expert panel report on diagnosis and management of asthma. U.S. Government Printing Office, Washington D.C. NIH Publication No. 92-2113A, 1992.

Neill, M, Martin, IR, Weir, R, et al. Community acquired pneumonia: aetiology and usefulness of severity criteria on admission. Thorax 1996;51:1010.

Nelson, HS. Adrenergic bronchodilators. N Engl J Med 1995;333:499.

Niederman, MS. Recent advances in community-acquired pneumonia: inpatient and outpatient. Chest 2007;131:1205.

Niewoehner, DE, Rice, K, Cote, C, et al. Prevention of exacerbations of chronic obstructive pulmonary disease with tiotropium, a once-daily inhaled anticholinergic bronchodilator: a randomized trial. Ann Intern Med 2005;143:317.

O'Brien, C, Guest, PJ, Hill, SL, Stockley, RA. Physiological and radiological characterisation of patients diagnosed with chronic obstructive pulmonary disease in primary care. Thorax 2000;55:635.

Obstructive lung disease. Med Clin North Am 1990;74:547.

O'Donnell, DE, Fluge, T, Gerken, F, et al. Effects of tiotropium on lung hyperinflation, dyspnoea and exercise tolerance in COPD. Eur Respir J 2004;23:832.

Olaechea, PM, Quintana, JM, Gallardo, MS, et al. A predictive model for the treatment approach to community-acquired pneumonia in patients needing ICU admission. Intensive Care Med 1996;22:1294.

Oosterheert, JJ, Bonten, MJ, Schneider, MM, et al. Effectiveness of early switch from intravenous to oral antibiotics in severe community acquired pneumonia: multicentre randomised trial. BMJ 2006;333:1193.

Oosterheert, JJ, van Loon, AM, Schuurman, R, et al. Impact of rapid detection of viral and atypical bacterial pathogens by real-time polymerase chain reaction for patients with lower respiratory tract infection. Clin Infect Dis 2005;41:1438.

Ortqvist, A, Hedlund, J, Grillner, L, et al. Aetiology, outcome and prognostic factors in community-acquired pneumonia requiring hospitalization. Eur Respir J 1990;3:1105.

Ortqvist, A, Sterner, G, Nilsson, JA. Severe community-acquired pneumonia: factors influencing need of intensive care treatment and prognosis. Scand J Infect Dis 1985;17:377.

Osborne, ML, Pedula, KL, O'Hollaren, M, et al. Assessing future need for acute care in adult asthmatics: the profile of asthma risk study: a prospective health maintenance organization-based study. Chest 2007;132:1151.

Ostergaard, L, Andersen, PL. Etiology of community-acquired pneumonia. Evaluation by transtracheal aspiration, blood culture, or serology. Chest 1993;104:1400.

Outbreak of group a streptococcal pneumonia among Marine Corps recruits – California, November 1-December 20, 2002. MMWR Morb Mortal Wkly Rep 2003;52:106.

Pachon, J, Prados, D, Capote, F, et al. Severe community-acquired pneumonia. Etiology, prognosis, and treatment. Am Rev Respir Dis 1990;142:369.

Paganin, F, Lilienthal, F, Bourdin, A, et al. Severe community-acquired pneumonia: assessment of microbial aetiology as mortality factor. Eur Respir J 2004;24:779.

Pareja, A, Bernal, C, Leyva, A, et al. Etiologic study of patients with community-acquired pneumonia. Chest 1992;101:1207.

Park, KJ, Bergin, CJ, Clausen, JL. Quantitation of emphysema with three-dimensional CT densitometry: comparison with two-dimensional analysis, visual emphysema scores, and pulmonary function test results. Radiology 1999;211:541.

Pennock, BE, Cottrell, JJ, Rodgers, RM. Pulmonary function testing. Arch Intern Med 1983;143:2123.

Petsky, HL, Kynaston, JA, Turner, C, et al. Tailored interventions based on sputum eosinophils versus clinical symptoms for asthma in children and adults. Cochrane Database Syst Rev 2007;CD005603.

Petty, RL, Nett, LM. COPD: Prevention in the primary care setting. The National Lung Health Education Program, 2001, 341.

Petty, TL, Silvers, GW, Stanford, RE. Mild emphysema is associated with reduced elastic recoil and increased lung size but not with air-flow limitation. Am Rev Respir Dis 1987;136:867.

Pierce, JA, Hocott, JB, Ebert, RV. The collagen and elastin content of the lung in emphysema. Ann Intern Med 1961;55:210.

Qaseem, A, Snow, V, Shekelle, P, et al. Diagnosis and management of stable chronic obstructive pulmonary disease: a clinical practice guideline from the American College of Physicians. Ann Intern Med 2007;147:633.

Rabe, KF. Treating COPD – the TORCH trial, P values, and the Dodo. N Engl J Med 2007;356:851.

Ram, FS, Jones, PW, Castro, AA, et al. Oral theophylline for chronic obstructive pulmonary disease. Cochrane Database Syst Rev 2002;CD003902.

Ramirez, JA, Srinath, L, Ahkee, S, et al. Early switch from intravenous to oral cephalosporins in the treatment of hospitalized patients with community-acquired pneumonia. Arch Intern Med 1995;155:1273.

Ramirez, JA, Vargas, S, Ritter, GW, et al. Early switch from intravenous to oral antibiotics and early hospital discharge: a prospective observational study of 200 consecutive patients with community-acquired pneumonia. Arch Intern Med 1999;159:2449.

Raschke, RA, Reilly, BM, Guidry, JR, et al. The weight-based heparin dosing nomogram compared with a "standard care" nomogram. Ann Intern Med 1993;119:874.

Read, RC. Evidence-based medicine: empiric antibiotic therapy in community-acquired pneumonia. J Infect 1999;39:171.

Rello, J, Quintana, E, Ausina, V, et al. A three-year study of severe community-acquired pneumonia with emphasis on outcome. Chest 1993;103:232.

Rennard, S, Decramer, M, Calverley, PM, et al. Impact of COPD in North America and Europe in 2000: subjects' perspective of Confronting COPD International Survey. Eur Respir J 2002;20:799.

Rennard, SI, Anderson, W, ZuWallack, R, et al. Use of a long-acting inhaled beta2-adrenergic agonist, salmeterol xinafoate, in patients with chronic obstructive pulmonary disease. Am J Respir Crit Care Med 2001;163:1087.

Rennard, SI. COPD: overview of definitions, epidemiology, and factors influencing its development. Chest 1998;113:235S.

Rennard, SI, Vestbo, J. COPD: the dangerous underestimate of 15%. Lancet 2006;367:1216.

Rodriguez, A, Mendia, A, Sirvent, JM, et al. Combination antibiotic therapy improves survival in patients with community-acquired pneumonia and shock. Crit Care Med 2007;35:1493.

Rosenberger, P, Shernan, SK, Mihaljevic, T, Eltzschig, HK. Transesophageal echocardiography for detecting extrapulmonary thrombi during pulmonary embolectomy. Ann Thorac Surg 2004;78:862.

Rosenbloom, J, Campbell, EJ, Mumford, R, et al. Biochemical/immunologic markers of emphysema. Ann N Y Acad Sci 1991;624 Suppl:7.

Roson, B, Carratala, J, Fernandez-Sabe, N, et al. Causes and factors associated with early failure in hospitalized patients with community-acquired pneumonia. Arch Intern Med 2004;164:502.

Sabatine, M, et al. Pocket Medicine, 2nd ed, Lippincott Williams & Wilkins, Philadelphia, PA, 2004.

Schmitz-Rode, T, Janssens, U, Duda, SH, et al. Massive pulmonary embolism: percutaneous emergency treatment by pigtail rotation catheter. J Am Coll Cardiol 2000;36:375.

Scott, JA, Hall, AJ, Muyodi, C, et al. Aetiology, outcome, and risk factors for mortality among adults with acute pneumonia in Kenya. Lancet 2000;355:1225.

Screening for chronic obstructive pulmonary disease using spirometry: U.S. Preventive Services Task Force recommendation statement. Ann Intern Med 2008;148:529.

Severe methicillin-resistant Staphylococcus aureus community-acquired pneumonia associated with influenza – Louisiana and Georgia, December 2006-January 2007. MMWR Morb Mortal Wkly Rep 2007;56:325.

Sharma, S. Chronic obstructive pulmonary disease; eMedicine Journal [serial online], 2004. Available from http://emedicine.medscape.com/article/297664-overview

Sharma, S. Pulmonary embolism; eMedicine Journal [serial online], 2006. Available from http://emedicine.medscape.com/article/300901-overview

Shaw, DE, Berry, MA, Thomas, M, et al. The use of exhaled nitric oxide to guide asthma management: a randomized controlled trial. Am J Respir Crit Care Med 2007;176:231.

Shefet, D, Robenshtock, E, Paul, M, Leibovici, L. Empiric antibiotic coverage of atypical pathogens for community acquired pneumonia in hospitalized adults. Cochrane Database Syst Rev 2005;CD004418.

Shim, C, Williams, MH Jr. Bronchial response to oral versus aerosol metaproterenol in asthma. Ann Intern Med 1980;93:428.

Shim, C, Williams, MH Jr. Comparison of oral aminophylline and aerosol metaproterenol in asthma. Am J Med 1981;71:452.

Shirtcliffe, P, Weatherall, M, Marsh, S, et al. COPD prevalence in a random population survey: a matter of definition. Eur Respir J 2007;30:232.

Siafakas, NM, Vermeire, P, Pride, NB, et al. Optimal assessmentand management of chronic obstructive pulmonary disease (COPD). The European Respiratory Society Task Force. Eur Respir J 1995;8:1398.

Silber, SH, Garrett, C, Singh, R, et al. Early administration of antibiotics does not shorten time to clinical stability in patients with moderate-to-severe community-acquired pneumonia. Chest 2003;124:1798.

Sin, DD, Paul Man, SF. Cooling the fire within: inhaled corticosteroids and cardiovascular mortality in COPD. Chest 2006;130:629.

Sin, DD, Tu, JV. Inhaled corticosteroid therapy reduces the risk of rehospitalization and all-cause mortality in elderly asthmatics. Eur Respir J 2001;17:380.

Sin, DD, Wu, L, Man, SF. The relationship between reduced lung function and cardiovascular mortality: a population-based study and a systematic review of the literature. Chest 2005;127:1952.

Smith, AD, Cowan, JO, Brassett, KP, Herbison, GP, Taylor, DR.Use of exhaled nitric oxide measurements to guide treatment in chronic asthma. N Engl J Med 2005;352:2163.

Smith, HJ, Oriol, A, Morch, J, McGregor, M. Hemodynamic studies in cardiogenic shock. Treatment with isoproterenol and metaraminol. Circulation 1967;35:1084.

Smith, HR, Irvin, CG, Cherniack, RM. The utility of spirometry in the diagnosis of reversible airways obstruction. Chest 1992;101:1577.

Snider, GL. Nosology for our day: its application to chronic obstructive pulmonary disease. Am J Respir Crit Care Med 2003;167:678.

Socan, M, Marinic-Fiser, N, Kraigher, A, et al. Microbial aetiology of community-acquired pneumonia in hospitalised patients. Eur J Clin Microbiol Infect Dis 1999;18:777.

Sorensen, J, Forsberg, P, Hakanson, E, et al. A new diagnostic approach to the patient with severe pneumonia. Scand J Infect Dis 1989;21:33.

Standards for the diagnosis and care of patients with chronic obstructive pulmonary disease. American Thoracic Society. Am J Respir Crit Care Med 1995;152:S77.

Stankovic, C, Mahajan, PV, Asmar, BI. Methicillin-resistant Staphylococcus aureus as a cause of community-acquired pneumonia. Curr Infect Dis Rep 2007;9:223.

Stein, PD, Hull, RD, Raskob, GE. Withholding treatment in patients with acute pulmonary embolism who have a high risk of bleeding and negative serial noninvasive leg tests. Am J Med 2000;109:301.

Stockley, RA, Chopra, N, Rice, L. Addition of salmeterol to existing treatment in patients with COPD: a 12 month study. Thorax 2006;61:122.

Strieter, RM, Belperio, JA, Keane, MP. Host innate defenses in the lung: the role of cytokines. Curr Opin Infect Dis 2003;16:193.

Sutherland, ER, Martin, RJ. Airway inflammation in chronic obstructive pulmonary disease: comparisons with asthma. J Allergy Clin Immunol 2003;112:819.

Swanney, MP, Jensen, RL, Crichton, DA, et al. FEV(6) is an acceptable surrogate for FVC in the spirometric diagnosis of airway obstruction and restriction. Am J Respir Crit Care Med 2000;162:917.

Tajima, H, Murata, S, Kumazaki, T, et al. Hybrid treatment of acute massive pulmonary thromboembolism: mechanical fragmentation with a modified rotating pigtail catheter, local fibrinolytic therapy, and clot aspiration followed by systemic fibrinolytic therapy. AJR Am J Roentgenol 2004;183:589.

Tanaka, H, Tajimi, K, Matsumoto, A, Kobayashi, K. Vasodilatory effects of milrinone on pulmonary vasculature in dogs with pulmonary hypertension due to pulmonary embolism: a comparison with those of dopamine and dobutamine. Clin Exp Pharmacol Physiol 1990;17:681.

Tapson, VF, Fulkerson, WJ, Saltzman, HA (Ed). Venous thromboembolism. Clin Chest Med 1995;16:229.

Templeton, KE, Scheltinga, SA, van den, Eeden, WC, et al. Improved diagnosis of the etiology of community-acquired pneumonia with real-time polymerase chain reaction. Clin Infect Dis 2005;41:345.

Thabut, G, Thabut, D, Myers, RP, et al. Thrombolytic therapy of pulmonary embolism: a meta-analysis. J Am Coll Cardiol 2002;40:1660.

The aetiology, management and outcome of severe community-acquired pneumonia on the intensive care unit. The British Thoracic Society Research Committee and The Public Health Laboratory Service. Respir Med 1992;86:7.

The urokinase pulmonary embolism trial. A national cooperative study. Circulation 1973;47:II1.

Torres, A, Serra-Batlles, J, Ferrer, A, et al. Severe community-acquired pneumonia. Epidemiology and prognostic factors. Am Rev Respir Dis 1991;144:312.

Turato, G, Zuin, R, Miniati, M, et al. Airway inflammation in severe chronic obstructive pulmonary disease: relationship with lung function and radiologic emphysema. Am J Respir Crit Care Med 2002;166:105.

Valdivia, L. Coccidioidomycosis as a Common Cause of Community-acquired Pneumonia. Emerg Infect Dis 2006;12:958.

Vandevoorde, J, Verbanck, S, Schuermans, D, et al. FEV1/FEV6 and FEV6 as an alternative for FEV1/FVC and FVC in the spirometric detection of airway obstruction and restriction. Chest 2005;127:1560.

van Noord, JA, Aumann, JL, Janssens, E, et al. Comparison of tiotropium once daily, formoterol twice daily and both combined once daily in patients with COPD. Eur Respir J 2005;26:214.

van Noord, JA, Aumann, JL, Janssens, E, et al. Effects of tiotropium with and without formoterol on airflow obstruction and resting hyperinflation in patients with COPD. Chest 2006;129:509.

Vasu, MA, O'Keefe, DD, Kapellakis, GZ, et al. Myocardial oxygen consumption: effects of epinephrine, isoproterenol, dopamine, norepinephrine, and dobutamine. Am J Physiol 1978;235:H237.

Vayalumkal, JV, Whittingham, H, Vanderkooi, O, et al. Necrotizing pneumonia and septic shock: suspecting CA-MRSA in patients presenting to Canadian emergency departments. CJEM 2007;9:300.

Vincken, W, van Noord, JA, Greefhorst, AP, et al. Improved health outcomes in patients with COPD during 1 yr's treatment with tiotropium. Eur Respir J 2002;19:209.

Vlahovic, G, Russell, ML, Mercer, RR, Crapo, JD. Cellular and connective tissue changes in alveolar septal walls in emphysema. Am J Respir Crit Care Med 1999;160:2086.

Vollmer, WM, Markson, LE, O'Connor, E, et al. Association of asthma control with health care utilization and quality of life. Am J Respir Crit Care Med 1999;160:1647.

Waterer, GW, Kessler, LA, Wunderink, RG. Delayed administration of antibiotics and atypicalpresentation in community-acquired pneumonia. Chest 2006;130:11.

Wattanathum, A, Chaoprason, C, Nunthapisud, P, et al. Community-acquired pneumonia in southeast Asia: the microbial differences between ambulatory and hospitalized patients. Chest 2003;123:1512.

Woo, PCY, Lau, SKP, Tsoi, H, et al. Clinical and molecular epidemiological features of coronavirus HKU1-associated community-acquired pneumonia. J Infect Dis 2005; 192:1898.

Woodhead, MA, Macfarlane, JT, Rodgers, FG, et al. Aetiology and outcome of severe community-acquired pneumonia. J Infect 1985;10:204.

Wunderink, RG, Waterer, GW. Community-acquired pneumonia: pathophysiology and host factors with focus on possible new approaches to management of lower respiratory tract infections. Infect Dis Clin North Am 2004;18:743.

Yalamanchili, K, Fleisher, AG, Lehrman, SG, et al. Open pulmonary embolectomy for treatment of major pulmonary embolism. Ann Thorac Surg 2004;77:819.

Yawn, BP, Enright, PL, Lemanske, RF Jr, et al. Spirometry can be done in family physicians' offices and alters clinical decisions in management of asthma and COPD. Chest 2007;132:1162.

GASTROENTEROLOGY

Abou-Assi, S, Craig, K, O'Keefe, SJ. Hypocaloric jejunal feeding is better than total parenteral nutrition in acute pancreatitis: results of a randomized comparative study. Am J Gastroenterol 2002;97:2255.

Agarwal, N, Pitchumoni, CS, Sivaprasad, AV. Evaluating tests for acute pancreatitis. Am J Gastroenterol 1990;85:356.

Al-Omran, M, Groof, A, Wilke, D. Enteral versus parenteral nutrition for acute pancreatitis. Cochrane Database Syst Rev 2003;CD002837.

Andriulli, A, Leandro, G, Clemente, R, et al. Meta-analysis of somatostatin, ocreotide and gabexate mesilate in the therapy of acute pancreatitis. Aliment Pharmacol Ther 1998;12:237.

Arvanitakis, M, Delhaye, M, De, Maertelaere, V, et al. Computed tomography and magnetic resonance imaging in the assessment of acute pancreatitis. Gastroenterology 2004;126:715.

Aubertin, JM, Levoir, D, Bouillot, JL, et al. Endoscopic ultrasonography immediately prior to laparoscopic cholecystectomy: a prospective evaluation. Endoscopy 1996; 28:667.

August, DA, Thorn, D, Fisher, RL, Welchek, CM. Home parenteral nutrition for patients with inoperable malignant bowel obstruction. JPEN J Parenter Enteral Nutr 1991;15:323.

Bai, Y, Gao, J, Zou, DW, Li, ZS. Prophylactic antibiotics cannot reduce infected pancreatic necrosis and mortality in acute necrotizing pancreatitis: evidence from a meta-analysis of randomized controlled trials. Am J Gastroenterol 2008;103:104.

Ballinger, AB, Barnes, E, Alstead, EM, Fairclough, PD. Is intervention necessary after first episode of idiopathic acute pancreatitis? Gut 1996;38:293.

Balthazar, EJ, Fisher, LA. Hemorrhagic complications of pancreatitis: radiologic evaluation with emphasis on CT imaging. Pancreatology 2001;1:306.

Balthazar, EJ, Freeny, PC. Contrast-enhanced computed tomography in acute pancreatitis: is it beneficial or harmful? Gastroenterology 1994;106:259.

Balthazar, EJ, Freeny, PC, van Sonnenberg, E. Imaging and intervention in acute pancreatitis. Radiology 1994;193:297.

Balthazar, EJ, Ranson, JH, Naidich, DP, et al. Acute pancreatitis: prognostic value of CT. Radiology 1985;156:767.

Balthazar, EJ, Robinson, DL, Megibow, AJ, Ranson, JH. Acute pancreatitis: value of CT in establishing prognosis. Radiology 1990;174:331.

Banks, PA, Freeman, ML. Practice guidelines in acute pancreatitis. Am J Gastroenterol 2006;101:2379.

Baron, TH, Morgan, DE. Endoscopic transgastric irrigation tube placement via PEG for debridement of organized pancreatic necrosis. Gastrointest Endosc 1999;50:574.

Bassi, C, Falconi, M, Talamini, G, et al. Controlled clinical trial of pefloxacin versus imipenem in severe acute pancreatitis. Gastroenterology 1998;115:1513.

Bassi, C, Larvin, M, Villatoro, E. Antibiotic therapy for prophylaxis against infection of pancreatic necrosis in acute pancreatitis. Cochrane Database Syst Rev 2003;CD002941.

Beck, DE, Cohen, Z, Fleshman, JW, et al. A prospective, randomized, multicenter, controlled study of the safety of seprafilm adhesion barrier in abdominopelvic surgery of the intestine. Dis Colon Rectum 2003;46:1310.

Becker, JM, Dayton, MT, Fazio, VW, et al. Prevention of postoperative abdominal adhesions by a sodium hyaluronate-based bioresorbable membrane: a prospective, randomized, double-blind multicenter study. J Am Coll Surg 1996;183:297.

Beger, HG, Bittner, R, Block, S, Buchler, M. Bacterial contamination of pancreatic necrosis. A prospective clinical study. Gastroenterology 1986;91:433.

Beger, HG, Buchler, M, Bittner, R, et al. Necrosectomy and postoperative local lavage in patients with necrotizing pancreatitis: results of a prospective clinical trial. World J Surg 1988;12:255.

Bennett, RG, Petrozzi, JW. Nodular subcutaneous fat necrosis. A manifestation of silent pancreatitis. Arch Dermatol 1975;111:896.

Bergstein, JM, Condon, RE. Obturator hernia: current diagnosis and treatment. Surgery 1996;119:133.

Besselink, MG, van Santvoort, HC, Buskens, E, et al. Probiotic prophylaxis in predicted severe acute pancreatitis: a randomised, double-blind, placebo-controlled trial. Lancet 2008;371:651.

Besselink, MG, Verwer, TJ, Schoenmaeckers, EJ, et al. Timing of surgical intervention in necrotizing pancreatitis. Arch Surg 2007;142:1194.

Bradley, EL III. A clinically based classification system for acute pancreatitis. Summary of the International Symposium on Acute Pancreatitis, Atlanta, Ga, September 11 through 13, 1992. Arch Surg 1993;128:586.

Bradley, EL III, Allen, K. A prospective longitudinal study of observation versus surgical intervention in the management of necrotizing pancreatitis. Am J Surg 1991;161:19.

Brolin, RE, Krasna, MJ, Mast, BA. Use of tubes and radiographs in the management of small bowel obstruction. Ann Surg 1987;206:126.

Brown, A, Baillargeon, JD, Hughes, MD, Banks, PA. Can fluid resuscitation prevent pancreatic necrosis in severe acute pancreatitis?. Pancreatology 2002;2:104.

Buchler, M, Malfertheiner, P, Friess, H, et al. Human pancreatic tissue concentration of bactericidal antibiotics. Gastroenterology 1992;103:1902.

Bulkley, GB, Zuidema, GD, Hamilton, SR, et al. Intraoperative determination of small intestinal viability following ischemic injury: a prospective, controlled trial of two adjuvant methods (Doppler and fluorescein) compared with standard clinical judgment. Ann Surg 1981;193:628.

Butler, JA, Cameron, BL, Morrow, M, et al. Small bowel obstruction in patients with a prior history of cancer. Am J Surg 1991;162:624.

Calvo, MM, Bujanda, L, Calderon, A, et al. Role of magnetic resonance cholangiopancreatography in patients with suspected choledocholithiasis. Mayo Clin Proc 2002;77:422.

Clancy, TE, Ashley, SW. Current management of necrotizing pancreatitis. Adv Surg 2002;36:103.

Clavien, PA, Richon, J, Burgan, S, Rohner, A. Gallstone ileus. Br J Surg 1990;77:737.

Connor, S, Alexakis, N, Raraty, MG, et al. Early and late complications after pancreatic necrosectomy. Surgery 2005;137:499.

Cooperman, M, Pace, WG, Martin, EW Jr, et al. Determination of viability of ischemic intestine by Doppler ultrasound. Surgery 1978;83:705.

Czyrko, C, Weltz, CR, Markowitz, RI, O'Neill, JA. Blunt abdominal trauma resulting in intestinal obstruction: when to operate?. J Trauma 1990;30:1567.

Dahl, PR, Su, WP, Cullimore, WC, Dicken, CH. Pancreatic panniculitis. J Am Acad Dermatol 1995;33:413.

Delcenserie, R, Yzet, T, Ducroix, JP. Prophylactic antibiotics in treatment of severe acute alcoholic pancreatitis. Pancreas 1996;13:198.

Dellinger, EP, Tellado, JM, Soto, NE, et al. Early antibiotic treatment for severe acute necrotizing pancreatitis: a randomized, double-blind, placebo-controlled study. Ann Surg 2007;245:674.

Dervenis, C, Johnson, CD, Bassi, C, et al. Diagnosis, objective assessment of severity, and management of acute pancreatitis. Santorini consensus conference. Int J Pancreatol 1999;25:195.

Eatock, FC, Chong, P, Menezes, N, et al. A randomized study of early nasogastric versus nasojejunal feeding in severe acute pancreatitis. Am J Gastroenterol 2005;100:432.

Elfstrom, J. The timing of cholecystectomy in patients with gallstine pancreatitis: a retrospective analysis of 89 patients. Acta Chir Scand 1978;144:487.

Ellis, CN, Boggs, HW Jr, Slagle, GW, Cole, PA. Small bowel obstruction after colon resection for benign and malignant diseases. Dis Colon Rectum 1991;34:367.

Fabri, PJ, Ellison, EC, Anderson, ED, Kudsk, KA. High molecular weight dextran – effect on adhesion formation and peritonitis in rats. Surgery 1983;94:336.

Fan, ST, Lai, EC, Mok, FP, et al. Early treatment of acute biliary pancreatitis by endoscopic papillotomy. N Engl J Med 1993;328:228.

Fazio, VW, Cohen, Z, Fleshman, JW, et al. Reduction in adhesive small-bowel obstruction by Seprafilm adhesion barrier after intestinal resection. Dis Colon Rectum 2006;49:1.

Fleshner, PR, Siegman, MG, Slater, GI, et al. A prospective, randomized trial of short versus long tubes in adhesive small-bowel obstruction. Am J Surg 1995;170:366.

Folsch, UR, Nitsche, R, Ludtke, R, et al. German study group on acute biliary pancreatitis: early ERCP and papillotomy compared with conservative treatment for acute biliary pancreatitis. N Engl J Med 1997;336:237.

Forsmark, CE, Baillie, J. AGA institute technical review on acute pancreatitis. Gastroenterology 2007;132:2022.

Fortson, MR, Freedman, SN, Webster, PD III. Clinical assessment of hyperlipidemic pancreatitis. Am J Gastroenterol 1995;90:2134.

Frager, D, Medwid, SW, Baer, JW, et al. CT of small-bowel obstruction: value in establishing the diagnosis and determining the degree and cause. AJR Am J Roentgenol 1994;162:37.

Franklin, ME Jr, Dorman, JP, Pharand, D. Laparoscopic surgery in acute small bowel obstruction. Surg Laparosc Endosc 1994;4:289.

Freeny, PC, Hauptmann, E, Althaus, AJ, et al. Percutaneous CT-guided catheter drainage of infected acute necrotizing pancreatitis: techniques and results. AJR Am J Roentgenol 1998;170:969.

Furuya, T, Komatsu, M, Takahashi, K, et al. Plasma exchange for hypertriglyceridemic acute necrotizing pancreatitis: report of two cases. Ther Apher 2002;6:454.

Galland, RB, Spencer, J. Surgical management of radiation enteritis. Surgery 1986;99:133.

Gallick, HL, Weaver, DW, Sachs, RJ, Bouwman, DL. Intestinal obstruction in cancer patients. An assessment of risk factors and outcome. Am Surg 1986;52:434.

Gemlo, B, Rayner, AA, Lewis, B, et al. Home support of patients with end-stage malignant bowel obstruction using hydration and venting gastrostomy. Am J Surg 1986;152:100.

Gerzof, SG, Banks, PA, Robbins, AH, et al. Early diagnosis of pancreatic infection by computer tomography guided aspiration. Gastroenterology 1987;93:1315.

Gloor, B, Muller, CA, Worni, M, et al. Pancreatic infection in severe pancreatitis: the role of fungus and multiresistant organisms. Arch Surg 2001;136:592.

Go, VL. Etiology of pancreatitis in the United States. In: Acute Pancreatitis: Diagnosis and Therapy, Bradley, EL (Ed), Raven, New York, 1994, p. 235.

Golub, R, Siddiqi, F, Pohl, D. Role of antibiotics in acute pancreatitis: a meta-analysis. J Gastrointest Surg 1998;2:496.

Greene, WL, Concato, J, Feinstein, AR. Claims of equivalence in medical research: are they supported by the evidence?. Ann Intern Med 2000;132:715.

Grendell, JH. Experimental pancreatitis. Curr Opin Gastroenterol 1991;7:702.

Grewe, M, Tsiotos, GG, Luque de-Leon, E, Sarr, MG. Fungal infection in acute necrotizing pancreatitis. J Am Coll Surg 1999;188:408.

Gumaste, VV, Dave, PB, Weissman, D, Messer, J. Lipase/amylase ratio. A new index that distinguishes acute episodes of alcoholic from nonalcoholic acute pancreatitis. Gastroenterology 1991;101:1361.

Gwozdz, GP, Steinberg, WM, Werner, M, et al. Comparative evaluation of the diagnosis of acute pancreatitis based on serum and urine enzyme assays. Clin Chim Acta 1990;187:243.

Hartwig, W, Maksan, SM, Foitzik, T, et al. Reduction in mortality with delayed surgical therapy of severe pancreatitis. J Gastrointest Surg 2002;6:481.

Hayashi, S, Takayama, T, Masuda, H, et al. Bioresorbable membrane to reduce postoperative small bowel obstruction in patients with gastric cancer: a randomized clinical trial. Ann Surg 2008;247:766.

Heider, TR, Azeem, S, Galanko, JA, Behrns, KE. The natural history of pancreatitis-induced splenic vein thrombosis. Ann Surg 2004;239:876.

Heinrich, S, Schafer, M, Rousson, V, Clavien, PA. Evidence-based treatment of acute pancreatitis: a look at established paradigms. Ann Surg 2006;243:154.

Helm, JF, Venu, RP, Geenen, JE, et al. Effects of morphine on the human sphincter of Oddi. Gut 1988;29:1402.

Hernandez, V, Pascual, I, Almela, P, et al. Recurrence of acute gallstone pancreatitis and relationship with cholecystectomy or endoscopic sphincterotomy. Am J Gastroenterol 2004;99:2417.

Horgan, PG, Gorey, TF. Operative assessment of intestinal viability. Surg Clin North Am 1992;72:143.

Horvath, KD, Kao, LS, Wherry, KL, et al. A technique for laparoscopic-assisted percutaneous drainage of infected pancreatic necrosis and pancreatic abscess. Surg endosc 2001;15:1221.

Ibrahim, IM, Wolodiger, F, Sussman, B, et al. Laparoscopic management of acute small-bowel obstruction. Surg Endosc 1996;10:1012.

Iovanna, JL, Keim, V, Nordback, I, et al. Serum levels of pancreatitis-associated protein as indicators of the course of acute pancreatitis. Gastroenterology 1994;106:728.

Isenmann, R, Ran, B, Berger, HG. Early severe acute pancreatitis: characteristics of a new subgroup. Pancreas 2001;22:274.

Isenmann, R, Runzi, M, Kron, M, et al. Prophylactic antibiotic treatment in patients with predicted severe acute pancreatitis: a placebo-controlled, double-blind trial. Gastroenterology 2004;126:997.

Isenmann, R, Schwarz, M, Rau, B, et al. Characteristics of infection with Candida species in patients with necrotizing pancreatitis. World J Surg 2002;26:372.

Jaakkola, M, Sillanaukee, P, Lof, K, et al. Blood tests for detection of alcoholic cause of acute pancreatitis. Lancet 1994;343:1328.

Jackson, BT. Bowel damage from radiation. Proc R Soc Med 1976;69:683.

Jacobson, BC, Baron, TH, Adler, DG, et al. ASGE guideline: the role of endoscopy in the diagnosis and the management of cystic lesions and inflammatory fluid collections of the pancreas. Gastrointest Endosc 2005;61:363.

Jacobson, BC, Vander Vliet, MB, Hughes, MD, et al. A prospective, randomized trial of clear liquids versus low-fat solid diet as the initial meal in mild acute pancreatitis. Clin Gastroenterol Hepatol 2007;5:946.

Johnson, C, Charnley, R, Rowlands, B, et al. UK guidelines for the management of acute pancreatitis. Gut 2005;54 Suppl 3:1.

Johnson, CD, Kingsnorth, AN, Imrie, CW, et al. Double blind, randomised, placebo controlled study of a platelet activating factor antagonist, lexipafant, in the treatment and prevention of organ failure in predicted severe acute pancreatitis. Gut 2001;48:62.

Johnson, SG, Ellis, CJ, Levitt, MD. Mechanism of increased renal clearance of amylase/creatinine in acute pancreatitis. N Engl J Med 1976;295:1214.

Kaiser, AM, Grady, T, Gerdes, D, et al. Intravenous contrast medium does not increase the severity of acute necrotizing pancreatitis in the opossum. Dig Dis Sci 1995;40:1547.

Kalfarentzos, F, Kehagias, J, Mead, N, et al. Enteral nutrition is superior to parenteral nutrition in severe acute pancreatitis – results of a randomized prospective trial. Br J Surg 1997;84:1665.

Kazmierczak, SC. Biochemical indicators of acute pancreatitis. In: Clinical Pathology of Pancreatic Disorders, Lott, JA (Ed), Humana Press, Totowa, 1997, p. 75.

Keim, V, Teich, Fiedler, F, et al. A comparison of lipase and amylase in the diagnosis of acute pancreatitis in patients with abdominal pain. Pancreas 1998;16:45.

Kemppainen, E, Hedstrom, J, Puolakkainen, P, et al. Increased serum trypsinogen 2 and trypsin 2-alpha 1 antitrypsin complex values identify endoscopic retrograde cholangiopancreatography induced pancreatitis with high accuracy. Gut 1997;41:690.

Kemppainen, E, Hedstrom, J, Puolakkainen, P, et al. Urinary trypsinogen-2 test strip in detecting ERCP-induced pancreatitis. Endoscopy 1997;29:247.

Khoo, D, Hall, E, Motson, R, et al. Palliation of malignant intestinal obstruction using octreotide. Eur J Cancer 1994;30A:28.

Kingsnorth, AN, Galloway, SW, Formela, LJ. Randomized, double-blind phase II trial of Lexipafant, a platelet-activating factor antagonist, in human acute pancreatitis. Br J Surg 1995;82:1414.

Konturek, SJ, Tasler, J, Obtulowicz, W. Localization of cholecystokinin release in intestine of the dog. Am J Physiol 1972;222:16.

Kudo, FA, Nishibe, T, Miyazaki, K, et al. Use of bioresorbable membrane to prevent postoperative small bowel obstruction in transabdominal aortic aneurysm surgery. Surg Today 2004;34:648.

Kylanpaa-Back, M, Kemppainen, E, Puolakkainen, P, et al. Reliable screening for acute pancreatitis with rapid urine trypsinogen-2 test strip. Br J Surg 2000;87:49.

Laws, HL, Kent, RB, III. Acute pancreatitis: management of complicating infection. Am Surg 2000;66:145.

Leach, SD, Gorelick, FS, Modlin, IM. New perspectives on acute pancreatitis. Scand J Gastroenterol 1992;27 Suppl 192:29.

Lecesne, R, Taourel, P, Bret, PM, et al. Acute pancreatitis: interobserver agreement and correlation of CT and MR cholangiopancreatography with outcome. Radiology 1999; 211:727.

Lessinger, JM, Ferard, G. Plasma pancreatic lipase activity: from analytical specificity to clinical efficiency for the diagnosis of acute pancreatitis. Eur J Clin Chem Clin Biochem 1994;32:377.

Levy, P, Heresbach, D, Pariente, EA, et al. Frequency and risk factors of recurrent pain during refeeding in patients with acute pancreatitis: a multivariate multicentre prospective study of 116 patients. Gut 1997;40:262.

Lo, CY, Lorentz, TG, Lau, PW. Obturator hernia presenting as small bowel obstruction. Am J Surg 1994;167:396.

Loo, CC, Tan, JY. Decreasing the plasma triglyceride level in hypertriglyceridemia-induced pancreatitis in pregnancy: a case report. Am J Obstet Gynecol 2002;187:241.

Luiten, EJ, Hop, WC, Lange, JF, Bruining, HA. Controlled clinical trial of selective decontamination for the treatment of severe acute pancreatitis. Ann Surg 1995;222:57.

McClave, SA, Chang, WK, Dhaliwal, R, Heyland, DK. Nutrition support in acute pancreatitis: a systematic review of the literature. JPEN J Parenter Enteral Nutr 2006;30:143.

McClave, SA, Greene, LM, Snider, HL, et al. Comparison of the safety of early enteral vs parenteral nutrition in mild acute pancreatitis. JPEN J Parenter Enteral Nutr 1997;21:14.

Manes, G, Uomo, I, Menchise, A, et al. timing of antibiotic prophylaxis in acute pancreatitis: a controlled randomized study with meropenem. Am J Gastroenterol 2006;101:1348.

Mann, WJ. Surgical management of radiation enteropathy. Surg Clin North Am 1991;71:977.

Marik, PE, Zaloga, GP. Meta-analysis of parenteral nutrition versus enteral nutrition in patients with acute pancreatitis. BMJ 2004;328:1407.

Martin, RG. Malignant tumors of the small intestine. Surg Clin North Am 1986;66:779.

Matulonis, UA, Seiden, MV, Roche, M, et al. Long-acting octreotide for the treatment and symptomatic relief of bowel obstruction in advanced ovarian cancer. J Pain Symptom Manage 2005;30:563.

Mendler, MH, Bouillet, P, Sautereau, D, et al. Value of MR cholangiography in the diagnosis of obstructive diseases of the biliary tree: a study of 58 cases. Am J Gastroenterol 1998;93:2482.

Messori, A, Rampazzo, R, Scroccaro, G, et al. Effectiveness of gabexate mesilate in acute pancreatitis. A metaanalysis. Dig Dis Sci 1995;40:734.

Mier, J, Leon, EL, Castillo, A, Robledo, F. Early versus late necrosectomy in severe necrotizing pancreatitis. Am J Surg 1997;173:71.

Mishler, JM, Durr, GH. Macroamylasemia induced by hydroxyethyl starch – confirmation by gel filtration analysis of serum and urine. Am J Clin Pathol 1980;74:387.

Moreau, JA, Zinsmeister, AR, Melton, LJ, DiMagno, EP. Gallstone pancreatitis and the effect of cholecystectomy. Mayo Clin Proc 1988;63:466.

Moreira, H Jr, Wexner, SD, Yamaguchi, T, et al. Use of bioresorbable membrane (sodium hyaluronate + carboxymethylcellulose) after controlled bowel injuries in a rabbit model. Dis Colon Rectum 2000;43:182.

Moretti, A, Papi, C, Aratari, A, et al. Is early endoscopic retrograde cholangiopancreatography useful in the management of acute biliary pancreatitis? A meta-analysis of randomized controlled trials. Dig Liver Dis 2008;40(5):379-85.

Morgan, DE, Baron, TH, Smith, JK, et al. Pancreatic fluid collections prior to intervention: evaluation with MR imaging compared with CT and US. Radiology 1997;203:773.

Mortele, KJ, Mergo, PJ, Taylor, HM, et al. Splenic and perisplenic involvement in acute pancreatitis: determination of prevalence and morphologic helical CT features. J Comput Assist Tomogr 2001;25:50.

Mukherjee, S. Ileus. eMedicine Journal [serial online], 2008. Available from http://emedicine.medscape.com/article/178948-overview

Nagorney, DM, Sarr, MG, McIlrath, DC. Surgical management of intussusception in the adult. Ann Surg 1981;193:230.

Neoptolemos, JP, Carr-Locke, DL, London, NJ, et al. Controlled trial of urgent endoscopic retrograde cholangiopancreatography and endoscopic sphincterotomy versus conservative treatment for acute pancreatitis due to gallstones. Lancet 1988;2:979.

Newsom, BD, Kukora, JS. Congenital and acquired internal hernias: unusual causes of small bowel obstruction. Am J Surg 1986;152:279.

Nieewenhuijs, VB, Besselink, MGH, van Minnen, LP, Gooszen, HG. Surgical management of acute necrotizing pancreatitis: a 13-year experience and systematic review. Scand J Gastroenterol 2003;38 Suppl 239:111.

Paloyan, D, Simonowitz, D, Skinner, DB. The timing of biliary tract operations in patients with pancreatitis associated with gallstones. Surg Gynecol Obstet 1975;141:737.

Pederzoli, P, Bassi, S, Vesentini, S, et al. A randomized multicenter clinical trial of antibiotic prophylaxis of septic complications in acute necrotizing pancreatitis with imipenem. Surg Gynecol Obstet 1993;176:480.

Petrov, MS, van Santvoort, HC, Besselink, MG, et al. Early endoscopic retrograde cholangiopancreatography versus conservative management in acute biliary pancreatitis without cholangitis: a meta-analysis of randomized trials. Ann Surg 2008;247:250.

Pezzilli, R, Billi, P, Migliori, M, Gullo, L. Clinical value of pancreatitis-associated protein in acute pancreatitis. Am J Gastroenterol 1997;92:1887.

Pickleman, J, Lee, RM. The management of patients with suspected early postoperative small bowel obstruction. Ann Surg 1989;210:216.

Ranson, JH. The timing of biliary surgery in acute pancreatitis. Ann Surg 1979;189:654.

Ranson, JH, Rifkind, KM, Roses, DF, Fink, SD, Eng, K, Spencer, FC. Prognostic signs and the role of operative management in acute pancreatitis. Surg Gynecol Obstet 1974;139(1):69-81.

Ranson, JH, Turner, JW, Roses, DF, et al. Respiratory complications in acute pancreatitis. Ann Surg 1974;179:557.

Redaelli, CA, Schilling, MK, Büchler, MW. Intraoperative laser Doppler flowmetry: a predictor of ischemic injury in acute mesenteric infarction. Dig Surg 1998;15:55.

Rhodes, M, Sussman, L, Cohen, L, Lewis, MP. Randomised trial of laparoscopic exploration of common bile duct versus postoperative endoscopic retrograde cholangiopathy for common bile duct stones. Lancet 1998;351:159.

Richards, WO, Williams, LF Jr. Obstruction of the large and small intestine. Surg Clin North Am 1988;68:355.

Ripamonti, C, De Conno, F, Ventafridda, V, et al. Management of bowel obstruction in advanced and terminal cancer patients. Ann Oncol 1993;4:15.

Ripamonti, C, Mercadante, S, Groff, L, et al. Role of octreotide, scopolamine butylbromide, and hydration in symptom control of patients with inoperable bowel obstruction and nasogastric tubes: a prospective randomized trial. J Pain Symptom Manage 2000;19:23.

Robles, R, Parrilla, P, Escamilla, C, Lujan, JA. Gastrointestinal bezoars. Br J Surg1994;81:1000.

Rodriguez, JR, Razo, AO, Targarona, J, et al. Debridement and closed packing for sterile or infected necrotizing pancreatitis: insights into indications and outcomes in 167 patients. Ann Surg 2008;247:294.

Rodriguez-Ruesga, R, Meagher, AP, Wolff, BG. Twelve-year experience with the long intestinal tube. World J Surg 1995;19:627.

Runzi, M, Niebel, W, Goebell, H, et al. Severe acute pancreatitis: nonsurgical treatment of infected necroses. Pancreas 2005;30:195.

Runzi, M, Saluja, A, Lerch, MM, et al. Early ductal decompression prevents the progression of biliary pancreatitis: an experimental study in the opossum. Gastroenterology 1993;105:157.

Sabatine, M, et al. Pocket Medicine, 2nd ed, Lippincott Williams & Wilkins, Philadelphia, PA, 2004

Sainio, V, Kemppainen, E, Puolakkainen, P, et al. Early antibiotic treatment in acute necrotising pancreatitis. Lancet 1995;346:663.

Sarr, MG, Bulkley, GB, Zuidema, GD. Preoperative recognition of intestinal strangulation obstruction. Prospective evaluation of diagnostic capability. Am J Surg 1983;145:176.

Schmidt, J, Hotz, HG, Foitzik, T, et al. Intravenous contrast medium aggravates the impairment of pancreatic microcirculation in necrotizing pancreatitis in the rat. Ann Surg 1995;221:257.

Seewald, S, Groth, S, Omar, S, et al. Aggressive endoscopic therapy for pancreatic necrosis and pancreatic abscess: a new safe and effective treatment algorithm (videos). Gastrointest Endosc 2005;62:92.

Sharma, VK, Howden, CW. Metaanalysis of randomized controlled trials of endoscopic retrograde cholangiography and endoscopic sphincterotomy for the treatment of acute biliary pancreatitis. Am J Gastroenterol 1999;94:3211.

Silen, W, Hein, MF, Goldman, L. Strangulation obstruction of the small intestine. Arch Surg 1962;85:121.

Smotkin, J, Tenner, S. Laboratory diagnostic tests in acute pancreatitis. J Clin Gastroenterol 2002;34:459.

Speed, CA, Bramble, MG, Corbett, WA, Haslock, I. Non-steroidal anti-inflammatory induced diaphragm disease of the small intestine: complexities of diagnosis and management. Br J Rheumatol 1994;33:778.

Steinberg, WA, Schlesselman, SE. Treatment of pancreatitis: comparison of animal and human studies. Gastroenterology 1987;93:1420.

Steinberg, WM, Geenen, JE, Bradley, EL III, Barkin, JS. Controversies in clinical pancreatology. Recurrent "idiopathic" acute pancreatitis: should a laparoscopic cholecystectomy be the first procedure of choice? Pancreas 1996;13:329.

Stewardson, RH, Bombeck, CT, Nyhus, LM. Critical operative management of small bowel obstruction. Ann Surg 1978;187:189.

Stewart, RM, Page, CP, Brender, J, et al. The incidence and risk of early postoperative small bowel obstruction. A cohort study. Am J Surg 1987;154:643.

Stimac, D, Lenac, T, Marusic, Z. A scoring system for early differentiation of the etiology of acute pancreatitis. Scand J Gastroenterol 1998;33:209.

Stitt, RB, Heslin, DJ, Currie, DJ. Gall-stone ileus. Br J Surg 1967;54:673.

Strickland, P, Lourie, DJ, Suddleson, EA, et al. Is laparoscopy safe and effective for treatment of acute small-bowel obstruction?. Surg Endosc 1999;13:695.

Stringer, MD, Pablot, SM, Brereton, RJ. Paediatric intussusception. Br J Surg 1992;79:867.

Sugiyama, M, Atomi, Y, Hachiya, J. Magnetic resonance cholangiography using half-Fourier acquisition for diagnosing choledocholithiasis. Am J Gastroenterol 1998;93:1886.

Swaroop, VS, Chari, ST, Clain, JE. Severe acute pancreatitis. JAMA 2004;291:2865.

Talamani, G, Uomo, G, Pezzilli, R, et al. Renal function and chest X-rays in the assessment of 539 acute pancreatitis patients. Gut 1997;41:A136.

Tandon, M, Topazian, M. Endoscopic ultrasound in idiopathic acute pancreatitis. Am J Gastroenterol 2001;96:705.

Tang, E, Davis, J, Silberman, H. Bowel obstruction in cancer patients. Arch Surg 1995;130:832.

Taylor, AC, Little, AF, Hennessy, OF, et al. Prospective assessment of magnetic resonance cholangiopancreatography for noninvasive imaging of the biliary tree. Gastrointest Endosc 2002;55:17.

Tenner, S. Initial management of acute pancreatitis: critical issues during the first 72 hours. Am J Gastroenterol 2004;99:2489.

Tenner, S, Dubner, H, Steinberg, W. Predicting gallstone pancreatitis with laboratory parameters. A meta-analysis. Am J Gastroenterol 1994;89:1863.

Tenner, S, Fernandez-del Castillo, C, Warshaw, A, et al. Urinary trypsinogen activation peptide (TAP) predicts severity in patients with acute pancreatitis. Int J Pancreatol 1997;21:105.

Tenner, SM, Steinberg, W. The admission serum lipase: amylase ratio differentiates alcoholic from nonalcoholic acute pancreatitis. Am J Gastroenterol 1992;87:1755.

Thaker, P, Weingarten, L, Friedman, IH. Stenosis of the small intestine due to nonocclusive ischemic disease. Arch Surg 1977;112:1216.

Tietz, NW, Shuey, DF. Lipase in serum – the elusive enzyme: an overview. Clin Chem 1993;39:746.

Toouli, J, Brooke-Smith, M, Bassi, C, et al. Working party report: guidelines for the management of acute pancreatitis. J Gastroenterol Hepatol 2002;17:S1.

Touloukian, RJ. Protocol for the nonoperative treatment of obstructing intramural duodenal hematoma during childhood. Am J Surg 1983;145:330.

Treacy, J, Williams, A, Bais, R, et al. Evaluation of amylase and lipase in the diagnosis of acute pancreatitis. ANZ J Surg 2001;71:577.

Uhl, W, Buchler, MW, Malfertheiner, P, et al. A randomised, double blind, multicentre trial of octreotide in moderate to severe acute pancreatitis. Gut 1999;45:97.

Uhl, W, Muller, CA, Krahenbuhl, L, et al. Acute gallstone pancreatitis: timing of laparoscopic cholecystectomy in mild and severe disease. Surg Endosc 1999;13:1070.

Vege, S, et al. Acute pancreatitis. Up to date online journal, 2008. Available from http://www.uptodate.com/patients/content/topic.do?topicKey=~W0TQKxLHotdLy1

Velasco, JM, Vallina, VL, Bonomo, SR, Hieken, TJ. Postlaparoscopic small bowel obstruction. Rethinking its management. Surg Endosc 1998;12:1043.

Villatoro, E, bassi, C, Larvin, M. Antibiotic therapy for prophylaxis against infection of pancreatic necrosis in acute pancreatitis. Cochrane database Syst Rev 2006;CD002941.

Vrijland, WW, Tseng, LN, Eijkman, HJ, et al. Fewer intraperitoneal adhesions with use of hyaluronic acid-carboxymethylcellulose membrane: a randomized clinical trial. Ann Surg 2002;235:193.

Vu, MK, van der, Veek, PP, Frolich, M, et al. Does jejunal feeding activate exocrine pancreatic secretion?. Eur J Clin Invest 1999;29:1053.

Weigelt, JA, Snyder, WH III, Norman, JL. Complications and results of 160 Baker tube plications. Am J Surg 1980;140:810.

Werner, J, Schmidt, J, Warshaw, AL, et al. The relative safety of MRI contrast agent in acute necrotizing pancreatitis. Ann Surg 1998;227:105.

Werner, M, Steinberg, WM, Pauley, C. Strategic use of individual and combined enzyme indicators for acute pancreatitis analyzed by receiver-operator characteristics. Clin Chem 1989;35:967.

Windsor, AC, Kanwar, S, Li, AG, et al. Compared with parenteral nutrition, enteral feeding attenuates the acute phase response and improves disease severity in acute pancreatitis. Gut 1998;42:431.

Wiseman, DM, Trout, JR, Franklin, RR, Diamond, MP. Metaanalysis of the safety and efficacy of an adhesion barrier (Interceed TC7) in laparotomy. J Reprod Med 1999;44:325.

Yadav, D, Agarwal, N, Pitchumoni, CS. A critical evaluation of laboratory tests in acute pancreatitis. Am J Gastroenterol 2002;97:1309.

Zollinger, RM Jr. Primary neoplasms of the small intestine. Am J Surg 1986;151:654.

NEPHROLOGY

Abraham, SC, Bhagavan, BS, Lee, LA, et al. Upper gastrointestinal tract injury in patients receiving kayexalate (sodium polystyrene sulfonate) in sorbitol: clinical, endoscopic, and histopathologic findings. Am J Surg Pathol 2001;25:637.

Abramson, E, Arky, R. Diabetic acidosis with initial hypokalemia. Therapeutic implications. JAMA 1966;196:401.

Adrogué, HJ, Lederer, ED, Suki, WN, Eknoyan, G. Determinants of plasma potassium levels in diabetic ketoacidosis. Medicine (Baltimore) 1986;65:163.

Adrogue, HJ, Madias, NE. Hypernatremia. N Engl J Med 2000;342:1493.

Adrogue, HJ, Madias, NE. Hyponatremia. N Engl J Med 2000;342:1581.

Ahmed, J, Weisberg, LS. Hyperkalemia in dialysis patients. Semin Dial 2001;14:348.

Alam, NH, Majumder, RH, Fuchs, GJ, and the CHOICE study group. Efficacy and safety of oral rehydration solution with reduced osmolarity in adults with cholera: a randomised double-blind clinical trial. Lancet 1999;354:296.

Allerton, JP, Strom, JA. Hypernatremia due to repeated doses of charcoal-sorbitol. Am J Kidney Dis 1991;17:581.

Allon, M. Hyperkalemia in end-stage renal disease: mechanisms and management. J Am Soc Nephrol 1995;6:1134.

Allon, M, Copkney, C. Albuterol and insulin for treatment of hyperkalemia in hemodialysis patients. Kidney Int 1990;38:869.

Allon, M, Shanklin, N. Adrenergic modulation of extrarenal potassium disposal in men with end-stage renal disease. Kidney Int 1991;40:1103.

Allon, M, Shanklin, N. Effect of albuterol treatment on subsequent dialytic potassium removal. Am J Kidney Dis 1995;26:607.

Allon, M, Takeshian, A, Shanklin, N. Effect of insulin-plus-glucose infusion with or without epinephrine on fasting hyperkalemia. Kidney Int 1993;43:212.

Allon, MA, Shanklin, N. Effect of bicarbonate administration of plasma potassium in dialysis patients: interactions with insulin and albuterol. Am J Kidney Dis 1996;28:508.

Alvestrand, A, Wahren, J, Smith, D, DeFronzo, RA. Insulin-mediated potassium uptake is normal in uremic and healthy subjects. Am J Physiol 1984;246:E174.

Appel, GB. Renal biopsy: how effective, what technique, and how safe. J Nephrol 1993;6:4.

Aselton, PJ, Jick, H. Short-term follow-up study of wax matrix potassium chloride in relation to gastrointestinal bleeding. Lancet 1983;1:184.

Ayus, JC, Wheeler, JM, Arieff, AI. Postoperative hyponatremic encephalopathy in menstruating women. Ann Intern Med 1992;117:891.

Bagshaw, SM, Langenberg, C, Haase, M, et al. Urinary biomarkers in septic acute kidney injury. Intensive Care Med 2007;33:1285.

Ballantyne, F III, Davis, LD, Reynolds, EW Jr. Cellular basis for reversal of hyperkalemic electrocardiographic changes by sodium. Am J Physiol 1975;229:935.

Barlow, ED, De Wardener, HE. Compulsive water drinking. Q J Med 1959;28:235.

Bashour, T, Hsu, I, Gorfinkel, HJ, et al. Atrioventricular and intraventricular conduction in hyperkalemia. Am J Cardiol 1975;35:199.

Bellomo, R, Ronco, C, Kellum, JA, et al. Acute renal failure – definition, outcome measures, animal models, fluid therapy and information technology needs: the Second

International Consensus Conference of the Acute Dialysis Quality Initiative (ADQI) Group. Crit Care 2004;8:R204.

Bennett, M, Dent, CL, Ma, Q, et al. Urine NGAL predicts severity of acute kidney injury after cardiac surgery: a prospective study. Clin J Am Soc Nephrol 2008;3:665.

Berl, T. Treating hyponatremia: damned if we do and damned if we don't. Kidney Int 1990;37:1006.

Berl, T, Linas, SL, Aisenbrey, GA, Anderson, RJ. On the mechanism of polyuria in potassium depletion. The role of polydipsia. J Clin Invest 1977;60:620.

Berne, RM, Levy, MN. Cardiovascular Physiology, 4th ed, Mosby, St Louis, 1981, pp. 7-17.

Bibl, D, Lampl, C, Gabriel, C, et al. Treatment of central pontine myelinolysis with therapeutic plasmapheresis (letter). Lancet 1999;353:1155.

Blum, D, Brasseur, D, Kahn, A, Brachet, E. Safe oral rehydration of hypertonic dehydration. J Pediatr Gastroenterol Nutr 1986;5:232.

Blumberg, A, Weidmann, P, Shaw, S, Gnadinger, M. Effect of various therapeutic approaches on plasma potassium and major regulating factors in terminal renal failure. Am J Med 1988;85:507.

Bonventre, JV. Diagnosis of acute kidney injury: from classic parameters to new biomarkers. Contrib Nephrol 2007;156:213.

Brunner, JE, Redmond, JM, Haggar, AM, et al. Central pontine myelinolysis and pontine lesions after rapid correction of hyponatremia: a prospective magnetic resonance imaging study. Ann Neurol 1990;27:61.

Capasso, G, Jaeger, P, Giebisch, G, et al. Renal bicarbonate reabsorption in the rat. II. Distal tubule load dependence and effect of hypokalemia. J Clin Invest 1987;80:409.

Castellino, P, Bia, M, DeFronzo, RA. Adrenergic modulation of potassium metabolism in uremia. Kidney Int 1990;37:793.

Chalasani, N, Clark, WS, Wilcox, CM. Blood urea nitrogen to creatinine concentration in gastrointestinal bleeding: a reappraisal. Am J Gastroenterol 1997;92:1796.

Charytan, D, Goldfarb, DS. Indications for hospitalization of patients with hyperkalemia. Arch Intern Med 2000;160:1605.

Cheng, JC, Zikos, D, Skopicki, HA, et al. Long-term neurologic outcome in psychogenic water drinkers with severe symptomatic hyponatremia: the effect of rapid correction. Am J Med 1990;88:561.

Cherney, DZ, Davids, MR, Halperin, ML. Acute hyponatraemia and "ecstasy": insights from a quantitative and integrative analysis. QJM 2002;95:475.

Chow, KM, Kwan, BC, Szeto, CC. Clinical studies of thiazide-induced hyponatremia. J Natl Med Assoc 2004;96:1305.

Chute, JP, Taylor, E, Williams, J, et al. A metabolic study of patients with lung cancer and hyponatremia of malignancy. Clin Cancer Res 2006;12:888.

Clausen, T, Everts, ME. Regulation of the Na,K-pump in skeletal muscle. Kidney Int 1989;35:1.

Clayton, JA, Le Jeune, IR, Hall, IP. Severe hyponatraemia in medical in-patients: aetiology, assessment and outcome. QJM 2006;99:505.

Craig, S. Hyponatremia: treatment and medication; eMedicine Journal [serial online], 2009. Available from http://emedicine.medscape.com/article/767624-overview

Davison, JM, Shiells, EA, Philips, PR, Lindheimer, MD. Influence of humoral and volume factors on altered osmoregulation of normal human pregnancy. Am J Physiol 1990;258:F900.

DeRubertis, FR, Michelis, MF, Beck, N, et al. "Essential" hypernatremia due to ineffective osmotic and intact volume regulation of vasopressin secretion. J Clin Invest 1971;50:97.

DeRubertis, FR, Michelis, MF, Davis, BB. "Essential" hypernatremia. Report of three cases and review of the literature. Arch Intern Med 1974;134:889.

Devarajan, P. Emerging biomarkers of acute kidney injury. Contrib Nephrol 2007;156:203.

Dixon, BS, Anderson, RJ. Nonoliguric acute renal failure. Am J Kidney Dis 1985;6:71.

Dominic, JA, Koch, M, Guthrie, GP, Galla, JH. Primary aldosteronism presenting as myoglobinuric acute renal failure. Arch Intern Med 1978;138:1433.

Eknoyan, G. Renal disorders in hepatic failure (letter). Br Med J 1974;2:670.

Espinel, CH, Gregory, AW. Differential diagnosis of acute renal failure. Clin Nephrol 1980;13:73.

Esposito, C, Bellotti, N, Fasoli, G, et al. Hyperkalemia-induced ECG abnormalities in patients with reduced renal function. Clin Nephrol 2004;62:465.

Esson, ML, Schrier, RW. Diagnosis and treatment of acute tubular necrosis. Ann Intern Med 2002;137:744.

Ferrannini, E, Taddei, S, Santoro, D, et al. Independent stimulation of glucose metabolism and Na+-K+ exchange by insulin in the human forearm. Am J Physiol 1988;255:E953.

Fichman, MP, Vorherr, H, Kleeman, CR, Telfer, N. Diuretic-induced hyponatremia. Ann Intern Med 1971;75:853.

Flinn, RB, Merrill, JP, Welzant, WR. Treatment of the oliguric patient with a new sodium-exchange resin and sorbitol: a preliminary report. N Engl J Med 1961;264:111.

Fox, BD. Crash diet potomania. Lancet 2002;359:942.

Fraley, DS, Adler, S. Correction of hyperkalemia by bicarbonate despite constant blood pH. Kidney Int 1977;12:354.

Gardiner, GW. Kayexalate (sodium polystyrene sulphonate) in sorbitol associated with intestinal necrosis in uremic patients. Can J Gastroenterol 1997;11:573.

Garth, D. Hypokalemia: differential diagnosis and workup; eMedicine Journal [serial online], 2009. Available from http://emedicine.medscape.com/article/767448-Overview

Garth, D. Hyperkalemia; eMedicine Journal [serial online], 2009. Available at http://emedicine.medscape.com/article/766479-overview

Gault, MH, Dixon, ME, Doyle, M, Cohen, WM. Hypernatremia, azotemia, and dehydration due to high-protein tube feeding. Ann Intern Med 1968;68:778.

Gennari, FJ. Hypokalemia. N Engl J Med 1998;339:451.

Gerstman, BB, Kirkman, R, Platt, R. Intestinal necrosis associated with postoperative orally administered sodium polystyrene sulfonate in sorbitol. Am J Kidney Dis 1992;20:159.

Gillum, DM, Linas, SL. Water intoxication in a psychotic patient with normal water excretion. Am J Med 1984;77:773.

Gipstein, RM, Boyle, JD. Hypernatremia complicating prolonged mannitol diuresis. N Engl JMed 1965;272:1116.

Goecke, IA, Bonilla, S, Marusic, Alvo, M. Enhanced insulin sensitivity in extrarenal potassium handling in uremic rats. Kidney Int 1991;39:39.

Greenberg, A, Verbalis, JG. Vasopressin receptor antagonists. Kidney Int 2006;69:2124.

Grimaldi, D, Cavalleri, F, Vallone, S, et al. Plasmapheresis improves the outcome of central pontine myelinolysis. J Neurol 2005;252:734.

Gross, P. Treatment of severe hyponatremia. Kidney Int 2001;60:2417.

Gruy-Kapral, C, Emmett, M, Santa Ana, CA, et al. Effect of single dose resin-cathartic therapy on serum potassium concentration in patients with end-stage renal disease. J Am Soc Nephrol 1998;9:1924.

Hamill, RJ, Robinson, LM, Wexler, HR, Moote, C. Efficacy and safety of potassium infusion therapy in hypokalemic critically ill patients. Crit Care Med 1991;19:694.

Hammond, DN, Moll, GW, Robertson, GL, Chelmicka-Schorr, E. Hypodipsic hypernatremia with normal osmoregulation of vasopressin. N Engl J Med 1986;315:433.

Han, WK, Bailly, V, Abichandani, R, et al. Kidney Injury Molecule-1 (KIM-1): a novel biomarker for human renal proximal tubule injury. Kidney Int 2002;62:237.

Han, WK, Waikar, SS, Johnson, A, et al. Urinary biomarkers in the early diagnosis of acute kidney injury. Kidney Int 2008;73:863.

Hariprasad, MK, Eisinger, RP, Nadler, IM, et al. Hyponatremia in psychogenic polydipsia. Arch Intern Med 1980;140:1639.

Henry, JA, Fallon, JK, Kicman, AT, et al. Low-dose MDMA ("ecstasy") induces vasopressin secretion. Lancet 1998;351:1784.

Herget-Rosenthal, S. One step forward in the early detection of acute renal failure. Lancet 2005;365:1205.

Herget-Rosenthal, S, Poppen, D, Hüsing, J, et al. Prognostic value of tubular proteinuria and enzymuria in nonoliguric acute tubular necrosis. Clin Chem 2004;50:552.

Hilden, T, Svendsen, TL. Electrolyte disturbances in beer drinkers. Lancet 1975;2:245.

Hillier, TA, Abbott, RD, Barrett, EJ. Hyponatremia: evaluating the correction factor for hyperglycemia. Am J Med 1999;106:399.

Hoes, AW, Grobbee, DE, Lubsen, JL, et al. Diuretics, beta blockers, and the risk for sudden cardiac death in hypertensive patients. Ann Intern Med 1995;123:481.

Holden, R, Jackson, MA. Near-fatal hyponatraemic coma due to vasopressin oversecretion after "ecstasy" (3,4-MDMA) [letter]. Lancet 1996;347:1052.

Holmes, SB, Banerjee, AK, Alexander, WD. Hyponatraemia and seizures after ecstasy use. Postgrad Med J 1999;75:32.

Hou, S, McElroy, PA, Nootens, J, Beach, M. Safety and efficacy of low-potassium dialysate. Am J Kidney Dis 1989;13:137.

Hou, SH, Bushinsky, DA, Wish, JB, et al. Hospital-acquired renal insufficiency: a prospective study. Am J Med 1983;74:243.

Hsu, CY, McCulloch, CE, Fan, D, et al. Community-based incidence of acute renal failure. Kidney Int 2007;72:208.

Johnson, BE, Chute, JP, Rushin, J, et al. A prospective study of patients with lung cancer and hyponatremia of malignancy. Am J Respir Crit Care Med 1997;156:1669.

Johnson, BE, Damodaran, A, Rushin, J, et al. Ectopic production and processing of atrial natriuretic peptide in a small cell lung carcinoma cell line and tumor from a patient with hyponatremia. Cancer 1997;79:35.

Kahn, A, Brachet, E, Blum, D. Controlled fall in natremia and risk of seizures in hypertonic dehydration. Intensive Care Med 1979;5:27.

Kamel, KS, Bear, RA. Treatment of hyponatremia: a quantitative analysis. Am J Kidney Dis 1993;21:439.

Kamel, KS, Wei, C. Controversial issues in the treatment of hyperkalaemia. Nephrol Dial Transplant 2003;18:2215.

Karp, BI, Laureno, R. Pontine and extrapontine myelinolysis: a neurologic disorder following rapid correction of hyponatremia. Medicine (Baltimore) 1993;72:359.

Katz, MA. Hyperglycemia-induced hyponatremia: calculation of expected serum sodium depression. N Engl J Med 1973;289:843.

Keith, NM, Osterberg, AE, Burchell, HB. Some effects of potassium salts in man. Ann Intern Med 1942;16:879.

Kjeldsen, L, Johnsen, AH, Sengelov, H, Borregaard, N. Isolation and primary structure of NGAL, a novel protein associated with human neutrophil gelatinase. J Biol Chem 1993;268:10425.

Kleeman, CR, Adams, DA, Maxwell, MH. An evaluation of maximal water diuresis in chronic renal disease. I. Normal solute intake. J Lab Clin Med 1961;58:169.

Klonoff, DC, Jurow, AH. Acute water intoxication as a complication of urine drug testing in the workplace. JAMA 1991;265:84.

Knoll, GA, Sahgal, A, Nair, RC, et al. Renin-angiotensin system blockade and the risk of hyperkalemia in chronic hemodialysis patients. Am J Med 2002;112:110.

Konig, R, Beeg, T, Tariverdian, G, et al. Holoprosencephaly, bilateral cleft lip and palate and ectrodactyly: another case and follow up. Clin Dysmorphol 2003;12:221.

Kopyt, N, Dalal, F, Narins, RG. Renal retention of potassium in fruit (letter). N Engl J Med 1985;313:582.

Kovacs, A, Chan, L, Hotrakitya, C, et al. Rotavirus gastroenteritis. Clinical and laboratory features and use of the Rotazyme test. Am J Dis Child 1987;141:161.

Krige, JE, Millar, AJ, Rode, H, Knobel, D. Fatal hypernatraemia after hypertonic saline irrigation of hepatic hydatid cysts. Pediatr Surg Int 2002;18:64.

Kruse, JA, Carlson, RW. Rapid correction of hypokalemia using concentrated intravenous potassium chloride infusions. Arch Intern Med 1990;150:613.

Kruse, JA, Clark, VL, Carlson, RW, Geheb, MA. Concentrated potassium chloride infusions in critically ill patients with hypokalemia. J Clin Pharmacol 1994;34:1077.

Kunin, AS, Surawicz, B, Sims, EA. Decrease in serum potassium concentration and appearance of cardiac arrhythmias during infusion of potassium with glucose in potassium-depleted patients. N Engl J Med 1962;266:228.

Lameire, N, Van Biesen, W, Vanholder, R. Acute renal failure. Lancet 2005;365:417.

Langgard, H, Smith, WO. Self-induced water intoxication without predisposing illness. N Engl J Med 1962;266:378.

Levin, A, Warnock, DG, Mehta, RL, et al. Improving outcomes from acute kidney injury: report of an initiative. Am J Kidney Dis 2007;50:1.

Levine, S, McManus, BM, Blackbourne, BD, Roberts, WC. Fatal water intoxication, schizophrenia, and diuretic therapy for systemic hypertension. Am J Med 1987;82:153.

Liangos, O, Wald, R, O'Bell, JW, et al. Epidemiology and outcomes of acute renal failure in hospitalized patients: a national survey. Clin J Am Soc Nephrol 2006;1:43.

Liano, F, Pascual, J, and the Madrid Acute Renal Failure Study Group. Epidemiology of acute renal failure: a prospective, multicenter, community-based study. Kidney Int 1996;50:811.

Lien, YH, Shapiro, JI, Chan, L. Effect of hypernatremia on organic brain osmoles. J Clin Invest 1990;85:1427.

Lien, YH, Shapiro, JI, Chan, L. Study of brain electrolytes and osmolytes during correction of chronic hyponatremia. Implications for the pathogenesis of central pontine myelinolysis. J Clin Invest 1991;88:303.

Lillemoe, KD, Romolo, JL, Hamilton, SR, et al. Intestinal necrosis due to sodium polystyrene (Kayexalate) in sorbitol enemas: clinical and experimental support for the hypothesis. Surgery 1987;101:267.

Lindinger, MI, Heigenhauser, GJF, McKelvie, RS, Jones, NL. Blood ion regulation during repeated maximal exercise and recovery in humans. Am J Physiol 1992;262:R126.

Lindner, G, Funk, GC, Schwarz, C, et al. Hypernatremia in the critically ill is an independent risk factor for mortality. Am J Kidney Dis 2007;50:952.

Liou, HH, Chiang, SS, Wu, SC, et al. Hypokalemic effects of intravenous infusion or nebulization of salbutamol in patients with chronic renal failure: comparative study. Am J Kidney Dis 1994;23:266.

Lipworth, BJ, McDevitt, DG, Struthers, AD. Prior treatment with diuretic augments the hypokalemic and electrocardiographic effects of inhaled albuterol. Am J Med 1989;86:653.

Liu, KD, Glidden, DV, Eisner, MD, et al. Predictive and pathogenetic value of plasma biomarkers for acute kidney injury in patients with acute lung injury. Crit Care Med 2007;35:2755.

Livingstone, IR, Cumming, WJ. Hyperkalaemic paralysis resembling Guillain-Barre syndrome. Lancet 1979;2:963.

Lu, KC, Hsu, YJ, Chiu, JS, et al. Effects of potassium supplementation on the recovery of thyrotoxic periodic paralysis. Am J Emerg Med 2004;22:544.

Madaio, MP. Renal biopsy. Kidney Int 1990;38:529.

Manganaro, R, Mami, C, Marrone, T, et al. Incidence of dehydration and hypernatremia in exclusively breast-fed infants. J Pediatr 2001;139:673.

Mange, K, Matsuura, D, Cizman, B, et al. Language guiding therapy: the case of dehydration versus volume depletion. Ann Intern Med 1997;127:848.

Mann, JF, Yi, QL, Sleight, P, et al. Serum potassium, cardiovascular risk, and effects of an ACE inhibitor: results of the HOPE study. Clin Nephrol 2005;63:181.

Mattar, JA, Weil, MH, Shubin, H, Stein, L. Cardiac arrest in the critically ill. II. Hyperosmolal states following cardiac arrest. Am J Med 1974;56:162.

McIver, B, Connacher, A, Whittle, I, et al. Adipsic hypothalamic diabetes insipidus after clipping of anterior communicating artery aneurysm. BMJ 1991;303:1465.

Meadow, R. Non-accidental salt poisoning. Arch Dis Child 1993;68:448.

Mehta, RL, Kellum, JA, Shah, SV, et al. Acute kidney injury network: report of an initiative to improve outcomes in acute kidney injury. Crit Care 2007;11:R31.

Mehta, RL, Pascual, MT, Soroko, S, et al. Spectrum of acute renal failure in the intensive care unit: the PICARD experience. Kidney Int 2004;66:1613.

Mendelssohn, DC, Cole, EH. Outcomes of percutaneous kidney biopsy, including those of solitary native kidneys. Am J Kidney Dis 1995;26:580.

Merrill, DC, Skelton, MM, Cowley, AC Jr. Humoral control of water and electrolyte excretion during water restriction. Kidney Int 1986;29:1152.

Miller, NL, Finberg, L. Peritoneal dialysis for salt poisoning. Report of a case. N Engl J Med 1960;263:1347.

Miller, TR, Anderson, RJ, Linas, SL, et al. Urinary diagnostic indices in acute renal failure: a prospective study. Ann Intern Med 1978;89:47.

Mishra, J, Dent, C, Tarabishi, R, et al. Neutrophil gelatinase-associated lipocalin (NGAL) as a biomarker for acute renal injury after cardiac surgery. Lancet 2005;365:1231.

Mishra, J, Ma, Q, Prada, A, et al. Identification of neutrophil gelatinase-associated lipocalin as a novel early urinary biomarker for ischemic renal injury. J Am Soc Nephrol 2003;14:2534.

Mishra, J, Mori, K, Ma, Q, et al. Amelioration of ischemic acute renal injury by neutrophil gelatinase-associated lipocalin. J Am Soc Nephrol 2004;15:3073.

Moder, KG, Hurley, DL. Fatal hypernatremia from exogenous salt intake: report of a case and review of the literature. Mayo Clin Proc 1990;65:1587.

Mohmand, HK, Issa, D, Ahmad, Z, et al. Hypertonic saline for hyponatremia: risk of inadvertent overcorrection. Clin J Am Soc Nephrol 2007;2:1110.

Montague, BT, Ouellette, JR, Buller, GK. Retrospective review of the frequency of ECG changes in hyperkalemia. Clin J Am Soc Nephrol 2008;3:324.

Mori, K, Lee, HT, Rapoport, D, et al. Endocytic delivery of lipocalin-siderophore-iron complex rescues the kidney from ischemia-reperfusion injury. J Clin Invest 2005;115:610.

Moritz, ML, Ayus, JC. The changing pattern of hypernatremia in hospitalized children. Pediatrics 1999;104:435.

Moritz, ML, Ayus, JC. Thepathophysiology and treatment of hyponatraemic encephalopathy: an update. Nephrol Dial Transplant 2003;18:2486.

Morrison, G, Michelson, EL, Brown, S, Morganroth, J. Mechanism and prevention of cardiac arrhythmias in chronic hemodialysis patients. Kidney Int 1980;17:811.

Muensterer, OJ. Hyperkalaemic paralysis. Age Ageing 2003;32:114.

Myers, BD, Miller, C, Mehigan, JT, et al. Nature of the renal injury following total renal ischemia in man. J Clin Invest 1984;73:329.

Nelson, DC, McGrew, WRG, Hoyumpa, AM. Hypernatremia and lactulose therapy. JAMA 1983;249:1295.

Nguyen, MT, Devarajan, P. Biomarkers for the early detection of acute kidney injury. Pediatr 2008;23(12):2151-7.

Nickolas, TL, O'Rourke, MJ, Yang, J, et al. Sensitivity and specificity of a single emergency department measurement of urinary neutrophil gelatinase-associated lipocalin for diagnosing acute kidney injury. Ann Intern Med 2008;148:810.

Nicolis, GL, Kahn, T, Sanchez, A, Gabrilove, JL. Glucose-induced hyperkalemia in diabetic subjects. Arch Intern Med 1981;141:49.

Nolan, CR, Anderson, RJ. Hospital-acquired acute renal failure. J Am Soc Nephrol 1998;9:710.

Nolph, KD, Popovich, RP, Ghods, AJ, Twardowski, Z. Determinants of low clearances of small solutes during peritoneal dialysis. Kidney Int 1978;13:117.

Nzerue, CM, Baffoe-Bonnie, H, You, W, et al. Predictors of outcome in hospitalized patients with severe hyponatremia. J Natl Med Assoc 2003;95:335.

Oddie, S, Richmond, S, Coulthard, M. Hypernatraemic dehydration and breast feeding: a population study. Arch Dis Child 2001;85:318.

Oh, MS, Uribarri, J, Barrido, D, et al. Danger of central pontine myelinolysis in hypotonic dehydration and recommendation for treatment. Am J Med Sci 1989;298:41.

Oster, JR, Singer, I. Hyponatremia, hyposmolality, and hypotonicity: tables and fables. Arch Intern Med 1999;159:333.

Oya, S, Tsutsumi, K, Ueki, K, Kirino, T. Reinduction of hyponatremia to treat central pontine myelinolysis. Neurology 2001;57:1931.

Palevsky, PM, Bhagrath, R, Greenberg, A. Hypernatremia in hospitalized patients. Ann Intern Med 1996;124:197.

Parikh, CR, Abraham, E, Ancukiewicz, M, Edelstein, CL. Urine IL-18 is an early diagnostic marker for acute kidney injury and predicts mortality in the intensive care unit. J Am Soc Nephrol 2005;16:3046.

Parikh, CR, Mishra, J, Thiessen-Philbrook, H, et al. Urinary IL-18 is an early predictive biomarker of acute kidney injury after cardiac surgery. Kidney Int 2006;70:199.

Part 10.1: Life-threatening electrolyte abnormalities. Circulation 2005;112:IV121.

Peacock, P, et al. Acute renal failure: differential diagnosis and workup; eMedicine Journal [serial online], 2008. Available from http://emedicine.medscape.com/article/777845-overview

Perianayagam, A, Sterns, RH, Silver, SM, et al. DDAVP is effective in preventing and reversing inadvertent overcorrection of hyponatremia. Clin J Am Soc Nephrol 2008;3:331.

Pham, PC, Pham, PM, Pham, PT, et al. Vasopressin excess and hyponatremia. Am J Kidney Dis 2006;47:727.

Pham, PC, Pham, PM, Pham, PT. Vasopressin excess and hyponatremia. Am J Kidney Dis 2006;47:727.

Phillips, PA, Bretherton, M, Johnston, CI, Gray, L. Reduced osmotic thirst in healthy elderly men. Am J Physiol 1991;261:R166.

Polderman, KH, Schreuder, WO, van Schijndel, S, Thijs, LG. Hypernatremia in the intensive care unit: an indicator of quality of care?. Crit Care Med 1999;27:1041.

Pollock, AS, Arieff, AI. Abnormalities of cell volume regulation and their functional consequences. Am J Physiol 1980;239:F195.

Prescott, GJ, Metcalfe, W, Baharani, J, et al. A prospective national study of acute renal failure treated with RRT: incidence, aetiology and outcomes. Nephrol Dial Transplant 2007;22:2513.

Rao, KJ, Miller, M, Moses, A. Water intoxication and thioridazine. Ann Intern Med 1975;82:61.

Rashid, A, Hamilton, SR. Necrosis of the gastrointestinal tract in uremic patients as a result of sodium polystyrene sulfonate (Kayexalate) in sorbitol: an underrecognized condition. Am J Surg Pathol 1997;21:60.

Renneboog, B, Musch, W, Vandemergel, X, et al. Mild chronic hyponatremia is associated with falls, unsteadiness, and attention deficits. Am J Med 2006;119:71.

Riemenschneider, T, Bohle, A. Morphologic aspects of low-potassium and low-sodium nephropathy. Clin Nephrol 1983;19:271.

Robertson, GL. Abnormalities of thirst regulation. Kidney Int 1984;25:460.

Robertson, GL, Aycinena, P, Zerbe, RL. Neurogenic disorders of osmoregulation. Am J Med 1982;72:339.

Robertson, GL, Shelton, RL, Athar, S. The osmoregulation of vasopressin. Kidney Int 1976;10:25.

Rogers, FB, Li, SC. Acute colonic necrosis associated with sodium polystyrene sulfonate (Kayexalate) enemas in a critically ill patient: case report and review of the literature. J Trauma 2001;51:395.

Rose, BD. New approach to disturbances in the plasma sodium concentration. Am J Med 1986;81:1033.

Rose, BD. Pathophysiology of Renal Disease, 2nd ed, McGraw-Hill, New York, 1987, p. 41.

Rosenson, J, Smollin, C, Sporer, KA, et al. Patterns of ecstasy-associated hyponatremia in California. Ann Emerg Med 2007;49:164.

Rubini, ME. Water excretion in potassium-deficient man. J Clin Invest 1961;40:2215.

Schaff-Blass, E, Robertson, GL, Rosenfield, RL. Chronic hypernatremia from a congenital defect in osmoregulation of thirst and vasopressin. J Pediatr1983;102:703.

Scherr, L, Ogden, DA, Mead, AW, et al. Management of hyperkalemia with a cation-exchange resin. N Engl J Med 1961;264:115.

Schow, DA, Vinson, RK, Morrisseau, PM. Percutaneous renal biopsy of the solitary kidney: a contraindication? J Urol 1992;147:1235.

Schrier, RW. An odyssey into the milieu intérieur: pondering the enigmas. J Am Soc Nephrol 1992;2:1549.

Schrier, RW, Gross, P, Gheorghiade, M, et al. Tolvaptan, a selective oral vasopressin V2-receptor antagonist, for hyponatremia. N Engl J Med 2006;355:2099.

Schwartz, WB, Van Ypersele, de Strihou, Kassirer, JP. Role of anions in metabolic alkalosis and potassium deficiency. N Engl J Med 1968;279:630.

Seftel, HC, Kew, MC. Early and intensive potassium replacement in diabetic acidosis. Diabetes 1966;15:694.

Shapiro, W, Taubert, K. Hypokalaemia and digoxin-induced arrhythmias. Lancet 1975; 2:604.

Shepard, KU. Cleansing enemas after sodium polystyrene sulfonate enemas (letter). Ann Intern Med 1990;112:711.

Shiau, YF, Feldman, GM, Resnick, MA, Coff, PM. Stool electrolyte and osmolality measurements in the evaluation of diarrheal disorders. Ann Intern Med 1985;102:773.

Shintani, S, Shliigai, T, Tsukagoshi, H. Marked hypokalemic rhabdomyolysis with myoglobinuria due to diuretic treatment. Eur Neurol 1991;31:396.

Siegel, D, Hulley, SB, Black, DM, et al. Diuretics, serum and intracellular electrolyte levels, and arrhythmias in hypertensive men. JAMA 1992;267:1083.

Snyder, NA, Feigal, DW, Arieff, AI. Hypernatremia in elderly patients. Ann Intern Med 1987;107:309.

Sopko, JA, Freeman, RM. Salt substitutes as a source of potassium. JAMA 1977;238:608.

Soupart, A, Ngassa, M, Decaux, G. Therapeutic relowering of the serum sodium in a patient after excessive correction of hyponatremia. Clin Nephrol 1999;51:383.

Soupart, A, Penninckx, R, Crenier, L, et al. Prevention of brain demyelination in rats after excessive correction of chronic hyponatremia by serum sodium lowering. Kidney Int 1994;45:193.

Soupart, A, Penninckx, R, Stenuit, A, et al. Treatment of chronic hyponatremia in rats by intravenous saline: comparison of rate versus magnitude of correction. Kidney Int 1992;41:1662.

Sowinski, KM, Cronin, D, Mueller, BA, Kraus, MA. Subcutaneous terbutaline use in CKD to reduce potassium concentrations. Am J Kidney Dis 2005;45:1040.

Steiner, RW. Interpretingthe fractional excretion of sodium. Am J Med 1984;77:699.

Stephanides, S. Hypernatremia: differential diagnosis and workup; eMedicine Journal [serial online], 2007. Available from http://emedicine.medscape.com/article/766683-overview

Sterns, RH. Severe symptomatic hyponatremia: treatment and outcome. A study of 64 cases. Ann Intern Med 1987;107:656.

Sterns, RH, Cappuccio, JD, Silver, SM, Cohen, EP. Neurologic sequelae after treatment of severe hyponatremia: a multicenter perspective. J Am Soc Nephrol 1994;4:1522.

Sterns, RH, Cox, M, Feig, PU, Singer, I. Internal potassium balance and the control of the plasma potassium concentration. Medicine (Baltimore) 1981;60:339.

Sterns, RH, Feig, PU, Pring, M, et al. Disposition of intravenous potassium in anuric man: a kinetic analysis. Kidney Int 1979;15:651.

Sterns, RH, Silver, SM. Brain volume regulation in response to hypo-osmolality and its correction. Am J Med 2006;119:S12.

Sterns, RH, Silver, SM. Hemodialysis in hyponatremia: is there a risk?. Semin Dial 1990;3:3.

Strange, K. Regulation of solute and water balance and cell volume in the central nervous system. J Am Soc Nephrol 1992;3:12.

Struthers, AD, Whitesmith, R, Reid, JL. Prior thiazide treatment increases adrenaline-induced hypokalemia. Lancet 1983;1:1358.

Stuart, CA, Neelon, FA, Lebovitz, HE. Disordered control of thirst in hypothalamic-pituitary sarcoidosis. N Engl J Med 1980;303:1078.

Sze, L, Ulrich, B, Brandle, M. Severe hypernatraemia due to nephrogenic diabetes insipidus – a life-threatening side effect of chronic lithium therapy. Exp Clin Endocrinol Diabetes 2006;114:596.

Tanneau, RS, Henry, A, Rouhart, F, et al. High incidence of neurologic complications following rapid correction of severe hyponatremia in polydipsic patients. J Clin Psychiatry 1994;55:349.

Tannen, RL, Regal, EM, Dunn, MJ, Schrier, RW. Vasopressin-resistant hyposthenuria in advanced chronic renal failure. N Engl J Med 1969;280:1135.

Thaler, SM, Teitelbaum, I, Berl, T. "Beer potomania" in non-beer drinkers: effect of low dietary solute intake. Am J Kidney Dis 1998;31:1028.

Thompson, CJ, Baylis, PH. Thirst in diabetes insipidus: clinical relevance of quantitative assessment. Q J Med 1987;65:853.

Tizianello, A, Garibotto, G, Robaudo, C, et al. Renal ammoniagenesis in humans with chronic potassium depletion. Kidney Int 1991;40:772.

Torres, VE, Young, WF Jr, Offord, KP, Hattery, RR. Association of hypokalemia, aldosteronism, and renal cysts. N Engl J Med 1990;322:345.

Trof, RJ, Di Maggio, F, Leemreis, J, Groeneveld, AB. Biomarkers of acute renal injury and renal failure. Shock 2006;26:245.

Tsuji, H, Venditti, FJ Jr, Evans, JC, et al. The associations of levels of serum potassium and magnesium with ventricular premature complexes (the Framingham Heart Study). Am J Cardiol 1994;74:237.

Uchida, K, Gotoh, A. Measurement of cystatin-C and creatinine in urine. Clin Chim Acta 2002;323:121.

Uchino, S, Kellum, JA, Bellomo, R, et al. Acute renal failure in critically ill patients: a multinational, multicenter study. JAMA 2005;294:813.

Vaidya, VS, Ramirez, V, Ichimura, T, et al. Urinary kidney injury molecule-1: a sensitive quantitative biomarker for early detection of kidney tubular injury. Am J Physiol Renal Physiol 2006;290:F517.

Verbalis, JG, Goldsmith, SR, Greenberg, A, et al. Hyponatremia treatment guidelines 2007: expert panel recommendations. Am J Med 2007;120:S1.

Villamil, MF, DeLand, EC, Henney, RP, Maloney, JV. Anion effects on cation movements during correction of potassium depletion. Am J Physiol 1975;229:161.

Wagener, G, Jan, M, Kim, M, et al. Association between increases in urinary neutrophil gelatinase-associated lipocalin and acute renal dysfunction after adult cardiac surgery. Anesthesiology 2006;105:485.

Wahr, JA, Parks, R, Boisvert, D, et al. Preoperative serum potassium levels and perioperative outcomes in cardiac surgery patients. Multicenter Study of Perioperative Ischemia Research Group. JAMA 1999;281:2203.

Waikar, SS, Curhan, GC, Wald, R, et al. Declining mortality in patients with acute renal failure, 1988 to 2002. J Am Soc Nephrol 2006;17:1143.

Weiner, ID, Wingo, CS. Hyperkalemia: a potential silent killer. J Am Soc Nephrol 1998; 9:1535.

Weisberg, LS. Pseudohyponatremia: a reappraisal. Am J Med 1989;86:315.

Wilkins, B. Cerebral oedema afterMDMA ("ecstasy") and unrestricted water intake. Hyponatraemia must be treated with low water input. BMJ 1996;313:689.

Wolff, K, Tsapakis, EM, Winstock, AR, et al. Vasopressin and oxytocin secretion in response to the consumption of ecstasy in a clubbing population. J Psychopharmacol 2006;20:400.

Xue, JL, Daniels, F, Star, RA, et al. Incidence and mortality of acute renal failure in Medicare beneficiaries, 1992 to 2001. J Am Soc Nephrol 2006;17:1135.

Yamamoto, T, Noiri, E, Ono, Y, et al. Renal L-type fatty acid – binding protein in acute ischemic injury. J Am Soc Nephrol 2007;18:2894.

Yeates, KE, Singer, M, Morton, AR. Salt and water: a simple approach to hyponatremia. CMAJ 2004;170:365.

Zappitelli, M, Washburn, KK, Arikan, AA, et al. Urine neutrophil gelatinase-associated lipocalin is an early marker of acute kidney injury in critically ill children: a prospective cohort study. Crit Care 2007;11:R84.

Zhang, L, Wang, M, Wang, H. Acute renal failure in chronic kidney disease – clinical and pathological analysis of 104 cases. Clin Nephrol 2005;63:346.

Zhou, H, Hewitt, SM, Yuen, PS, Star, RA. Acute kidney injury biomarkers – Needs, present, status, and future promise. Neph SAP 2006;5:63.

NEUROLOGY

A randomised, blinded, trial of clopidogrel versus aspirin in patients at risk of ischaemic events (CAPRIE). CAPRIE Steering Committee. Lancet 1996;348:1329.

Adams, G, Deaver, KA, Cochi, SL, et al. Decline of childhood Haemophilus influenzae type b (Hib) disease in the Hib vaccine era. JAMA 1993;269:221.

Adams, HP Jr, Bendixen, BH, Leira, E, et al. Antithrombotic treatment of ischemic stroke among patients with occlusion or severe stenosis of the internal carotid artery. Neurology 1999;53:122.

Adams, HP Jr, del Zoppo, G, Alberts, MJ, et al. Guidelines for the early management of adults with ischemic stroke: a guideline from the American Heart Association/American Stroke Association Stroke Council, Clinical Cardiology Council, Cardiovascular Radiology and Intervention Council, and the Atherosclerotic Peripheral Vascular Disease and Quality of Care Outcomes in Research Interdisciplinary Working Groups:

the American Academy of Neurology affirms the value of this guideline as an educational tool for neurologists. Stroke 2007;38:1655.

Adams, HP Jr, Effron, MB, Torner, J, et al. Emergency administration of abciximab for treatment of patients with acute ischemic stroke: results of an international phaseIII trial: Abciximab in Emergency Treatment of Stroke Trial (AbESTT-II). Stroke 2008;39:87.

Adams, HP, Brott, TG, Furlan, AJ, et al. Guidelines for thrombolytic therapy of acute stroke: a supplement to the guidelines for the management of patients with acute ischemic stroke. Stroke 1996;27:1711.

Adams, RJ, Chimowitz, MI, Alpert, JS, et al. Coronary risk evaluation in patients with transient ischemic attack and ischemic stroke: a scientific statement for healthcare professionals from the Stroke Council and the Council on Clinical Cardiology of the American Heart Association/American Stroke Association. Stroke 2003;34:2310.

Aktekin, B, Dogan, EA, Oguz, Y, Senol, Y. Withdrawal of antiepileptic drugs in adult patients free of seizures for 4 years: a prospective study. Epilepsy Behav 2006;8:616.

Alberico, RA, Patel, M, Casey, S, et al. Evaluation of the circle of Willis with three-dimensional CT angiography in patients with suspected intracranial aneurysms. AJNR Am J Neuroradiol 1995;16:1571.

Albers, GW, Amarenco, P, Easton, JD, et al. Antithrombotic andthrombolytic therapy for ischemic stroke: the Seventh ACCP Conference on Antithrombotic and Thrombolytic Therapy. Chest 2004;126:483S.

Albers, GW, Comess, KA, DeRook, FA, et al. Transesophageal echocardiographic findings in stroke subtypes. Stroke 1994;25:23.

Aldenkamp, AP. Effect of seizures and epileptiform discharges on cognitive function. Epilepsia 1997;38 Suppl 1:S52.

American Academy of Pediatrics. Committee on Drugs: behavioral and cognitive effects of anticonvulsant therapy. Pediatrics 1985;76:644.

American Academy of Pediatrics. Haemophilus influenzae infections. In: Red Book: 2006 Report of the Committee on Infectious Diseases, 27th ed, Pickering, LK (Ed), American Academy of Pediatrics, Elk Grove Village, IL 2006, p. 310.

Andrade, DM, Zumsteg, D, Hamani, C, et al. Long-term follow-up of patients with thalamic deep brain stimulation for epilepsy. Neurology 2006;66:1571.

Arnold, M, Nedeltchev, K, Brekenfeld, C, et al. Outcome of acute stroke patients without visible occlusion on early arteriography. Stroke 2004;35:1135.

Aronin, SI, Peduzzi, P, Quagliarello, VJ. Community-acquired bacterial meningitis: risk stratification for adverse clinical outcome and effect of antibiotic timing. Ann Intern Med 1998;129:862.

Attia, J, Hatala, R, Cook, DJ, Wong, JG. The rational clinical examination. Does this adult patient have acute meningitis?. JAMA 1999;282:175.

Aubert, G, Jacquemond, G, Pozzetto, B, et al. Pharmacokinetic evidence of imipenem efficacy in the treatment of Klebsiella pneumoniae nosocomial meningitis. J Antimicrob Chemother 1991;28:316.

Auburtin, M, Wolff, M, Charpentier, J, et al. Detrimental role of delayed antibiotic administration and penicillin-nonsusceptible strains in adult intensive care unit patients with pneumococcal meningitis: the PNEUMOREA prospective multicenter study. Crit Care Med 2006;34:2758.

Babikian, VL, Wechsler, LR (Eds). Transcranial Doppler Ultrasonography, CV Mosby, St Louis, 1993.

Band, JD, Fraser, DW, Ajello, G. Prevention of Hemophilus influenzae type b disease. JAMA 1984;251:2381.

Barber, M, Langhorne, P, Rumley, A, et al. Hemostatic function and progressing ischemic stroke: D-dimer predicts early clinical progression. Stroke 2004;35:1421.

Barnett, HJ, Gunton, RW, Eliasziw, M, et al. Causes and severity of ischemic stroke in patients with internal carotid artery stenosis. JAMA 2000;283:1429.

Bartels, E. Color-Coded Duplex Ultrasonography of the Cerebral Vessels. Schattauer, Stuttgart, 1998.

Bath, PM, Lindenstrom, E, Boysen, G, et al. Tinzaparin in acute ischaemic stroke (TAIST): a randomised aspirin-controlled trial. Lancet 2001;358:702.

Beamer, N, Coull, BM, Sexton, G, et al. Fibrinogen and the albumin-globulin ratio in recurrent stroke. Stroke 1993;24:1133.

Beauchamp, NJ, Bryan, RN. Neuroimaging of stroke. In: Primer on Cerebrovascular Diseases, Welch, KM, Caplan, LR, Reis, DJ, et al (Eds), Academic Press, San Diego, 1997, p. 599.

Berge, E, Sandercock, P. Anticoagulants versus antiplatelet agents for acute ischaemic stroke. Cochrane Database Syst Rev 2002;CD003242.

Bladin, CF, Alexandrov, AV, Bellavance, A, et al. Seizures after stroke: a prospective multi-center study. Arch Neurol 2000;57:1617.

Blazer, S, Berant, M. Bacterial meningitis: effect of antibiotic treatment on cerebrospinal fluid. Am J Clin Pathol 1983;80:386.

Brant-Zawadzki, M, Atkinson, D, Detrick, M, et al. Fluid-attenuated inversion recovery (FLAIR) for assessment of cerebral infarction. Initial clinical experience in 50 patients. Stroke 1996;27:1187.

Briley, DP, Coull, BM, Goodnight, SH Jr. Neurological disease associated with antiphospholipid antibodies. Ann Neurol 1989;25:221.

Britton, JW. Antiepileptic drug withdrawal: literature review. Mayo Clin Proc 2002;77:1378.

Britton, JW, Ghearing, GR, Benarroch, EE, Cascino, GD. The ictal bradycardia syndrome: localization and lateralization. Epilepsia 2006;47:737.

Brodie, MJ, Perucca, E, Ryvlin, P, et al. Comparison of levetiracetam and controlled-release carbamazepine in newly diagnosed epilepsy. Neurology 2007;68:402.

Brouwer, MC, van de, Beek, D, Heckenberg, SG, et al. Hyponatraemia in adults with community-acquired bacterial meningitis. QJM 2007;100:37.

Bula, CJ, Bille, J, Glauser, MP. An epidemic of food-borne listeriosis in western Switzerland: description of 57 cases involving adults. Clin Infect Dis 1995;20:66.

Bushnell, CD, Goldstein, LB. Diagnostic testing for coagulopathies in patients with ischemic stroke. Stroke 2000;31:3067.

Cabellos, C, Viladrich, PF, Verdaguer, R, et al. A single daily dose of ceftriaxone for bacterial meningitis in adults: experience with 84 patients and review of the literature. Clin Infect Dis 1995;20:1164.

Calandra, G, Lydick, E, Carrigan, J, et al. Factors predisposing to seizures in seriously ill infected patients receiving antibiotics: experience with imipenem/cilastatin. Am J Med 1988;84:911.

Callaghan, N, Garrett, A, Goggin, T. Withdrawal of anticonvulsant drugs in patients free of seizures for two years. A prospective study. N Engl J Med 1988;318:942.

Camerlingo, M, Salvi, P, Belloni, G, et al. Intravenous heparin started within the first 3 hours after onset of symptoms as a treatment for acute nonlacunar hemispheric cerebral infarctions. Stroke 2005;36:2415.

Camilo, O, Goldstein, LB. Seizures and epilepsy after ischemic stroke. Stroke 2004;35:1769.

Caplan, LR, Brass, LM, DeWitt, LD, et al. Transcranial Doppler ultrasound: present status. Neurology 1990;40:696.

Caplan, LR, DeWitt, LD, Breen, JC. Neuroimaging in patients with cerebrovascular disease. In: Neuroimaging, Greenberg, J (Ed), McGraw-Hill, New York, 1995, p. 435.

Caplan, LR, Flamm, ES, Mohr, JP, et al. Lumbar puncture and stroke. A statement for physicians by a Committee of the Stroke Council, American Heart Association. Circulation 1987;75:505A.

Caplan, LR, Gorelick, PB, Hier, DB. Race, sex, and occlusive vascular disease: a review. Stroke 1986;17:648.

Caplan, LR, Mohr, JP, Kistler, JP, Koroshetz, W. Should thrombolytic therapy be the first-line treatment for acute ischemic stroke? Thrombolysis – not a panacea for ischemic stroke. N Engl J Med 1997;337:1309.

Caplan, LR. Brain embolism. In: Practical Clinical Neurocardiology, Caplan, LR, Chimowitz, M, Hurst, JW (Eds). Marcel Dekker, New York, 1999.

Caplan, LR. Computed tomography and stroke. In: Cerebrovascular Survey Report for the National Institute of Neurological and Communicative Disorders and Stroke (NINCDS), McDowell, F, Caplan, L (Eds), Washington, DC (revised), 1985, p. 61.

Caplan, LR. Laboratory investigations. In: Stroke: A Clinical Approach, 3rd ed, Caplan, LR, Butterworth-Heinemann, Boston, 2000.

Caplan, LR. Posterior Circulation Disease. Clinical Findings, Diagnosis, and Management, Blackwell Science, Boston, 1996.

Caplan, LR. Stroke: A Clinical Approach, 3rd ed, Butterworth-Heinemann, Boston, 2000, p. 59.

Caplan, LR. Terms describing brain ischemia by tempo are no longer useful: a polemic (with apologies to Shakespeare). Surg Neurol 1993;40:91.

Caplan, LR. TIAs – we need to return to the question What is wrong with Mr Jones (editorial). Neurology 1988;38:791.

Cardoso, TA, Coan, AC, Kobayashi, E, et al. Hippocampal abnormalities and seizure recurrence after antiepileptic drug withdrawal. Neurology 2006;67:134.

CAST: randomised placebo-controlled trial of early aspirin use in 20,000 patients with acute ischaemic stroke. CAST (Chinese Acute Stroke Trial) Collaborative Group. Lancet 1997;349:1641.

Cavazon, J. et al. Seizures and epilepsy, overview and classification; eMedicine Journal [serial online], 2009. Available from http://emedicine.medscape.com/article/1184846-overview

Cestari, DM, Weine, DM, Panageas, KS, et al. Stroke in patients with cancer: incidence and etiology. Neurology 2004;62:2025.

Charpentier, E, Gerbaud, G, Jacquet, C, et al. Incidence of antibiotic resistance in Listeria species. J Infect Dis 1995;172:277.

Cheitlin, MD, Armstrong, WF, Aurigemma, GP, et al. ACC/AHA/ASE 2003 guideline update for the clinical application of echocardiography: summary article: a report of the American College of Cardiology/American Heart Association Task Force on Practice Guidelines (ACC/AHA/ASE Committee to Update the 1997 Guidelines for the Clinical Application of Echocardiography). Circulation 2003;108:1146.

Chen, Z, Sandercock, P, Pan, H, et al. Indications for early aspirin use in acute ischemic stroke: a combined analysis of 40 000 randomized patients from the Chinese Acute Stroke Trial and the International Stroke Trial. Stroke 2000;31:1240.

Cherubin, CE, Appleman, MD, Heseltine, PN, et al. Epidemiological spectrum and current treatment of listeriosis. Rev Infect Dis 1991;13:1108.

Cherubin, CE, Eng, RHK, Norrby, R, et al. Penetration of newer cephalosporins into cerebrospinal fluid. Rev Infect Dis 1989;11:526.

Cherubin, CE, Marr, JS, Sierra, MF, Becker, S. Listeria and gram-negative bacillary meningitis in New York City, 1972-1979;frequent causes of meningitis in adults. Am J Med 1981;71:199.

Collins, R, Peto, R, MacMahon, S, et al. Blood pressure, stroke, and coronary heart disease. Part 2, Short-term reductions in blood pressure: overview of randomised drug trials in their epidemiological context. Lancet 1990;335:827.

Cottagnoud, P, Acosta, F, Cottagnoud, M, Tauber, MG. Gemifloxacin is efficacious against penicillin-resistant and quinolone-resistant pneumococci in experimental meningitis. Antimicrob Agents Chemother 2002;46:1607.

Coull, AJ, Lovett, JK, Rothwell, PM. Population based study of early risk of stroke after transient ischaemic attack or minor stroke: implications for public education and organisation of services. BMJ 2004;328:326.

Coull, BM, Beamer, NB, deGarmo, PL, et al. Chronic blood hyperviscosity in subjects with acute stroke, transient ischemic attack, and risk factors for stroke. Stroke 1991;22:162.

Coull, BM, Goodnight, SH. Antiphospholipid antibodies, prothrombotic states, and stroke. Stroke 1990;21:1370.

Daffertshofer, M, Mielke, O, Pullwitt, A, et al. Transient ischemic attacks are more than "ministrokes." Stroke 2004;35:2453.

Davis, SM, Donnan, GA. The stroke-prone state: rapid assessment of transient ischemic attacks. Stroke 2006;37:1140.

de Gans, J, van de Beek, D. Dexamethasone in adults with bacterial meningitis. N Engl J Med 2002;347:1549.

Dee, RR, Lorber, B. Brain abscess due to Listeria monocytogenes: case report and literature review. Rev Infect Dis 1986;8:968.

Demchuk, AM, Morgenstern, LB, Krieger, DW, et al. Serum glucose level and diabetes predict tissue plasminogen activator-related intracerebral hemorrhage in acute ischemic stroke. Stroke 1999;30:34.

Dennis, MS, Bamford, JM, Sandercock, PA, Warlow, CP. A comparison of risk factors and prognosis for transient ischemic attacks and minor ischemic strokes. The Oxfordshire Community Stroke Project. Stroke 1989;20:1494.

Derex, L, Tomsick, TA, Brott, TG, et al. Outcome of stroke patients without angiographically revealed arterial occlusion within four hours of symptom onset. AJNR Am J Neuroradiol 2001;22:685.

DeRook, FA, Comess, KA, Albers, GW, Popp, RL. Transesophageal echocardiography in the evaluation of stroke. Ann Intern Med 1992;117:922.

Diener, HC, Ringelstein, EB, von Kummer, R, et al. Treatment of acute ischemic stroke with the low-molecular-weight heparin certoparin: results of the TOPAS trial. Stroke 2001;32:22.

Domingo, P, Mancebo, J, Blanch, L, et al. Fever in adult patients with acute bacterial meningitis. J Infect Dis 1988;158:496.

Donnan, GA, Davis, SM, Hill, MD, Gladstone, DJ. Patients with transient ischemic attack or minor stroke should be admitted to hospital: for. Stroke 2006;37:1137.

Dul, K, Drayer, BP. CT and MR imaging of intracerebral hemorrhage. In: Intracerebral Hemorrhage, Kase, CS, Caplan, LR (Eds), Butterworth-Heinemann, Boston, 1994, p. 73.

Durack, DT, Spanos, A. End-of-treatment spinal tap in bacterial meningitis: is it worthwhile? JAMA 1982;248:75.

Durand, ML, Calderwood, SB, Weber, DJ, et al. Acute bacterial meningitis in adults. N Engl J Med 1993;328:21.

Eckert, B, Zeumer, H. Brain computed tomography. In: Cerebrovascular Disease: Pathophysiology, Diagnosis, and Management, vol 2, Ginsberg, MD, Bogousslavsky, J (Eds), Blackwell Science, Boston, 1998, p. 1241.

Edelman, RR, Mattle, HP, Atkinson, DJ, Hoodgewoud, HM. MR angiography. AJR Am J Roentgenol 1990;154:937.

Elmore, JG, Horwitz, RI, Quagliarello, VJ. Acute meningitis with a negative Gram's stain: clinical and management outcomes in 171 episodes. Am J Med 1996;100:78.

Emergency administration of abciximab for treatment of patients with acute ischemic stroke: results of a randomized phase 2 trial. Stroke 2005;36:880.

Ernst, E, Resch, KL. Fibrinogen as a cardiovascular risk factor: a meta-analysis and review of the literature. Ann Intern Med 1993;118:956.

Finberg, RW, Moellering, RC, Tally, FP, et al. The importance of bactericidal drugs: future directions in infectious disease. Clin Infect Dis 2004;39:1314.

Fisher, M. Occlusion of the internal carotid artery. AMA Arch Neurol Psychiatry 1951; 65:346.

Fitch, MT, van de Beek, D. Emergency diagnosis and treatment of adult meningitis. Lancet Infect Dis 2007;7:191.

Flemming, KD, Brown, RD Jr, Petty, GW, et al. Evaluation and management of transient ischemic attack and minor cerebral infarction. Mayo Clin Proc 2004;79:1071.

Flossmann, E, Rothwell, PM. Prognosis of vertebrobasilar transient ischaemic attack and minor stroke. Brain 2003;126:1940.

Fong, IW, Tomkins, KB. Review of Pseudomonas aeruginosa meningitis with special emphasis on treatment with ceftazidime. Rev Infect Dis 1985;7:604.

Fregni, F, Otachi, PT, Do Valle, A, et al. A randomized clinical trial of repetitive transcranial magnetic stimulation in patients with refractory epilepsy. Ann Neurol 2006;60:447.

Friedland, IR, Klugman, KP. Failure of chloramphenicol therapy in penicillin-resistant pneumococcal meningitis. Lancet 1992;339:405.

Gallmetzer, P, Leutmezer, F, Serles, W, et al. Postictal paresis in focal epilepsies – incidence, duration, and causes: a video-EEG monitoring study. Neurology 2004;62:2160.

Gamble, C, Williamson, PR, Chadwick, DW, Marson, AG. A meta-analysis of individual patient responses to lamotrigine or carbamazepine monotherapy. Neurology 2006;66:1310.

Geiseler, PJ, Nelson, KE, Levin, S, et al. Community-acquired purulent meningitis: a review of 1,316 cases during the antibiotic era, 1954-1976. Rev Infect Dis 1980;2:725.

Geroulakos, G, Hobson, RW, Nicolaides, AW. Ultrasonic carotid plaque morphology. In: Cerebrovascular Ischaemia, Investigation and Management, Caplan, LR, Shifrin, EG, Nicolaides, AN, Moore, WS (Eds), Med-Orion, London, 1996, p. 25.

Gerraty, RP, Parsons, MW, Barber, PA, et al. Examining the lacunar hypothesis with diffusion and perfusion magnetic resonance imaging. Stroke 2002;33:2019.

Giles, MF, Rothwell, PM. Risk of stroke early after transient ischaemic attack: a systematic review and meta-analysis. Lancet Neurol 2007;6:1063.

Ginsberg, MD, Busto, R. Combating hyperthermia in acute stroke: a significant clinical concern. Stroke 1998;29:529.

Glass, TA, Hennessey, PM, Pazdera, L, et al. Outcome at 30 days in the New England Medical Center posterior circulation registry. Arch Neurol 2002;59:369.

Glauser, T, Ben-Menachem, E, Bourgeois, B, et al. ILAE treatment guidelines: evidence-based analysis of antiepileptic drug efficacy and effectiveness as initial monotherapy for epileptic seizures and syndromes. Epilepsia 2006;47:1094.

Goldstein, J. Transient ischemic attack; eMedicine Journal [serial online], 2008. Available at http://emedicine.medscape.com/article/794281-overview

Gopal, AK, Whitehouse, JD, Simel, DL, Corey, GR. Cranial computed tomography before lumbar puncture. A prospective clinical evaluation. Arch Intern Med 1999;159:2681.

Gorelick, PB, Caplan, LR. Calcium, hypercalcemia, and stroke. Current Concepts of Cerebrovascular Disease (Stroke) 1985;20:13.

Gorelick, PB, Hier, DB, Caplan, LR, Langenberg, P. Headache in acute cerebrovascular disease. Neurology 1986;36:1445.

Gronholdt, ML, Nordestgaard, BG, Nielsen, TG, Sillesen, H. Echolucent carotid artery plaques are associated with elevated levels of fasting and postprandial triglyceride-rich lipoproteins. Stroke 1996;27:2166.

Gubitz, G, Sandercock, P, Counsell, C. Anticoagulants for acute ischaemic stroke. Cochrane Database Syst Rev 2004;CD000024.

Hacke, W, Kaste, M, Fieschi, C, et al. Intravenous thrombolysis with recombinant tissue plasminogen activator for acute hemispheric stroke. The European Cooperative Acute Stroke Study (ECASS). JAMA 1995;274:1017.

Hankey, GJ, Eikelboom, JW, van Bockxmeer, FM, et al. Inherited thrombophilia in ischemic stroke and its pathogenic subtypes. Stroke 2001;32:1793.

Harloff, A, Handke, M, Reinhard, M, et al. Therapeutic strategies after examination by transesophageal echocardiography in 503 patients with ischemic stroke. Stroke 2006;37:859.

Hart, C, Cuevas, L. Meningococcal disease in Africa. Ann Trop Med Parasitol 1997;91:777.

Hart, YM, Sander, JW, Johnson, AL, Shorvon, SD. National General Practice Study of Epilepsy: Recurrence after a first unprovoked seizure. Lancet 1990;336:1271.

Hasbun, R, Abrahams, J, Jekel, J, Quagliarello, VJ. Computed tomography of the head before lumbar puncture in adults with suspected meningitis. N Engl J Med 2001;345:1727.

Hauser, WA, Annegers, JF, Kurland, LT. Incidence of epilepsy and unprovoked seizures in Rochester, Minnesota: 1935-1984. Epilepsia 1993;34:453.

Hauser, WA, Rich, SS, Annegers, JF, et al. Seizure recurrence after a first unprovoked seizure: an extended follow-up. Neurology 1990;40:1163.

Hauser, WA, Rich, SS, Jacobs, MP, et al. Patterns of seizure occurrence and recurrence risks in patients with newly diagnosed epilepsy. Epilepsia 1983;24:516.

Hauw, JJ, Seilhean, D, Duyckaerts, C. Cerebral amyloid angiopathy. In: Cerebrovascular Disease: Pathophysiology, Diagnosis, and Management, vol 2, Ginsberg, MD, Bogousslavsky, J (Eds), Blackwell Science, Boston, 1998, p. 1772.

Hieber, JP, Nelson, JD. A pharmacologic evaluation ofpenicillin in children with purulent meningitis. N Engl J Med 1977;297:410.

Hill, MD, Yiannakoulias, N, Jeerakathil, T, et al. The high risk of stroke immediately after transient ischemic attack: a population-based study. Neurology 2004;62:2015.

Hillbom, M, Erila, T, Sotaniemi, K, et al. Enoxaparin vs heparin for prevention of deep-vein thrombosis in acute ischaemic stroke: a randomized, double-blind study. Acta Neurol Scand 2002;106:84.

Hirsch, LJ, Hauser, WA. Can sudden unexplained death in epilepsy be prevented?. Lancet 2004;364:2157.

Horowitz, DR, Tuhrim, S, Weinberger, J, et al. Transesophageal echocardiography: diagnostic and clinical applications in the evaluation of the stroke patient. J Stroke Cerebrovasc Dis 1997;6:332.

Intracerebral hemorrhage after intravenous t-PA therapy for ischemic stroke. The NINDS t-PA Stroke Study Group. Stroke 1997;28:2109.

Jackson, LA, Tenover, FC, Baker, C. Prevalence of Neisseria meningitidis relatively resistant to penicillin in the Unites States, 1991. J Infect Dis 1994;169:438.

Jacoby, A, Gamble, C, Doughty, J, et al. Quality of life outcomes of immediate or delayed treatment of early epilepsy and single seizures. Neurology 2007;68:1188.

Janardhan, V, Wolf, PA, Kase, CS, et al. Anticardiolipin antibodies and risk of ischemic stroke and transient ischemic attack: the Framingham cohort and offspring study. Stroke 2004;35:736.

Jauch, E. Acute stroke management: treatment and medication; eMedicine Journal [serial online], 2009. Available from http://emedicine.medscape.com/article/1159752-treatment

John, CC. Treatment failure with use of a third-generation cephalosporin for penicillin-resistant pneumococcal meningitis: case report and review. Clin Infect Dis 1994;18:188.

Johnson, BA, Heiserman, JE, Drayer, BP, Keller, PJ. Intracranial MR angiography: its role in the integrated approach to brain infarction. AJNR Am J Neuroradiol 1994;15:901.

Johnston, KC, Li, JY, Lyden, PD, et al. Medical and neurological complications of ischemic stroke: experience from the RANTTAS trial. RANTTAS Investigators. Stroke 1998;29:447.

Johnston, SC, Gress, DR, Browner, WS, Sidney, S. Short-term prognosis after emergency department diagnosis of TIA. JAMA 2000;284:2901.

Johnston, SC, Nguyen-Huynh, MN, Schwarz, ME, et al. National Stroke Association guidelines for the management of transient ischemic attacks. Ann Neurol 2006;60:301.

Johnston, SC, Rothwell, PM, Nguyen-Huynh, MN, et al. Validation and refinement of scores to predict very early stroke risk after transient ischaemic attack. Lancet 2007;369:283.

Johnston, SC, Smith, WS. Practice variability in management of transient ischemic attacks. Eur Neurol 1999;42:105.

Kanegaye, JT, Soliemanzadeh, P, Bradley, JS. Lumbar puncture in pediatric bacterial meningitis: defining the time interval for recovery of cerebrospinal fluid pathogens after parenteral antibiotic pre-treatment. Pediatrics 2001;108:1169.

Kase, CS, Caplan, LR. Intracerebral hemorrhage. Butterworth-Heinemann, Boston, 1996.

Kase, CS, Robinson, RK, Stein, RW, et al. Anticoagulant-related intracerebral hemorrhages. Neurology 1985;35:943.

Kase, CS. Bleeding disorders. In: Intracerebral Hemorrhage, Kase, CS, Caplan, LR (Eds), Butterworth-Heinemann, Boston, 1994, p. 117.

Kase, CS. Cerebral amyloid angiopathy. In: Intracerebral Hemorrhage, Kase, CS, Caplan, LR (Eds), Butterworth-Heinemann, Boston, 1994, p. 179.

Kastenbauer, S, Pfister, HW. Pneumococcal meningitis in adults: spectrum of complications and prognostic factors in a series of 87 cases. Brain 2003;126:1015.

Kawachi, I, Colditz, GA, Stampfer, MJ, et al. Smoking cessation and the decreased risk of stroke in women. JAMA 1993;269:232.

Kay, R, Wong, KS, Yu, YL, et al. Low-molecular-weight heparin for the treatment of acute ischemic stroke. N Engl J Med 1995;333:1588.

Kernan, WN, Schindler, JL. Rapid intervention for TIA: a new standard emerges. Lancet Neurol 2007;6:940.

Kho, LK, Lawn, ND, Dunne, JW, Linto, J. First seizure presentation: do multiple seizures within 24 hours predict recurrence?. Neurology 2006;67:1047.

Kidwell, CS, Alger, JR, Di Salle, F, et al. Diffusion MRI in patients with transient ischemic attacks. Stroke 1999;30:1174.

Kilpi, T, Anttila, M, Kallio, MJ, Peltola, H. Length of prediagnostic history related to the course and sequelae of childhood bacterial meningitis. Pediatr Infect Dis J 1993;12:184.

Kim, LG, Johnson, TL, Marson, AG, Chadwick, DW. Prediction of risk of seizure recurrence after a single seizure and early epilepsy: further results from the MESS trial. Lancet Neurol 2006;5:317.

Klotzsch, C, Janssen, G, Berlit, P. Transesophageal echocardiography and contrast-TCD in thedetection of a patent foramen ovale: experiences with 111 patients. Neurology 1994;44:1603.

Klugman, KP, Dagan, R, the Meropenem Meningitis Study Group. Randomized comparison of meropenem with cefotaxime for treatment of bacterial meningitis. Antimicrob Agents Chemother 1995;39:1140.

Klugman, KP, Friedland, IR, Bradley, JS. Bactericidal activity against cephalosporin-resistant Streptococcus pneumoniae in cerebrospinal fluid of children with acute bacterial meningitis. Antimicrob Agents Chemother 1995;39:1988.

Korinek, AM, Baugnon, T, Golmard, JL, et al. Risk factors for adult nosocomial meningitis after craniotomy: role of antibiotic prophylaxis. Neurosurgery 2006;59:126.

Kothari, R, Jauch, E, Broderick, et al. Acutestroke: delays to presentation and emergency department evaluation. Ann Emerg Med 1999;33:3.

Kramer, G, Biraben, A, Carreno, M, et al. Current approaches to the use of generic antiepileptic drugs. Epilepsy Behav 2007;11:46.

Kwan, P, Brodie, MJ. Early identification of refractory epilepsy. N Engl J Med 2000;342:314.

Kwan, P, Brodie, MJ. Effectiveness of first antiepileptic drug. Epilepsia 2001;42:1255.

Labovitz, DL, Hauser, WA, Sacco, RL. Prevalence and predictors of early seizure and status epilepticus after first stroke. Neurology 2001;57:200.

Langan, Y, Nashef, L, Sander, JW. Case-control study of SUDEP. Neurology 2005;64:1131.

Lazoff, M. Meningitis; eMedicine Journal [serial online], 2009. Available at http://emedicine.medscape.com/article/784389-overview

Lavallee, PC, Meseguer, E, Abboud, H, et al. A transient ischaemic attack clinic with round-the-clock access (SOS-TIA): feasibility and effects. Lancet Neurol 2007;6:953.

Lebel, MH, Freij, BJ, Syrogiannopoulos, GA, et al. Dexamethasone therapy for bacterial meningitis. N Engl J Med 1988;319:964.

Leonardi-Bee, J, Bath, PM, Bousser, MG, et al. Dipyridamole for preventing recurrent ischemic stroke and other vascular events: a meta-analysis of individual patient data from randomized controlled trials. Stroke 2005;36:162.

Leone, M, Franzini, A, Broggi, G, et al. Acute hypothalamic stimulation and ongoing cluster headache attacks. Neurology 2006;67:1844.

Leung, DY, Davidson, PM, Cranney, GB, Walsh, WF. Thromboembolic risks of left atrial thrombus detected by transesophageal echocardiogram. Am J Cardiol 1997;79:626.

Levine, SR, Brey, RL, Tilley, BC, et al. Antiphospholipid antibodies and subsequent thrombo-occlusive events in patients with ischemic stroke. JAMA 2004;291:576.

Lewington, S, Clarke, R, Qizilbash, N, et al. Age-specific relevance of usual blood pressure to vascular mortality: a meta-analysis of individual data for one million adults in 61 prospective studies. Lancet 2002;360:1903.

Lindley, RI. Patients with transient ischemic attack do not need to be admitted to hospital for urgent evaluation and treatment: against. Stroke 2006;37:1139.

Linfante, I, Llinas, RH, Caplan, LR, Warach, S. MRI features of intracerebral hemorrhage within 2 hours from symptom onset. Stroke 1999;30:2263.

Lossius, MI, Hessen, E, Mowinckel, P, et al. Consequences of antiepileptic drug withdrawal: a randomized, double-blind study (Akershus Study). Epilepsia 2008;49:455.

Lossius, MI, Ronning, OM, Slapo, GD, et al. Poststroke epilepsy: occurrence and predictors – a long-term prospective controlled study (Akershus Stroke Study). Epilepsia 2005;46:1246.

Lovblad, KO, Laubach, HJ, Baird, AE, et al. Clinical experience with diffusion-weighted MR in patients with acute stroke. AJNR Am J Neuroradiol 1998;19:1061.

Low molecular weight heparinoid, ORG 10172 (danaparoid), and outcome after acute ischemic stroke: a randomized controlled trial. The Publications Committee for the Trial of ORG 10172 in Acute Stroke Treatment (TOAST) Investigators. JAMA 1998; 279:1265.

MacMahon, S, Peto, R, Cutler, J, et al. Blood pressure, stroke, and coronary heart disease. Part 1, Prolonged differences in blood pressure: prospective observational studies corrected for the regression dilution bias. Lancet 1990;335:765.

Marhoum El Filali, K, Noun, M, Chakib, A, et al. Ceftriaxone versus penicillin G in the short-term treatment of meningococcal meningitis in adults. Eur J Clin Microbiol Infect Dis 1993;12:766.

Markus, HS, Hambley, H. Neurology and the blood: haematological abnormalities in ischaemic stroke. J Neurol Neurosurg Psychiatry 1998;64:150.

Markus, HS, Harrison, MJ. Microembolic signal detection using ultrasound. Stroke 1995;26:1517.

Markus, HS. Transcranial Doppler detection of circulating cerebral emboli. A review. Stroke 1993;24:1246.

Marson, A, Jacoby, A, Johnson, A, et al. Immediate versus deferred antiepileptic drug treatment for early epilepsy and single seizures: a randomised controlled trial. Lancet 2005;365:2007.

McMillan, DA, Lin, CY, Aronin, SI, Quagliarello, VJ. Community-acquired bacterial meningitis in adults: categorization of causes and timing of death. Clin Infect Dis 2001;33:969.

McNamara, RL, Lima, JA, Whelton, PK, Powe, NR. Echocardiographic identification of cardiovascular sources of emboli to guide clinical management of stroke: a cost effectiveness analysis. Ann Intern Med 1997;127:775.

Meadow, WL, Lantos, J, Tanz, RR, et al. Ought "standard care" be the "standard of care"? A study of the time to administration of antibiotics in children with meningitis. Am J Dis Child 1993;147:40.

Menkes, DL, Gruenthal, M. Slow-frequency repetitive transcranial magnetic stimulation in a patient with focal cortical dysplasia. Epilepsia 2000;41:240.

Metersky, ML, Williams, A, Rafanan, AL. Retrospective analysis: are fever and altered mental status indications for lumbar puncture in a hospitalized patient who has not undergone neurosurgery?. Clin Infect Dis 1997;25:285.

Meuli, RA, Maeder, P, Uske, A. Magnetic resonance imaging. In: Cerebrovascular Disease: Pathophysiology, Diagnosis, and Management, vol 2, Ginsberg, MD, Bogousslavsky, J (Eds), Blackwell Science, Boston, 1998, p. 1265.

Mohr, JP, Caplan, LR, Melski, JW, et al. The Harvard Cooperative Stroke Registry: a prospective registry. Neurology 1978;28:754.

Moncayo, J, Devuyst, G, Van Melle, G, Bogousslavsky, J. Coexisting causes of ischemic stroke. Arch Neurol 2000;57:1139.

Muller, M, Marson, AG, Williamson, PR. Oxcarbazepine versus phenytoin monotherapy for epilepsy. Cochrane Database Syst Rev 2006;CD003615.

Musicco, M, Beghi, E, Solari, A, Viani, F. Treatment of first tonic-clonic seizures does not improve the prognosis of epilepsy: First Seizure Trial Group. Neurology 1997;49:991.

Nathan, N, Borel, T, Djibo, A, et al. Ceftriaxone as effective as long-acting chloramphenicol in short-course treatment of meningococcal meningitis during epidemics: a randomised non-inferiority study. Lancet 2005;366:308.

National Institute for Clinical Excellence. Newer drugs for epilepsy in adults, full guidance. Technology Appraisal Guidance 76, March 2004, www.nice.org.uk/TA076guidance (Accessed March 7, 2005).

Negrini, B, Kelleher, KJ, Wald, ER. Cerebrospinal fluid findings in aseptic versus bacterial meningitis. Pediatrics 2000;105:316.

Nguyen-Huynh, MN, Johnston, SC. Is hospitalization after TIA cost-effective on the basis of treatment with tPA?. Neurology 2005;65:1799.

Nojima, J, Kuratsune, H, Suehisa, E, et al. Strong correlation between the prevalence of cerebral infarction and the presence of anti-cardiolipin/beta2-glycoprotein I and anti-phosphatidylserine/prothrombin antibodies – coexistence of these antibodies enhances ADP-induced platelet activation in vitro. Thromb Haemost 2004;91:967.

Oates-Whitehead, R, Maconochie, I, Baumer, H, Stewart, M. Fluid therapy for acute bacterial meningitis. Cochrane Database Syst Rev 2005;CD004786.

O'Connor, RE, McGraw, P, Edelsohn, L. Thrombolytic therapy for acute ischemic stroke: why the majority of patients remain ineligible for treatment. Ann Emerg Med 1999;33:9.

Oral contraceptives and stroke in young women. Associated risk factors. JAMA 1975; 231:718.

Ostergaard, C, Brandt, C, Konradsen, HB, Samuelsson, S. Differences in survival, brain damage, and cerebrospinal fluid cytokine kinetics due to meningitis caused by 3 different Streptococcus pneumoniae serotypes: evaluation in humans and in 2 experimental models. J Infect Dis 2004;190:1212.

Otis, SM, Ringelstein, EB. The transcranial Doppler examination: principles and applications of transcranial Doppler sonography. In: Neurosonology, Tegeler, CH, Babikian, VL, Gomez, CR (Eds), Mosby, St Louis 1996, p. 113.

Paciaroni, M, Agnelli, G, Micheli, S, Caso, V. Efficacy and safety of anticoagulant treatment in acute cardioembolic stroke: a meta-analysis of randomized controlled trials. Stroke 2007;38:423.

Pappas, DG, Hammerschlag, PE, Hammerschlag, M. Cerebrospinal fluid rhinorrhea and recurrent meningitis. Clin Infect Dis 1993;17:364.

Paris, MM, Ramilo, O, McCracken, GH. Management of meningitis caused by penicillin-resistant Streptococcus pneumoniae. Antimicrob Agents Chemother 1995;39:2171.

Patel, MR, Edelman, RR, Warach, S. Detection of hyperacute primary intraparenchymal hemorrhage by magnetic resonance imaging. Stroke 1996;27:2321.

Pearson, AC, Labovitz, AJ, Tatineni, S, Gomez, CR. Superiority of transesophageal echocardiography in detecting cardiac source of embolism in patients with cerebral ischemia of uncertain etiology. J Am Coll Cardiol 1991;17:66.

Pedley, TA, Hauser, WA. Sudden death in epilepsy: a wake-up call for management. Lancet 2002;359:1790.

Perucca, E. NICE guidance on newer drugs for epilepsy in adults. BMJ 2004;328:1273.

Pessin, MS, Hinton, RC, Davis, KR, et al. Mechanisms of acute carotid stroke. Ann Neurol 1979;6:245.

Petitti, DB, Sidney, S, Bernstein, A, et al. Stroke in users of low-dose oral contraceptives. N Engl J Med 1996;335:8.

Petty, GW, Brown, RD, Whisnant, JP, et al. Ischemic stroke subtypes. A population-based study of incidence and risk factors. Stroke 1999;30:2513.

Practice Advisory: thrombolytic therapy for acute ischemic stroke – Summary statement: report of the Quality Standards Subcommittee of the American Academy of Neurology. Neurology 1996;47:835.

Prevention of stroke by antihypertensive drug treatment in older persons with isolated systolic hypertension. Final results of the Systolic Hypertension in the Elderly Program (SHEP). SHEP Cooperative Research Group. JAMA 1991;265:3255.

Proposal for revised classification of epilepsies and epileptic syndromes. Commission on Classification and Terminology of the International League Against Epilepsy. Epilepsia 1989;30:389.

Proulx, N, Frechette, D, Toye, B, et al. Delays in the administration of antibiotics are associated with mortality from adult acute bacterial meningitis. QJM 2005;98:291.

Purroy, F, Montaner, J, Molina, CA, et al. Patterns and predictors of early risk of recurrence after transient ischemic attack with respect to etiologic subtypes. Stroke 2007;38:3225.

Quagliarello, VJ, Scheld, WM. Treatment of bacterial meningitis. N Engl J Med 1997;336:708.

Randomised study of antiepileptic drug withdrawal in patients in remission. Medical Research Council Antiepileptic Drug Withdrawal Study Group. Lancet 1991;337:1175.

Ratilal, B, Costa, J, Sampaio, C. Antibiotic prophylaxis for preventing meningitis in patients with basilar skull fractures. Cochrane Database Syst Rev 2006;CD004884.

Rauh, R, Fischereder, M, Spengel, FA. Transesophageal echocardiography in patients with focal cerebral ischemia of unknown cause. Stroke 1996;27:691.

Roden-Jullig, A, Britton, M. Effectiveness of heparin treatment for progressing ischaemic stroke: before and after study. J Intern Med 2000;248:287.

Rokey, R, Rolak, LA, Harati, Y, et al. Coronary artery disease in patients with cerebrovascular disease: a prospective study. Ann Neurol 1984;16:50.

Ropper, AH. A preliminary MRI study of the geometry of brain displacement and level of consciousness with acute intracranial masses. Neurology 1989;39:622.

Ropper, AH. Lateral displacement of the brain and level of consciousness in patients with an acute hemispheral mass. N Engl J Med 1986;314:953.

Rothwell, PM, Eliasziw, M, Gutnikov, SA, et al. Endarterectomy for symptomatic carotid stenosis in relation to clinical subgroups and timing of surgery. Lancet 2004; 363:915.

Rothwell, PM, Giles, MF, Chandratheva, A, et al. Effect of urgent treatment of transient ischaemic attack and minor stroke on early recurrent stroke (EXPRESS study): a prospective population-based sequential comparison. Lancet 2007;370:1432.

Rothwell, PM, Giles, MF, Flossmann, E, et al. A simple score (ABCD) to identify individuals at high early risk of stroke after transient ischaemic attack. Lancet 2005;366:29.

Rothwell, PM, Howard, SC, Power, DA, et al. Fibrinogen concentration and risk of ischemic stroke and acute coronary events in 5113 patients with transient ischemic attack and minor ischemic stroke. Stroke 2004;35:2300.

Rothwell, PM, Warlow, CP. Timing of TIAs preceding stroke: time window for prevention is very short. Neurology 2005;64:817.

Rubboli, G, Bisulli, F, Michelucci, R, et al. Sudden falls due to seizure-induced cardiac asystole in drug-resistant focal epilepsy. Neurology 2008;70:1933.

Rugg-Gunn, FJ, Simister, RJ, Squirrell, M, et al. Cardiac arrhythmias in focal epilepsy: a prospective long-term study. Lancet 2004;364:2212.

Russo, LS Jr. Carotid system transient ischemic attacks: clinical, racial, and angiographic correlations. Stroke 1981;12:470.

Saez-Llorens, X, McCoig, C, Feris, JM, et al. Quinolone treatment for pediatric bacterial meningitis: a comparative study of trovafloxacin and ceftriaxone with or without vancomycin. Pediatr Infect Dis J 2002;21:14.

Saito, K, Kimura, K, Nagatsuka, K, et al. Vertebral artery occlusion in duplex color-coded ultrasonography. Stroke 2004;35:1068.

Sandercock, P, Gubitz, G, Foley, P, Counsell, C. Antiplatelet therapy for acute ischaemic stroke. Cochrane Database Syst Rev 2003;CD000029.

Schaad, UB, Suter, S, Gianella-Borradori, A. A comparison of ceftriaxone and cefuroxime for the treatment of bacterial meningitis in children. N Engl J Med 1990;322:141.

Schachter, SC. Advances in the assessment of refractory epilepsy. Epilepsia 1993;34:S24.

Schachter, SC. Brainstorms: Epilepsy in Our Words. Raven Press, New York, 1993.

Schachter, SC. Update in the treatment of epilepsy. Compr Ther 1995;21:473.

Scheld, WM, Koedel, U, Nathan, B, Pfister, HW. Pathophysiology of bacterial meningitis: mechanism(s) of neuronal injury. J Infect Dis 2002;186 Suppl 2:S225.

Scheld, WM, Sande, MA. Bactericidal versus bacteriostatic antibiotic therapy of experimental pneumococcal meningitis in rabbits. J Clin Invest 1983;71:411.

Scheld, WM. Quinolone therapy for infections of the central nervous system. Rev Infect Dis 1989;11 Suppl 5:S1194.

Schellinger, PD, Fiebach, J, Mohr, A, et al. [Value of MRI in intracerebral and subarachnoid hemorrhage]. Nervenarzt 2001;72:907.

Schellinger, PD, Fiebach, JB, Gass, A et al. Accuracy of Stroke MRI in hyperacute intracerebral hemorrhage <6hrs: a prospective standardized blinded multicenter study (abstract). Stroke 2003;34:239.

Schellinger, PD, Jansen, O, Fiebach, JB, et al. A standardized MRI stroke protocol: comparison with CT in hyperacute intracerebral hemorrhage. Stroke 1999;30:765.

Schellinger, PD. Editorial comment – outcome of acute stroke patients without visible occlusion on early arteriography. Stroke 2004;35:1139.

Schenk, EA, Bond, MG, Aretz, TH, et al. Multicenter validation study real-time ultrasonography, arteriography and pathology: pathologic evaluation of carotid endarterectomy specimens. Stroke 1988;19:289.

Schuchat, A, Robinson, K, Wenger, JD, et al. Bacterial meningitis in the United States in 1995. N Engl J Med 1997;337:970.

Schuele, SU, Bermeo, AC, Alexopoulos, AV, et al. Video-electrographic and clinical features in patients with ictal asystole. Neurology 2007;69:434.

Schuele, SU, Bermeo, AC, Locatelli, E, et al. Ictal asystole: a benign condition?. Epilepsia 2008;49:168.

Schulz, UG, Briley, D, Meagher, T, et al. Abnormalities on diffusion weighted magnetic resonance imaging performed several weeks after a minor stroke or transient ischaemic attack. J Neurol Neurosurg Psychiatry 2003;74:734.

Schwartz, SM, Siscovick, DS, Longstreth, WT Jr, et al. Use of low-dose oral contraceptives and stroke in young women. Ann Intern Med 1997;127:596.

Sen, S, Laowatana, S, Lima, J, Oppenheimer, SM. Risk factors for intracardiac thrombus in patients with recent ischaemic cerebrovascular events. J Neurol Neurosurg Psychiatry 2004;75:1421.

Shah, KH, Kleckner, K, Edlow, JA. Short-term prognosis of stroke among patients diagnosed in the emergency department with a transient ischemic attack. Ann Emerg Med 2008;51:316.

Silverman, IE, Restrepo, L, Mathews, GC. Poststroke seizures. Arch Neurol 2002;59:195.

Sirna, S, Biller, J, Skorton, DJ, Seabold, JE. Cardiac evaluation of the patient with stroke. Stroke 1990;21:14.

Skogberg, K, Syrjanen, J, Jahkola, M. Clinical presentation and outcome of listeriosis in patients with and without immunosuppressive therapy. Clin Infect Dis 1992;14:815.

Spangler, SC, Jacobs, MR, Appelbaum, PC. Susceptibilities of 177 penicillin-susceptible and – resistant pneumococci to FK 037, cefpirome, cefepime, ceftriaxone, cefotaxime, ceftazidime, imipenem, biapenem, meropenem, and vancomycin. Antimicrob Agents Chemother 1994;34:898.

Spanos, A, Harrell, FE, Durack, DT. Differential diagnosis of acute meningitis, an analysis of the predictive value of initial observations. JAMA 1989;262:2700.

Specchio, LM, Tramacere, L, La Neve, A, Beghi, E. Discontinuing antiepileptic drugs in patients who are seizure free on monotherapy. J Neurol Neurosurg Psychiatry 2002;72:22.

Spitzer, PG, Hammer, SM, Karchmer, AW. Treatment of Listeria monocytogenes infection with trimethoprim-sulfamethoxazole: case report and review of the literature. Rev Infect Dis 1986;8:427.

Steinke, W, Kloetzsch, C, Hennerici, M. Carotid artery disease assessed by color Doppler flow imaging: correlation with standard Doppler sonography and angiography. AJNR Am J Neuroradiol 1990;11:259.

Steinke, W, Ries, S, Artemis, N, et al. Power Doppler imaging of carotid artery stenosis. Comparison with color Doppler flow imaging and angiography. Stroke 1997;28:1981.

Stratton, JR, Lighty, GW Jr, Pearlman, AS, Ritchie, JL. Detection of left ventricular thrombus by two-dimensional echocardiography: sensitivity, specificity, and causes of uncertainty. Circulation 1982;66:156.

Streifler, JY, Eliasziw, M, Benavente, OR, et al. The risk of stroke in patients with first-ever retinal vs hemispheric transient ischemic attacks and high-grade carotid stenosis. North American Symptomatic Carotid Endarterectomy Trial. Arch Neurol 1995; 52:246.

Sung, CY, Chu, NS. Epileptic seizures in thrombotic stroke. J Neurol 1990;237:166.

Talan, DA, Hoffman, JR, Yoshikawa, TT, Overturf, GD. Role of empiric antibiotics prior to lumbar puncture in suspected bacterial meningitis: state of the art. Rev Infect Dis 1988;10:365.

Tan, TQ, Schutze, GE, Mason, EO Jr, et al. Antibiotic therapy and acute outcome of meningitis due to Streptococcus pneumoniae considered intermediately susceptible to broad-spectrum cephalosporins. Antimicrob Agents Chemother 1994;38:918.

Tauber, MG, Doroshow, CA, Hackbarth, CJ, et al. Antibacterial activity of beta-lactam antibiotics in experimental meningitis due to Streptococcus pneumoniae. J Infect Dis 1984;149:568.

Tergau, F, Naumann, U, Paulus, W, Steinhoff, BJ. Low-frequency repetitive transcranial magnetic stimulation improves intractable epilepsy. Lancet 1999;353:2209.

The International Stroke Trial (IST): a randomised trial of aspirin, subcutaneous heparin, both, or neither among 19435 patients with acute ischaemic stroke. International Stroke Trial Collaborative Group. Lancet 1997;349:1569.

The management of neurosurgical patients with postoperative bacterial or aseptic meningitis or external ventricular drain-associated ventriculitis. Infection in Neurosurgery Working Party of the British Society for Antimicrobial Chemotherapy. Br J Neurosurg 2000;14:7.

Theodore, WH, Hunter, K, Chen, R, et al. Transcranial magnetic stimulation for the treatment of seizures: a controlled study. Neurology 2002;59:560.

Thijs, VN, Lansberg, MG, Beaulieu, C, et al. Is early ischemic lesion volume on diffusion-weighted imaging an independent predictor of stroke outcome? A multivariable analysis. Stroke 2000;31:2597.

Thomas, KE, Hasbun, R, Jekel, J, Quagliarello, VJ. The diagnostic accuracy of Kernig's sign, Brudzinski's sign, and nuchal rigidity in adults with suspected meningitis. Clin Infect Dis 2002;35:46.

Tissue plasminogen activator for acute ischemic stroke. The National Institute of Neurological Disorders and Stroke rt-PA Stroke Study Group. N Engl J Med 1995;333:1581.

Toth, C, Voll, C. Validation of a weight-based nomogram for the use of intravenous heparin in transient ischemic attack or stroke. Stroke 2002;33:670.

Touze, E, Varenne, O, Chatellier, G, et al. Risk of myocardial infarction and vascular death after transient ischemic attack and ischemic stroke: a systematic review and meta-analysis. Stroke 2005;36:2748.

Trouillas, P, Derex, L, Philippeau, F, et al. Early fibrinogen degradation coagulopathy is predictive of parenchymal hematomas in cerebral rt-PA thrombolysis: a study of 157 cases. Stroke 2004;35:1323.

Truwit, CL, Barkovich, AJ, Gean-Marton, A, et al. Loss of the insular ribbon: another early sign of acute MCA infarction. Radiology 1990;176:801.

Tunkel, AR, Hartman, BJ, Kaplan, SL, et al. Practice guidelines for the management of bacterial meningitis. Clin Infect Dis 2004;39:1267.

Tuomanen, E, Hengstler, B, Rich, R, et al. Nonsteroidal anti-inflammatory agents in the therapy of experimental pneumococcal meningitis. J Infect Dis 1987;155:985.

Uchihara, T, Tsukagoshi, H. Jolt accentuation of headache: the most sensitive sign of CSF pleocytosis. Headache 1991;31:167.

van de Beek, D, de Gans, J, Spanjaard, L, et al. Clinical features and prognostic factors in adults with bacterial meningitis. N Engl J Med 2004;351:1849.

van de, Beek, D, de Gans, J, Tunkel, AR, Wijdicks, EF. Community-acquired bacterial meningitis in adults. N Engl J Med 2006;354:44.

van Wijk, I, Kappelle, LJ, van Gijn, J, et al. Long-term survival and vascular event risk after transient ischaemic attack or minor ischaemic stroke: a cohort study. Lancet 2005;365:2098.

Vazquez, B. Monotherapy in epilepsy: role of the newer antiepileptic drugs. Arch Neurol 2004;61:1361.

Viladrich, PF, Gudiol, F, Linares, J, et al. Evaluation of vancomycin for therapy of adult pneumococcal meningitis. Antimicrob Agents Chemother 1991;35:2467.

Von Kummer, R, Meyding-Lamad'e, U, Forsting, M, et al. Sensitivity and prognostic value of early CT in occlusion of the middle cerebral artery trunk. AJNR Am J Neuroradiol 1994;15:9.

von Reutern, GM, von Budingen, HJ. Ultrasound Diagnosis of Cerebrovascular Disease, Thieme, New York, 1993.

Warach, S, Gaa, J, Siewert, B, et al. Acute human stroke studied by whole brain echo planar diffusion-weighted magnetic resonance imaging. Ann Neurol 1995;37:231.

Ward, JI, Fraser, DW, Baraff, LJ, Plikaytis, BD. Haemophilus influenzae meningitis: a national study of secondary spread in household contacts. N Engl J Med 1979;301:122.

Weisfelt, M, van de, Beek, D, Spanjaard, L, de Gans, J. Arthritis in adults with community-acquired bacterial meningitis: a prospective cohort study. BMC Infect Dis 2006;6:64.

WHO. Control of epidemic meningococcal disease. WHO practical guidelines, 1995; Foundation Marcel Merieux, Lyon

Winbeck, K, Bruckmaier, K, Etgen, T, et al. Transient ischemic attack and stroke can be differentiated by analyzing early diffusion-weighted imaging signal intensity changes. Stroke 2004;35:1095.

Woessner, R, Grauer, M, Bianchi, O, et al. Treatment with anticoagulants in cerebral events (TRACE). Thromb Haemost 2004;91:690.

Wong, KS, Chen, C, Ng, PW, et al. Low-molecular-weight heparin compared with aspirin for the treatment of acute ischaemic stroke in Asian patients with large artery occlusive disease: a randomised study. Lancet Neurol 2007;6:407.

Wong, KS, Liang, EY, Lam, WW, et al. Spiral computed tomography angiography in the assessment of middle cerebral artery occlusive disease. J Neurol Neurosurg Psychiatry 1995;59:537.

Wu, CM, McLaughlin, K, Lorenzetti, DL, et al. Early risk of stroke after transient ischemic attack: a systematic review and meta-analysis. Arch Intern Med 2007;167:2417.

Zarrouk, V, Vassor, I, Bert, F, et al. Evaluation of the management of postoperative aseptic meningitis. Clin Infect Dis 2007;44:1555.

Zeller, JA, Tschoepe, D, Kessler, C. Circulating platelets show increased activation in patients with acute cerebral ischemia. Thromb Haemost 1999;81:373.

Zoons, E. Neurology 2008;70:2109.

HEMATOLOGY

Agnihotri, P, Telfer, M, Butt, Z, et al. Chronic anemia and fatigue in elderly patients: results of a randomized, double-blind, placebo-controlled, crossover exploratory study with epoetin alfa. J Am Geriatr Soc 2007;55:1557.

Alikhan, R, Cohen, AT, Combe, S, et al. Risk factors for venous thromboembolism in hospitalized patients with acute medical illness: analysis of the MEDENOX Study. Arch Intern Med 2004;164:963.

Ansell, J, Hirsh, J, Dalen, J, et al. Managing oral anticoagulant therapy. Chest 2001;119 Suppl:22S-38S.

Artz, AS, Fergusson, D, Drinka, PJ, et al. Mechanisms of unexplained anemia in the nursing home. J Am Geriatr Soc 2004;52:423.

ATS website. Click on section dealing with Statements and Guidelines. (Accessed February 28, 2008).

Balducci, L. Epidemiology of anemia in the elderly: information on diagnostic evaluation. J Am Geriatr Soc 2003;51:2.

Baldwin, JG. Hematopoietic function in the elderly. Arch Intern Med 1988;148:2544.

Beard, J, Tobin, B. Iron status and exercise. Am J Clin Nutr 2000;72:594S.

Berglund, B. High-altitude training. Aspects of haematological adaptation. Sports Med 1992;14:289.

Bergstrome Jones, AK, Poon, A. Evaluation of a single-tube multiplex polymerase chain reaction screen for detection of common alpha-thalassemia genotypes in a clinical laboratory. Am J Clin Pathol 2002;118:18.

Beutler, E, Waalen, J. The definition of anemia: what is the lower limit of normal of the blood hemoglobin concentration? Blood 2006;107:1747.

Beutler, E, West, C. Hematologic differences between African-Americans and whites: the roles of iron deficiency and alpha-thalassemia on hemoglobin levels and mean corpuscular volume. Blood 2005;106:740.

Birdwell, BG, Raskob, GE, Whitsett, TL, et al. The clinical validity of normal compression ultrasonography in outpatients suspected of having deep venous thrombosis. Ann Intern Med 1998;128:1.

Ble, A, Fink, JC, Woodman, RC, et al. Renal function, erythropoietin, and anemia of older persons: the InCHIANTI study. Arch Intern Med 2005;165:2222.

Brouwer, JL, Veeger, NJ, Kluin-Nelemans, HC, van der, Meer J. The pathogenesis of venous thromboembolism: evidence for multiple interrelated causes. Ann Intern Med 2006;145:807.

Bull, BS, Breton-Gorius, J. Morphology of the erythron. In: Williams' Hematology, 5th ed, Beutler, E, Lichtman, MA, Coller, BS, Kipps, TJ (Eds), McGraw-Hill, New York, p. 349.

Buller, HR, Agnelli, G, Hull, RD, et al. Antithrombotic therapy for venous thromboembolic disease: the Seventh ACCP Conference on Antithrombotic and Thrombolytic Therapy. Chest 2004;126:401S.

Chaves, PH, Xue, QL, Guralnik, JM, et al. What constitutes normal hemoglobin concentration in community-dwelling disabled older women?. J Am Geriatr Soc 2004;52:1811.

Conrad, M. Anemia; eMedicine Journal [serial online], 2008. Available from http://emedicine.medscape.com/article/198475-diagnosis

Constans, J, Boutinet, C, Salmi, LR, et al. Comparison of four clinical prediction scores for the diagnosis of lower limb deep venous thrombosis in outpatients. Am J Med 2003;115:436.

Culleton, BF, Manns, BJ, Zhang, J, et al. Impact of anemia on hospitalization and mortality in older adults. Blood 2006;107:3841.

Cushman, M, Tsai, AW, White, RH, et al. Deep vein thrombosis and pulmonary embolism in two cohorts: the longitudinal investigation of thromboembolism etiology. Am J Med 2004;117:19.

Davenport, J. Macrocytic anemia. Am Fam Physician 1996;53:155.

Denny, SD, Kuchibhatla, MN, Cohen, HJ. Impact of anemia on mortality, cognition, and function in community-dwelling elderly. Am J Med 2006;119:327.

Dufaux, B, Hoederath, A, Streitberger, I, et al. Serum ferritin, transferrin, haptoglobin and iron in middle-and long-distance runners, elite rowers and professional racing cyclists. Int J Sports Med 1981;2:43.

Erslev, AJ. Reticulocyte enumeration. In: Williams' Hematology, 5th ed, Beutler, E, Lichtman, MA, Coller, BS, et al (Eds), McGraw-Hill, New York 1995, p. L28.

Ferrucci, L, Guralnik, JM, Bandinelli, S, et al. Unexplained anaemia in older persons is characterised by low erythropoietin and low levels of pro-inflammatory markers. Br J Haematol 2007;136:849.

Ferrucci, L, Maggio, M, Bandinelli, S, et al. Low testosterone levels and the risk of anemia in older men and women. Arch Intern Med 2006;166:1380.

Galen, RS. Application of the predictive value model in the analysis of test effectiveness. Clin Lab Med 1982;2:685.

Garn, SM, Ryan, AS, Abraham, S, Owen, G. Suggested sex and age appropriate values for "low" and "deficient" hemoglobin levels. Am J Clin Nutr 1981;34:1648.

Gjorup, T, Bugge, PM, Hendriksen, C, Jensen, AM. A critical evaluation of the clinical diagnosis of anemia. Am J Epidemiol 1986;124:657.

Gomes, ME, Deinum, J, Timmers, HJ, Lenders, JW. Occam's razor; anaemia and ortho-static hypotension. Lancet 2003;362:1282.

Gonzalez, C, Penado, S, Llata, L, et al. The clinical spectrum of retroperitoneal hematoma in anticoagulated patients. Medicine (Baltimore) 2003;82:257.

Gorman, WP, Davis, KR, Donnelly, R. ABC of arterial and venous disease. Swollen lower limb-1: general assessment and deep vein thrombosis. BMJ 2000;320:1453.

Greydanus, DE, Patel, DR.The female athlete. Before and beyond puberty. Pediatr Clin North Am 2002;49:553.

Guralnik, JM, Eisenstaedt, RS, Ferrucci, L, et al. Prevalence of anemia in persons 65 years and older in the United States: evidence for a high rate of unexplained anemia. Blood 2004;104:2263.

Hillman, RS, Ault, KA (Eds). Clinical approach to anemia. In: Hematology in Clinical Practice, McGraw-Hill, New York 2001, p. 29.

Hillman, RS, Ault, KA (Eds). Normal erythropoiesis. In: Hematology in Clinical Practice, McGraw-Hill, New York 2001, p. 3.

Hirsh, J, Fuster, V, Ansell, J, Halperin, JL. American Heart Association/American College of Cardiology Foundation guide to warfarin therapy. J Am Coll Cardiol 2003;41:1633.

Hirsh, J, Lee, AY. How we diagnose and treat deep vein thrombosis. Blood 2002;99:3102.

Huisman, MV, Buller, HR, Ten Cate, JW, Vreeken, J. Serial impedance plethysmography for suspected deep-vein thrombosis in outpatients. N Engl J Med 1986;314:823.

Hull, RD, Hirsh, J, Sackett, DL, et al. Clinical validity of a negative venogram in patients with clinically suspected venous thrombosis. Circulation 1981;64:622.

Hung, OL, Kwon, NS, Cole, AE, et al. Evaluation of the physician's ability to recognize the presence or absence of anemia, fever, and jaundice. Acad Emerg Med 2000;7:146.

Inelmen, EM, D'Alessio, M, Gatto, MR, et al. Descriptive analysis of the prevalence of anemia in a randomly selected sample of elderly people living at home: some results of an Italian multicentric study. Aging (Milano) 1994; 6:81.

Izaks, GJ, Westendorp, RGJ, Knook, DL. The definition of anemia in older persons. JAMA 1999;281:1714.

Jacob, G, Raj, SR, Ketch, T, et al. Postural pseudoanemia: posture-dependent change in hematocrit. Mayo Clin Proc 2005;80:611.

Jones, J. Transfusion in oligemia. In: Blood Transfusion in Clinical Medicine, 8th ed, Mollison, PL, Engelfriet, CP, Contreras, M (Eds), Blackwell, Oxford 1987, p. 41.

Kehat, I, Shupak, A, Goldenberg, I, Shoshani, O. Long-term hematological effects in Special Forces trainees. Mil Med 2003;168:116.

Marchand, A, Galen, RS, Van Lente, F. The predictive value of serum haptoglobin in hemolytic disease. JAMA 1980;243:1909.

Mohandas, N, Schrier, SL. Mechanisms of red cell destruction in hemolytic anemias. In: The Hereditary Hemolytic Anemias, Mentzer, WC, Wagner, GM (Eds), Churchill Livingstone, New York, 1989, p. 391.

Morris, MW, Williams, WJ, Nelson, DA. Automated blood cell counting. In: Williams' Hematology, 5th ed, Beutler, E, Lichtman, MA, Coller, BS, et al (Eds), McGraw-Hill, New York, 1995, p. L3.

Nardone, DA, Roth, KM, Mazur, DJ, et al. Usefulness of physical examination in detecting the presence or absence of anemia. Arch Intern Med 1990;150:201.

Nilsson-Ehle, H, Jagenburg, R, Landahl, S, et al. Decline of blood haemoglobin in the aged: a longitudinal study of an urban Swedish population from age 70 to 81. Br J Haematol 1989;71:437.

Nilsson-Ehle, H, Jagenburg, R, Landahl, S, et al. Haematological abnormalities and reference intervals in the elderly. A cross-sectional comparative study of three urban Swedish population samples aged 70, 75 and 81 years. Acta Med Scand 1988;224:595.

Nissenson, AR, Goodnough, LT, Dubois, RW. Anemia: not just an innocent bystander?. Arch Intern Med 2003;163:1400.

Nordenberg, D, Yip, R, Binkin, NJ. The effect of cigarette smoking on hemoglobin levels and anemia screening. JAMA 1990;264:1556.

Patel, KV, Harris, TB, Faulhaber, M, et al. Racial variation in the relationship of anemia with mortality and mobility disability among older adults. Blood 2007; 109(11): 4663-70.

Patel, KV, Harris, TB, Faulhaber, M, et al. Racial variation in the relationship of anemia with mortality and mobility disability among older adults. Blood 2007;109:4663.

Penninx, BW, Guralnik, JM, Onder, G, et al. Anemia and decline in physical performance among older persons. Am J Med 2003;115:104.

Perera, R, Isola, L, Kaufmann, H. Effect of recombinant erythropoietin on anemia and orthostatic hypotension in primary autonomic failure. Clin Auton Res 1995;5:211.

Perry, GS, Byers, T, Yip, R, Margen, S. Iron nutrition does not account for the hemoglobin differences between blacks and whites. J Nutr 1992;122:1417.

Reed, WW, Diehl, LF. Leukopenia, neutropenia, and reduced hemoglobin levels in healthy American blacks. Arch Intern Med 1991;151:501.

Robins, EB, Blum, S. Hematologic reference values for African American children and adolescents. Am J Hematol 2007;82:611.

Rudzki, SJ, Hazard, H, Collinson, D. Gastrointestinal blood loss in triathletes: its etiology and relationship to sports anaemia. Aust J Sci Med Sport 1995;27:3.

Ruiz, MA, Saab, S, Rickman, LS. The clinical detection of scleral icterus: Observations of multiple examiners. Mil Med 1997;162:560.

Ruiz-Arguelles, GJ, Beutler, E, Waalen, J. Altitude above sea level as a variable for definition of anemia. Blood 2006;108:2131.

Sabatine, M, et al. Pocket Medicine, 2nd ed, Lippincott Williams Wilkins, Philadelphia, PA, 2004.

Sandler, DA, Martin, JF, Duncan, JS, et al. Diagnosis of deep vein thrombosis: comparison of clinical evaluation, ultrasound, plethysmography and venoscan with X-ray venogram. Lancet 1984;2:716.

Sawka, MN, Convertino, VA, Eichner, ER, et al. Blood volume: importance and adaptations to exercise training, environmental stresses, and trauma/sickness. Med Sci Sports Exerc 2000;32:332.

Selby, GB, Eichner, ER. Endurance swimming, intravascular hemolysis, anemia and iron depletion. Am J Med 1986;81:791.

Schreiber, D. Deep venous thrombosis and thrombophlebitis; eMedicine Journal [serial online], 2008. Available from http://emedicine.medscape.com/article/758140-overview

Serjeant, GR, Serjeant, GE, Thomas, PW, et al. Human parvovirus infection in homozygous sickle cell disease. Lancet 1993;341:1237.

Shaskey, DJ, Green, GA. Sports haematology. Sports Med 2000;29:27.

Sheth, TN, Choudhry, NK, Bowes, M, Detsky, AS. The relation of conjunctival pallor to the presence of anemia. J Gen Intern Med 1997;12:102.

Silverberg, DS, Wexler, D, Iaina, A, Schwartz, D. The interaction between heart failure and other heart diseases, renal failure, and anemia. Semin Nephrol 2006;26:296.

Stachon, A, Sondermann, N, Imohl, M, Krieg, M. Nucleated red blood cells indicate high risk of in-hospital mortality. J Lab Clin Med 2002;140:407.

Steensma, DP, Hoyer, JD, Fairbanks, VF. Hereditary red blood cell disorders in Middle Eastern patients. Mayo Clin Proc 2001;76:285.

Steensma, DP, Tefferi, A. Anemia in the elderly: How should we define it, when does it matter, and what can be done?. Mayo Clin Proc 2007;82:958.

Stewart, RD, Baretta, ED, Platte, LR, et al. Carboxyhemoglobin levels in American blood donors. JAMA 1974; 229:1187.

Subramaniam, RM, Snyder, B, Heath, R, et al. Diagnosis of lower limb deep venous thrombosis in emergency department patients: performance of Hamilton and modified Wells scores. Ann Emerg Med 2006;48:678.

Tamariz, LJ, Eng, J, Segal, JB, et al. Usefulness of clinical prediction rules for the diagnosis of venous thromboembolism: a systematic review. Am J Med 2004;117:676.

Tefferi, A. Anemia in adults: a contemporary approach to diagnosis. Mayo Clin Proc 2003;78:1274.

Valeri, CR, Dennis, RC, Ragno, G, et al. Limitations of the hematocrit level to assess the need for red blood cell transfusion in hypovolemic anemic patients. Transfusion 2006;46:365.

Weiskopf, RB, Viele, MK, Feiner, J, et al. Human cardiovascular and metabolic response to acute, severe isovolemic anemia. JAMA 1998;279:217.

Weiss, GB, Bessman, JD. Spurious automated red cell values in warm autoimmune hemolytic anemia. Am J Hematol 1984;17:433.

Wells, PS, Anderson, DR, Bormanis, J, et al. Value of assessment of pretest probability of deep-vein thrombosis in clinical management. Lancet 1997;350:1795.

Westerman, DA, Evans, D, Metz, J. Neutrophil hypersegmentation in iron deficiency anaemia: a case-control study. Br J Haematol 1999;107:512.

Williams, WJ, Morris, MW, Nelson, DA. Examination of the blood. In: Williams' Hematology, 5th ed, Beutler, E, Lichtman, MA, Coller, BS, et al (Eds), McGraw-Hill, New York, 1995, p. 8.

World Health Organization. Nutritional Anaemias: Report of a WHO Scientific Group. Geneva, World Health Organizatio, 1968.

ENDOCRINE

Abramson, E, Arky, R. Diabetic acidosis with initial hypokalemia. JAMA 1966;196:401.

Adler, D, Voide, C, Thorens, JB, Desmeules, J. SIADH consecutive to ciprofloxacin intake. Eur J Intern Med 2004;15:463.

Adrogué, HJ, Eknoyan, G, Suki, WN. Diabetic ketoacidosis: role of the kidney in the acid-base homeostasis re-evaluated. Kidney Int 1984;25:591.

Adrogué, HJ, Lederer, ED, Suki, WN, Eknoyan, G. Determinants of plasma potassium levels in diabetic ketoacidosis. Medicine (Baltimore) 1986;65:163.

Adrogue, HJ, Madias, NE. Hyponatremia. N Engl J Med 2000;342:1581.

Adrogué, HJ, Wilson, H, Boyd, AE III, et al. Plasma acid-base patterns in diabetic ketoacidosis. N Engl J Med 1982;307:1603.

Anderson, RJ. Hospital-associated hyponatremia. Kidney Int 1986;29:1237.

Arieff, AI, Carroll, HJ. Nonketotic hyperosmolar coma with hyperglycemia: clinical features, pathophysiology, renal function, acid-base balance, plasma-cerebrospinal fluid equilibria and the effects of therapy in 37 cases. Medicine (Baltimore) 1972; 51:73.

Aronson, D, Dragu, RE, Nakhoul, F, et al. Hyponatremia as a complication of cardiac catheterization: a prospective study. Am J Kidney Dis 2002;40:940.

Barrett, EJ, DeFronzo, RA. Diabetic ketoacidosis: diagnosis and treatment. Hosp Pract (Off Ed) 1984;19:89.

Barsotti, MM. Potassium phosphate and potassium chloride in the treatment of DKA. Diabetes Care 1980;3:569.

Beigelman, PM. Potassium in severe diabetic ketoacidosis. Am J Med 1973;54:419.

Bratusch-Marrain, PR, Komajati, M, Waldhausal, W. The effect of hyperosmolarity on glucose metabolism. Pract Cardiol 1985;11:153.

Bressler, RB, Huston, DP. Water intoxication following moderate dose intravenous cyclophosphamide. Arch Intern Med 1985;145:548.

Brown, PM, Tompkins, CV, Juul, S, Sonksen, PH. Mechanism of action of insulin in diabetic patients: a dose-related effect on glucose production and utilisation. Br Med J 1978;1:1239.

Brun-Buisson, CJ, Bonnet, F, Bergeret, S, et al. Recurrent high-permeability pulmonary edema associated with diabetic ketoacidosis. Crit Care Med 1985;13:55.

Casteels, K, Beckers, D, Wouters, C, Van Geet, C. Rhabdomyolysis in diabetic ketoacidosis. Pediatr Diabetes 2003;4:29.

Cooke, CR, Turin, MD, Walker, WD. The syndrome of inappropriate antidiuretic hormone secretion: pathophysiologic mechanisms in solute and volume regulation. Medicine (Baltimore) 1979;58:240.

Covyeou, JA, Jackson, CW. Hyponatremia associated with escitalopram. N Engl J Med 2007;356:94.

Cruz, J, Spitler, D, Blyer, A, et al. Hyponatremia secondary to inappropriate antidiuretic hormone (SIADH) in association with high dose chemotherapy and bone marrow rescue (abstract). Proc Annu Meet Am Soc Clin Oncol 1994;13:A1530.

Daugirdas, JT, Kronfol, NO, Tzalaloukas, AH, Ing, TS. Hyperosmolar coma: cellular dehydration and the serum sodium concentration. Ann Intern Med 1989;110:855.

Decaux, G, Brimioulle, S, Genette, F, Mockel, J. Treatment of the syndrome of inappropriate secretion of antidiuretic hormone by urea. Am J Med 1980;69:99.

Decaux, G, Genette F. Urea for long-term treatment of syndrome of inappropriate secretion of antidiuretic hormone. Br Med J 1981;2:1081.

Decaux, G, Vandergheynst, F, Bouko, Y, et al. Nephrogenic syndrome of inappropriate antidiuresis in adults: high phenotypic variability in men and women from a large pedigree. J Am Soc Nephrol 2007;18:606.

Decaux, G, Waterlot, Y, Genette, F, Mockel, J. Treatment of the syndrome of inappropriate secretion of antidiuretic hormone with furosemide. N Engl J Med 1981;304:329.

DeFronzo, RA, Matzuda, M, Barret, E. Diabetic ketoacidosis: a combined metabolic-nephrologic approach to therapy. Diabetes Rev 1994;2:209.

Dunn, AL, Powers, JR, Ribeiro, MJ, et al. Adverse events during use of intranasal desmopressin acetate for haemophilia A and von Willebrand disease: a case report and review of 40 patients. Haemophilia 2000;6:11.

Ellison, DH, Berl, T. The syndrome of inappropriate antidiuresis. N Engl J Med 2007; 356:2064.

Ennis, ED, Stahl, EJ, Kreisberg, RA. The hyperosmolar hyperglycemic syndrome. Diabetes Rev 1994;2:115.

Fabian, TJ, Amico, JA, Kroboth, PD, et al. Paroxetine-induced hyponatremia in older adults: a 12-week prospective study. Arch Intern Med 2004;164:327.

Feeney, JG. Water intoxication and oxytocin [editorial]. Br Med J (Clin Res Ed) 1982;285:243.

Feldman, BJ, Rosenthal, SM, Vargas, GA, et al. Nephrogenic syndrome of inappropriate antidiuresis. N Engl J Med 2005;352:1884.

Ferlito, A, Rinaldo, A, Devaney, KO. Syndrome of inappropriate antidiuretic hormone secretion associated with head neck cancers: review of the literature. Ann Otol Rhinol Laryngol 1997;106:878.

Fieldman, NR, Forsling, ML, Le Quesne, LP. The effect of vasopressin on solute and water excretion during and after surgical operations. Ann Surg 1985;201:383.

Fisher, JN, Kitabchi, AE. A randomized study of phosphate therapy in the treatment of diabetic ketoacidosis. J Clin Endocrinol Metab 1983;57:177.

Fisher, JN, Shahshahani, MM, Kitabshi, AE. Diabetic ketoacidosis: low-dose insulin therapy by various routes. N Engl J Med 1977;297:238.

Forrest, JN Jr, Cox, M, Hong, C, et al. Superiority of demeclocycline over lithium in the treatment of chronic syndrome of inappropriate secretion of antidiuretic hormone. N Engl J Med 1978;298:173.

Fraley, DS, Adler, S. Correction of hyperkalemia by bicarbonate despite constant blood pH. Kidney Int 1977;12:354.

Fulop, M, Tannenbaum, H, Dreyer, N. Ketotic hyperosmolar coma. Lancet 1973;2:635.

Gentric, A, Baccino, E, Mottier, D, et al. Temporal arteritis revealed by a syndrome of inappropriate secretion of antidiuretic hormone. Am J Med 1988;85:559.

Gold, PW, Robertson, GL, Ballenger, JC, et al. Carbamazepine diminishes the sensitivity of the plasma arginine vasopressin response to osmotic stimulation. J Clin Endocrinol Metab 1983;57:952.

Gowrishankar, M, Lin, SH, Mallie, JP, et al. Acute hyponatremia in the perioperative period: insights into its pathophysiology and recommendations for management. Clin Nephrol 1998;50:352.

Greenberg, A, Verbalis, JG. Vasopressin receptor antagonists. Kidney Int 2006;69:2124.

Hensen, J, Haenelt, M, Gross, P. Water retention after oral chlorpropamide is associated with an increase in renal papillary arginine vasopressin receptors. Eur J Endocrinol 1995;132:459.

Hill, AR, Uribarri, J, Mann, J, Berl, T. Altered water metabolism in tuberculosis. Role of vasopressin. Am J Med 1990;88:357.

Hillier, TA, Abbott, RD, Barrett, EJ. Hyponatremia: evaluating the correction factor for hyperglycemia. Am J Med 1999;106:399.

Hillman, K. Fluid resuscitation in diabetic emergencies – a reappraisal. Intensive Care Med 1987;13:4.

Holden, R, Jackson, MA. Near-fatal hyponatremic coma due to vasopressin over-secretion after "ecstasy" (3,4-MDMA). Lancet 1996;347:1052.

Humphries, JE, Siragy, H. Significant hyponatremia following DDAVP administration in a healthy adult. Am J Hematol 1993;44:12.

Inappropriate antidiuretic hormone secretion of unknown origin. Kidney Int 1980;17:554.

Johnson, BE, Chute, JP, Rushin, J, et al. A prospective study of patients with lung cancer and hyponatremia of malignancy. Am J Respir Crit Care Med 1997;156:1669.

Kahn, T. Reset osmostat and salt and water retention in the course of severe hyponatremia. Medicine (Baltimore) 2003;82:170.

Kamiyama, T, Iseki, K, Kawazoe, N, et al. Carbamazepine-induced hyponatremia in a patient with partial central diabetes insipidus. Nephron 1993;64:142.

Kebler, R, McDonald, FD, Cadnapaphornchai, P. Dynamic changes in serum phosphorus levels in diabetic ketoacidosis. Am J Med 1985;79:571.

Keller, V, Berger, W. Prevention of hypophosphalemia by phosphate infusion during treatment of diabetic ketoacidosis and hyperosmolar coma. Diabetes 1980;29:87.

Kim, JK, Summer, SN, Wood, WM, et al. Osmotic and non-osmotic regulation of arginine vasopressin (AVP) release, mRNA, and promoter activity in small cell lung carcinoma (SCLC) cells. Mol Cell Endocrinol 1996;123:179.

Kitabchi, AE, Ayyagari, V, Guerra, SM, et al. The efficacy of low-dose versus conventional therapy of insulin for treatment of diabetic ketoacidosis. Ann Intern Med 1976;84:633.

Kitabchi, AE, Fisher, JN, Murphy, MB, Rumbak, MJ. Diabetic ketoacidosis and the hyperglycemic hyperosmolar nonketotic state. In: Joslin's Diabetes Mellitus, 13th ed, Kahn, CR, Weir, GC (Eds), Lea & Febiger, Philadelphia 1994, p. 738.

Kitabchi, AE, Umpierrez, GE, Murphy, MB, et al. Management of hyperglycemic crises in patients with diabetes. Diabetes Care 2001;24:131.

Kitabchi, AE, Umpierrez, GE, Murphy, MB, Kreisberg, RA. Hyperglycemic crises in adult patients with diabetes: a consensus statement from the American Diabetes Association. Diabetes Care 2006;29:2739.

Kitabchi, AE, Umpierrez, GE, Murphy, MB. Diabetic ketoacidosis and hyperglycemic hyperosmolar state. In: International Textbook of Diabetes Mellitus, 3rd ed, DeFronzo, RA, Ferrannini, E, Keen, H, Zimmet, P (Eds), John Wiley & Sons, Ltd, Chichester, UK, 2004, p. 1101.

Kreisberg, RA. Diabetic ketoacidosis: new concepts and trends in pathogenesis and treatment. Ann Intern Med 1978;88:681.

Kreisberg, RA. Phosphorus deficiency and hypophosphatemia. Hosp Pract 1977;12:121.

Li, C, Wang, W, Summer, SN, et al. Molecular mechanisms of antidiuretic effect of oxytocin. J Am Soc Nephrol 2008;19:225.

Liu, BA, Mittmann, N, Knowles, SR, Shear, NH. Hyponatremia and the syndrome of inappropriate secretion of antidiuretic hormone associated with the use of selective serotonin reuptake inhibitors: a review of spontaneous reports [published erratum appears in Can Med Assoc J 1996 Oct 15;155(8):1043]. CMAJ 1996;155:519.

Middleton, P, Kelly, AM, Brown, J, Robertson, M. Agreement between arterial and central venous values for pH, bicarbonate, base excess, and lactate. Emerg Med J 2006;23:622.

Molitch, ME, Rodman, E, Hirsch, CA, Dubinsky, E. Spurious serum creatinine elevations in ketoacidosis. Ann Intern Med 1980;93:280.

Morris, LR, Murphy, MB, Kitabchi, AE. Bicarbonate therapy in diabetic ketoacidosis. Ann Intern Med 1986;105:836.

Narins, RG, Cohen JJ. Bicarbonate therapy for organic acidosis: the case for its continued use. Ann Intern Med 1987;106:615.

Nielsen, OA, Johannessen, AC, Bardrum, B. Oxcarbazepine-induced hyponatremia, a cross-sectional study. Epilepsy Res 1988;2:269.

Oh, MS, Carroll, HJ, Goldstein, DA, Fein, IA. Hyperchloremic acidosis during the recovery phase of diabetic ketosis. Ann Intern Med 1978;89:925.

Oh, MS, Carroll, HJ, Uribarri, J. Mechanism of normochloremic and hyperchloremic acidosis in diabetic ketoacidosis. Nephron 1990;54:1.

Okuda, Y, Adrogué, HJ, Field, JB, et al. Counterproductive effects of sodium bicarbonate in diabetic ketoacidosis. J Clin Endocrinol Metab 1996;81:314.

Olson, BR, Rubino, D, Gumowski, J, Oldfield, EH. Isolated hyponatremia after transsphenoidal pituitary surgery. J Clin Endocrinol Metab 1995;80:85.

Owen, OE, Licht, JH, Sapir, DG. Renal function and effects of partial rehydration during diabetic ketoacidosis. Diabetes 1981;30:510.

Ozturk, S, Ozsenel, EB, Kazancioglu, R, Turkmen, A. A case of fluoxetine-induced syndrome of inappropriate antidiuretic hormone secretion. Nat Clin Pract Nephrol 2008;4:278.

Padilla, AJ, Loeb, JN. "Low dose" versus "high dose" insulin regimens in the management of uncontrolled diabetes. A survey. Am J Med 1977;63:843.

Page, MM, Alberti, KG, Greenwood, R, et al. Treatment of diabetic coma with continuous low-dose insulin infusion. Br Med J 1974;2:687.

Powner, D, Snyder, JV, Grenvik, A. Altered pulmonary capillary permeability complicating recovery from diabetic ketoacidosis. Chest 1975;68:253.

Raghavan, V, et al. Hypoglycemia; eMedicine Journal [serial online], 2007. Available from http://emedicine.medscape.com/article/122122-diagnosis

Rainey, RL, Estes, PW, Neely, CL, Amick, LD. Myoglobinuria following diabetic acidosis with electromyographic evaluation. Arch Intern Med 1963;111:564.

Renneboog, B, Musch, W, Vandemergel, X, et al. Mild chronic hyponatremia is associated with falls, unsteadiness, and attention deficits. Am J Med 2006;119:71.

Robertson, GL, Aycinena, P, Zerbe, RL. Neurogenic disorders of osmoregulation. Am J Med 1982;72:339.

Robertson, GL, Shelton, RL, Athar, S. The osmoregulation of vasopressin. Kidney Int 1976;10:25.

Rofallov, A. Syndrome of inappropriate antidiuretic hormone secretion: treatment and medication; eMedicine Journal [serial online]. Available from http://emedicine.medscape.com/article/768380-treatment

Rose, BD. New approach to disturbances in the plasma sodium concentration. Am J Med 1986;81:1033.

Rose, BD, Post, TW. Clinical Physiology of Acid-Base and Electrolyte Disorders, 5th ed, McGraw-Hill, New York, 2001, pp. 809-815.

Rosenthal, NR, Barrett, EJ. An assessment of insulin action in hyperosmolar hyperglycemic nonketotic diabetic patients. J Clin Endocrinol Metab 1985;60:607.

Rucker, D. Diabetic ketoacidosis; eMedicine Journal [serial online], 2009. Available from http://emedicine.medscape.com/article/766275-overview

Sachdeo, RC, Wasserstein, A, Mesenbrink, PJ, D'Souza, J. Effects of oxcarbazepine on sodium concentration and water handling. Ann Neurol 2002;51:613.

Saito, T, Ishikawa, S, Abe, K, et al. Acute aquaresis by the nonpeptide arginine vasopressin (AVP) antagonist OPC-31260 improves hyponatremia in patients with syndrome of inappropriate secretion of antidiuretic hormone (SIADH). J Clin Endocrinol Metab 1997;82:1054.

Sane, T, Rantakari, K, Poranen, A, et al. Hyponatremia after transsphenoidal surgery for pituitary tumors. J Clin Endocrinol Metab 1994;79:1395.

Schrier, RW, Gross, P, Gheorghiade, M, et al. Tolvaptan, a selective oral vasopressin V2-receptor antagonist, for hyponatremia. N Engl J Med 2006;355:2099.

Serradeil-Le Gal, C, Lacour, C, Valette, G, et al. Characterization of SR 121463A, a highly potent and selective vasopressin V2 receptor antagonist. J Clin Invest 1996;98:2729.

Shepherd, LL, Hutchinson, RJ, Worden, EK, et al. Hyponatremia and seizures after intravenous administration of desmopressin acetate for surgical hemostasis. J Pediatr 1989;114:470.

Shilo, S, Werner, D, Hershko, C. Acute hemolytic anemia caused by severe hypophosphatemia in diabetic ketoacidosis. Acta Haematol 1985;73:55.

Sorensen, JB, Andersen, MK, Hansen, HH. Syndrome of inappropriate secretion of antidiuretic hormone (SIADH) in malignant disease. J Intern Med 1995;238:97.

Soupart, A, Gross, P, Legros, JJ, et al. Successful long-term treatment of hyponatremia in syndrome of inappropriate antidiuretic hormone secretion with stavaptan (SR121463B), an orally active nonpeptide vasopressin V2-receptor antagonist. Clin J Am Soc Nephrol 2006;1:1154.

Sprung, CL, Rackow, EC, Fein, IA. Pulmonary edema: a complication of diabetic ketoacidosis. Chest 1980;77:687.

Steele, A, Gowrishankar, M, Abrahamson, S, et al. Postoperative hyponatremia despite near-isotonic saline infusion: a phenomenon of desalination. Ann Intern Med 1997;126:20.

Sulway, MJ, Malins, JM. Acetone in diabetic ketoacidosis. Lancet 1970;2:736.

Talmi, YP, Wolf, GT, Hoffman, HT, Krause, CJ. Elevated arginine vasopressin levels in squamous cell cancer of the head and neck. Laryngoscope 1996;106:317.

Thumfart, J, Roehr, CC, Kapelari, K, Querfeld, U. Desmopressin associated symptomatic hyponatremic hypervolemia in children. are there predictive factors?. J Urol 2005;174:294.

Umpierrez, GE, Cuervo, R, Karabell, A, et al. Treatment of diabetic ketoacidosis with subcutaneous insulin aspart. Diabetes Care 2004;27:1873.

Umpierrez, GE, Latif, K, Stoever, J, et al. Efficacy of subcutaneous insulin lispro versus continuous intravenous regular insulin for the treatment of patients with diabetic ketoacidosis. Am J Med 2004;117:291.

Van Amelsvoort, T, Bakshi, R, Devaux, CB, Schwabe, S. Hyponatremia associated with carbamazepine and oxcarbazepine therapy: a review. Epilepsia 1994;35:181.

Verbalis, JG, Goldsmith, SR, Greenberg, A, et al. Hyponatremia treatment guidelines 2007: expert panel recommendations. Am J Med 2007;120:S1.

Verbalis, JG. Pathogenesis of hyponatremia in an experimental model of the syndrome of inappropriate antidiuresis. Am J Physiol 1994;267:R1617.

Viallon, A, Zeni, F, Lafond, P, et al. Does bicarbonate therapy improve the management of severe diabetic ketoacidosis? Crit Care Med 1999;27:2690.

Vitting, KE, Gardenswartz, MH, Zabetakis, PM, et al. Frequency of hyponatremia and nonosmolar vasopressin release in the acquired immune deficiency syndrome. JAMA 1990;263:973.

Wachtel, TJ. The diabetic hyperosmolar state. Clin Geriatr Med 1990;6:797.

Weatherall, M. The risk of hyponatremia in older adults using desmopressin for nocturia: a systematic review and meta-analysis. Neurourol Urodyn 2004;23:302.

Weissman, PN, Shenkman, L, Gregerman, RI. Chlorpropamide hyponatremia: drug-induced inappropriate antidiuretic-hormone activity. N Engl J Med 1971;284:65.

Wiggam, MI, O'Kane, MJ, Harper, R, et al. Treatment of diabetic ketoacidosis using normalization of blood 3-hydroxybutyrate concentration as the endpoint of emergency management. A randomized controlled study. Diabetes Care 1997;20:1347.

Wijdicks, EF, Vermeulen, M, Murray, GD, et al. The effects of treating hypertension following aneurysmal subarachnoid hemorrhage. Clin Neurol Neurosurg 1990;92:111.

Wilkins, B. Cerebral oedema after MDMA ("ecstasy") and unrestricted water intake. Hyponatraemia must be treated with low water input. BMJ 1996;313:689.

Wilson, HK, Keuer, SP, Lea, AS, et al. Phosphate therapy in diabetic ketoacidosis. Arch Intern Med 1982;142:517.

Winter, RJ, Harris, CJ, Phillips, LS, Green, OC. Diabetic ketoacidosis. Induction of hypocalcemia and hypomagnesemia by phosphate therapy. Am J Med 1979;67:897.

Wolfsdorf, J, Glaser, N, Sperling, MA. Diabetic ketoacidosis in infants, children, and adolescents: a consensus statement from the American Diabetes Association. Diabetes Care 2006;29:1150.

Zeltser, D, Rosansky, S, van Rensburg, H, et al. Assessment of the efficacy and safety of conivaptan in euvolemic and hypervolemic hyponatremia. Am J Nephrol 2007;27:447.

Zipf, WB, Bacon, GE, Spencer, ML, et al. Hypocalcemia, hypomagnesemia, and transient hypoparathyroidism during therapy with potassium phosphate in diabetic ketoacidosis. Diabetes Care 1979;2:265.

INFECTIONS/INFECTIOUS DISEASES

Allman, R, LaPrade, C, Noel, L, et al. Pressure sores among hospitalized patients. Ann Intern Med 1986;105:337.

Allman, RM, Goode, PS, Patrick, MM, et al. Pressure ulcer risk factors among hospitalized patients with activity limitation. JAMA 1995;273:865.

Allman, RM, Walker, JM, Hart, MK, et al. Air-fluidized beds or conventional therapy for pressure sores. A randomized trial. Ann Intern Med 1987;107:641.

Alm, A, Hornmark, AM, Fall, PA, et al. Care of pressure sores: a controlled study of the use of hydrocolloid dressing compared with wet saline gauze compresses. Acta Derm Venereol (Stockh) 1983;35:142.

Argenta, LC, Morykwas, MJ. Vacuum-assisted closure: a new method for wound control and treatment: clinical experience. Ann Plast Surg 1997;38:563.

Baier, RR, Gifford, DR, Lyder, CH, et al. Quality improvement for pressure ulcer care in the nursing home setting: the Northeast Pressure Ulcer Project. J Am Med Dir Assoc 2003;4:291.

Barbenel, J, Ferguson-Pell, M, Kennedy, R. Mobility of elderly patients in bed. J Am Geriatr Soc 1986;34:633.

Barbenel, JC, Jordan, MM, Nicol, SM, et al. Incidence of pressure sores in the greater Glasgow health board area. Lancet 1977;2:548.

Bates-Jensen, BM. The Pressure Sore Status Tool a few thousand assessments later. Adv Wound Care 1997;10:65.

Baumgarten, M, Margolis, DJ, Localio, AR, et al. Pressure ulcers among elderly patients early in the hospital stay. J Gerontol A Biol Sci Med Sci 2006;61:749.

Bello, YM, Phillips, TJ. Recent advances in wound healing. JAMA 2000;283:716.

Belmin, J, Meaume, S, Rabus, MT, Bohbot, S. Sequential treatment with calcium alginate dressings and hydrocolloid dressings accelerates pressure ulcer healing in older subjects: a multicenter randomized trial of sequential versus nonsequential treatment with hydrocolloid dressings alone. J Am Geriatr Soc 2002;50:269.

Bennett, L, Lee, BY. Vertical shear existence in animal pressure threshold experiments. Decubitus 1988;1:18.

Bennett, RG, Bellatoni, MF, Ouslander, JG. Air-fluidized bed treatment of nursing home patients with pressure sores. J Am Geriatr Soc 1989;37:235.

Bennett, RG, O'Sullivan, J, DeVito, EM, Remsburg, R. The increasing medical malpractice risk related topressure ulcers in the United States. J Am Geriatr Soc 2000;48:73.

Bergstrom, N, Braden, B. A prospective study of pressure sore risk among institutionalized elderly. J Am Geriatr Soc 1992;40:747.

Bergstrom, N, Braden, B, Kemp, M, et al. Multi-site study of incidence of pressure ulcers andthe relationship between risk level, demographic characteristics, diagnoses, and prescription of preventive interventions. J Am Geriatr Soc 1996;44:22.

Bergstrom, N, Braden, BJ, Laguzza, A, Holman, V. The Braden scale for predicting pressure sore risk. Nurs Res 1987;36:205.

Bergstrom, N, Demuth, PJ, Braden, BJ. A clinical trial of the Braden Scale for predicting pressure sore risk. Nursing Clinics of North America 1987;22:417.

Bergstrom, N, Horn, SD, Smout, RJ, et al. The national pressure ulcer long-term care study: outcomes of pressure ulcer treatments in long-term care. J Am Geriatr Soc 2005;53:1721.

Berlowitz, DR, Ash, AS, Brandeis, GH, et al. Rating long-term care facilities on pressure ulcer development: importance of case-mix adjustment. Ann Intern Med 1996;124:557.

Berlowitz, DR, Brandeis, GH, Anderson, J, Du, W. Effect of pressure ulcers on the survival of long-term care residents. J Gerontol A Biol Sci Med Sci 1997;52:M106.

Berlowitz, DR, Brandeis, GH, Anderson, JJ, Brand, HK. Predictors of pressure ulcer healing among long-term care residents. J Am Geriatr Soc 1997;45:30.

Berlowitz, DR, Brandeis, GH, Anderson, JJ, et al. Evaluation of a risk-adjustment model for pressure ulcer development using the Minimum Data Set. J Am Geriatr Soc 2001;49:872.

Berlowitz, DR, Brandeis, GH, Morris, JN, et al. Deriving a risk-adjustment model for pressure ulcer development using the Minimum Data Set. J Am Geriatr Soc 2001;49:866.

Berlowitz, DR, Wilking, SV. Risk factors for pressure sores. J Am Geriatr Soc 1989;37:1043.

Berlowitz, DR, Wilking, SV. The short-term outcome of pressure sores. J Am Geriatr Soc 1990;38:748.

Berlowitz, DR, Young, GJ, Hickey, EC, et al. Quality improvement implementation in the nursing home. Health Serv Res 2003;38:65.

Black, JM. Moving Toward Consensus on Deep Tissue Injury and Pressure Ulcer Staging. Adv Skin Wound Care 2005;18:415.

Black, J, Baharestani, M, et al. National Pressure Ulcer Advisory Panel's updated pressure ulcer staging system. Adv Skin Wound Care 2007 May;20(5):269-274.

Bliss, M, Simini, B. When are the seeds of postoperative pressure sores sown?. Often during surgery. BMJ 1999;319:863.

Bourdel-Marchasson, I, Barateau, M, Rondeau, V, et al. A multi-center trial of the effects of oral nutritional supplementation in critically ill older inpatients. GAGE Group. Groupe Aquitain Geriatrique d'Evaluation. Nutrition 2000;16:1.

Brandeis, GH, Berlowitz, DR, Katz, P. Are pressure ulcers preventable? A survey of experts. Adv Skin Wound Care 2001;14:244.

Brandeis, GH, Morris, JN, Nash, DJ, Lipsitz, LA. The epidemiology and natural history of pressure ulcers in elderly nursing home residents. JAMA 1990;264:2905.

Brandeis, GH, Ooi, WL, Hossain, M, et al. A longitudinal study of risk factors associated with the formation of pressure ulcers in nursing homes. J Am Geriatr Soc 1994;42:388.

Breslow, RA, Hallfrisch, J, Guy, DG, et al. The importance of dietary protein in healing pressure ulcers. J Am Geriatr Soc 1993;41:357.

Cooney, LM Jr. Pressure sores and urinary incontinence. J Am Geriatr Soc 1997;45:1278.

Cullum, N, McInnes, E, Bell-Syer, SE, Legood, R. Support surfaces for pressure ulcer prevention. Cochrane Database Syst Rev 2004;CD001735.

Curtis, D. Cellulitis; eMedicine Journal [serial online], 2009. Available from http://emedicine.medscape.com/article/781412-overview

Deshmukh, GR, Barkel, DC, Sevo, D, Hergenroeder, P. Use or misuse of colostomy to heal pressure ulcers. Dis Colon Rectum 1996;39:737.

Disa, JJ, Carlton, JM, Goldberg, NH. Efficacy of operative cure in pressure sore patients. Plast Reconstr Surg 1992;89:272.

Ellis, SL, Finn, P, Noone, M, Leaper, DJ. Eradication of methicillin-resistant Staphylococcus aureus from pressure sores using warming therapy. Surg Infect (Larchmt) 2003;4:53.

Evans, D, Land, L. Topical negative pressure for treating chronic wounds. Cochrane Database Syst Rev 2001;CD001898.

Exton-Smith, AN, Sherwin, RW. The prevention of pressure sores. Significance of spontaneous bodily movements. Lancet 1961;2:1124.

Feedar, JA, Kloth, LC, Gentzkow, GD. Chronic dermal ulcer healing enhanced with monophasic pulsed electrical stimulation. Phys Ther 1991;71:639.

Ferrell, BA, Josephson, K, Norvid, P, Alcorn, H. Pressure ulcers among patients admitted to home care. J Am Geriatr Soc 2000;48:1042.

Ferrell, BA, Osterweil, D, Christenson, P. A randomized trial of low-air-loss beds for treatment of pressure ulcers. JAMA 1993;269:494.

Ferrell, BA. The sessing scale for measurement of pressure ulcer healing. Adv Wound Care 1997;10:78.

Finucane, TE. Malnutrition, tube feeding, and pressure sores: data are incomplete. J Am Geriatr Soc 1995;43:447.

Flemming, K, Cullum, N. Electromagnetic therapy for the treatment of pressure sores. Cochrane Database Syst Rev 2001;CD002930.

Flemming, K, Cullum, N. Therapeutic ultrasound for pressure sores. Cochrane Database Syst Rev 2000;CD001275.

Flock, P. Pilot study to determine the effectiveness of diamorphine gel to control pressure ulcer pain. J Pain Symptom Manage 2003;25:547.

Gardner, SE, Frantz, RA, Schmidt, FL. Effect of electrical stimulation on chronic wound healing: a meta-analysis. Wound Repair Regen 1999;7:495.

Gaynes, RP, Weinstein, RA, Chamberlin, W, Kabins, SA. Antibiotic-resistant flora in nursing home patients admitted to the hospital. Arch Intern Med 1985;145:1804.

Goldstone, LA, Roberts, BV. A preliminary discriminant function analysis of elderly orthopaedic patients who will or will not contract a pressure sore. Int J Nurs Stud 1980;17:17.

Goode, PS, Thomas, DR.Pressure ulcers local wound care. Clin Geriatr Med 1997;13:543.

Gorse, GJ, Messner, RL. Improved pressure sore healing with hydrocolloid dressings. Arch Dermatol 1987;123:766.

Graumlich, JF, Blough, LS, McLaughlin, RG, Milbrandt, JC. Healing pressure ulcers with collagen or hydrocolloid: a randomized, controlled trial. J Am Geriatr Soc 2003;51:147.

Griffin, JW, Tooms, RE, Mendius, RA, et al. Efficacy of high voltage pulsed current for healing of pressure ulcers in patients with spinal cord injury. Phys Ther 1991;71:433.

Guralnik, J, Harris, T, White, L, et al. Occurrence and predictors of pressure sores in the National Health and Nutrition Examination Survey follow-up. J Am Geriatr Soc 1988;36:807.

Hing, E. Characteristics of nursing home residents, health status and care received; National Nursing Home Survey, United States, May-December 1977. Hyattsville, MD: US Department of Health and Human Services; Public Health Service; Office of Health Research, Statistics, and Technology; National Center for Health Statistics, 1981.

Hofman, A, Geelkerken, RH, Wille, J, et al. Pressure sores and pressure-decreasing mattresses: controlled clinical trial. Lancet 1994;343:568.

Horn, SD, Bender, SA, Ferguson, ML, et al. The national pressure ulcer long-term care study: pressure ulcer development in long-term care residents. J Am Geriatr Soc 2004;52:359.

Iglesias, C, Nixon, J, Cranny, G, et al. Pressure relieving support surfaces (PRESSURE) trial: cost effectiveness analysis. BMJ 2006;332:1416.

Inman, KJ, Sibbald, WJ, Rutledge, FS, Clark, BJ. Clinical utility and cost-effectiveness of an air suspension bed in the prevention of pressure ulcers. JAMA 1993;269:1139.

Jay, R. Other considerations in selecting a support surface. Adv Wound Care 1997;10:37.

Joseph, E, Hamori, CA, Bergman, S, et al. A prospective randomized trial of vacuum-assisted closure versus standard therapy of chronic nonhealing wounds. Wounds 2000;12:60.

Kloth, LC, Berman, JE, Dumit-Minkel, S, et al. Effects of a normothermic dressing on pressure ulcer healing. Adv Skin Wound Care 2000;13:69.

Kloth, LC, Berman, JE, Nett, M, et al. A randomized controlled clinical trial to evaluate the effects of noncontact normothermic wound therapy on chronic full-thickness pressure ulcers. Adv Skin Wound Care 2002;15:270.

Knox, DM, Anderson, TM, Anderson, PS. Effects of different turn intervals on skin of healthy older adults. Adv Wound Care 1994;7:48.

Koretz, RL, Avenell, A, Lipman, TO, et al. Does enteral nutrition affect clinical outcome? A systematic review of the randomized trials. Am J Gastroenterol 2007;102:412.

Kosiak, M. Etiology and pathology of ischemic ulcers. Arch Phys Med Rehabil 1959;40:62.

Kosiak, M. Etiology of decubitus ulcers. Arch Phys Med Rehabil 1961;42:19.

Kraft, MR, Lawson, L, Pohlmann, B, et al. A comparison of Epi-Lock and saline dressings in the treatment of pressure ulcers. Decubitus 1993;6:42.

Krasner, D. Wound healing scale, version 1.0: a proposal. Adv Wound Care 1997;10:82.

Landi, F, Aloe, L, Russo, A, et al. Topical treatment of pressure ulcers with nerve growth factor: a randomized clinical trial. Ann Intern Med 2003;139:635.

Langer, G, Schloemer, G, Knerr, A, et al. Nutritional interventions for preventing and treating pressure ulcers. Cochrane Database Syst Rev 2003;CD003216.

Lee, LK, Ambrus, JL. Collagenase therapy for decubitus ulcers. Geriatrics 1975;30:91.

Lowthian, PT. Underpads in the prevention of decubiti. In: Bedsore biomechanics, Kenedi, RM, Cowden, JM, Scales, JT (Eds), University Park Press, Baltimore, MD 1976, p. 141.

Mandrekas, AD, Mastorakos, DP. The management of decubitus ulcers by musculocutaneous flaps: a five-year experience. Ann Plast Surg 1992;28:167.

Mawson, AR, Biundo, JJ, Neville, P, et al. Risk factors for early occurring pressure ulcers following spinal cord injury. Am J Phys Med Rehabil 1988;67:123.

McKenna, MJ, Moyers, J, Feuerberg, M. Review of Non-regulatory Quality Improvement Interventions, pp. 339-384 in HCFA Report to Congress: Study of Private Accreditation (Deeming) Nursing Homes, Regulatory Incentives and Non-regulatory Initiatives, and Effectiveness of the Survey and Certification System, Vol II, HCFA, Washington, DC 1998.

Mendez-Eastman, S. Guidelines for using negative pressure wound therapy. Adv Skin Wound Care 2001;14:314.

Moody, B, Fanale, J, Thompson, M, et al. Impact of staff education on pressure sore development in elderly hospitalized patients. Arch Intern Med 1988;148:2241.

Moss, RJ, La Puma, J. The ethics of pressure sore evaluation and treatment in the elderly: a practical approach. J Am Geriatr Soc 1991;39:905.

Murphy, S, Denman, S, Bennett, RG, et al. Methicillin-resistant staphylococcus aureus colonization in a long-term-care facility. J Am Geriatr Soc 1992;40:213.

Mustoe, TA, Gutter, NR, Allman, RM, et al. A phase II study to evaluate recombinant platelet-derived growth factor B in the treatment of stage 3 and 4 pressure ulcers. Arch Surg 1994;129:213.

National Pressure Ulcer Advisory Panel. NPUAP position on reverse staging of pressure ulcers. Adv Wound Care 1998;8:32.

National Pressure Ulcer Advisory Panel. Updated staging system. www.npuap.org/pr2.htm. (Accessed August 22, 2007).

Niazi, ZB, Salzberg, CA, Byrne, DW, Viehbeck, M. Recurrence of initial pressure ulcer in persons with spinal cord injuries. Adv Wound Care 1997;10:38.

Niazi, ZB, Salzberg, CA. Surgical management of pressure ulcers. Ostomy Wound Manage 1997;43:44.

Nixon, J, Cranny, G, Iglesias, C, et al. Randomised, controlled trial of alternating pressure mattresses compared with alternating pressure overlays forthe prevention of pressure ulcers: PRESSURE (pressure relieving support surfaces) trial. BMJ 2006;332:1413.

Nola, GT, Vistnes, LM. Differential response of skin and muscle in the experimental production of pressure sores. Plast Reconstr Surg 1980;66:728.

Norton, D, McLaren, R, Exton-Smith, AN. An Investigation of Geriatric Nursing Problems in Hospital, Churchill Livingston, London, 1975.

Norton, D. Calculating the risk: reflections on the Norton scale. Decubitus 1989;2:24.

Perneger, TV, Gaspoz, JM, Rae, AC, et al. Contribution of individual items to the performance of the Norton pressure ulcer prediction scale. J Am Geriatr Soc 1998;46:1282.

Pressure ulcers in adults: prediction and prevention. Clinical Practice Guideline Number 3, AHCPR Publication no. 92-0047, May 1992.

Pressure ulcers in America: prevalence, incidence, and implications for the future. An executive summary of the National Pressure Ulcer Advisory Panel monograph. Adv Skin Wound Care 2001;14:208.

Pressure ulcers prevalence, cost and risk assessment: consensus development conference statement – the National Pressure Ulcer Advisory Panel. Decubitus 1989;2:24.

Preventing pressure sores. Lancet 1990;335:1311.

Price, P, Bale, S, Crook, H, Harding, KG. The effect of a radiant heat dressing on pressure ulcers. J Wound Care 2000;9:201.

Pullen, R, Popp, R, Volkers, P, Fusgen, I. Prospective randomized double-blind study of the wound-debriding effects of collagenase and fibrinolysin/deoxyribonuclease in pressure ulcers. Age Ageing 2002;31:126.

Rao, DB, Sane, PG, Georgiev, EL. Collagenase in the treatment of dermal and decubitus ulcers. J Am Geriatr Soc 1975;23:22.

Reddy, M, Gill, SS, Rochon, PA. Preventing pressure ulcers: a systematic review. JAMA 2006;296:974.

Reed, JW. Pressure ulcers in the elderly: prevention and treatment utilizing the team approach. MD State Med J 1981;45.

Rees, RS, Robson, MC, Smiell, JM, Perry, BH. Becaplermin gel in the treatment of pressure ulcers: a phase II randomized, double-blind, placebo-controlled study. Wound Repair Regen 1999;7:141.

Reuler, JB, Cooney, T. The pressure sore: pathophysiology and principles of management. Ann Intern Med 1981;94:661.

Revis, D. Decubitus ulcers; eMedicine Journal [serial online], 2008. Available from http://emedicine.medscape.com/article/190115-overview

Robson, MC, Phillips, LG, Lawrence, WT, et al. The safety and effect of topically applied recombinant basic fibroblast growth factor on healing of chronic pressure sores. Ann Surg 1992;216:401.

Robson, MC, Phillips, LG, Thomason, A, et al. Platelet-derived growth factorB for the treatment of chronic pressure ulcers. Lancet 1992;339:23.

Rosen, J, Mittal, V, Degenholtz, H, et al. Ability, incentives, and management feedback: organizational change to reduce pressure ulcers in a nursing home. J Am Med Dir Assoc 2006;7:141.

Salvadalena, GD, Snyder, ML, Brogdon, KE. Clinical trial of the Braden Scale on an acute care medical unit. J ET Nurs 1992;19:160.

Sanada, H, Nagakawa, T, Yamamoto, M, et al. The role of skin blood flow in pressure ulcer development during surgery. Adv Wound Care 1997;10:29.

Scheckler, WE, Peterson, PJ. Infections and infection control among residents of eight rural Wisconsin nursing homes. Arch Intern Med 1986;146:1981.

Schoonhoven, L, Haalboom, JR, Bousema, MT, et al. Prospective cohort study of routine use of risk assessment scales for prediction of pressure ulcers. BMJ 2002;325:797.

Schubert, V. Hypotension as a risk factor for the development of pressure sores in elderly subjects. Age Ageing 1991;20:255.

Sebern, MD. Pressure ulcer management in home health care: efficacy and cost effectiveness of moisture vapor permeable dressing. Arch Phys Med Rehabil 1986;67:726.

Shea, JD. Pressure sores. Clin Orthop Relat Res 1998;112:89.

Shekelle, PG, Ortiz, E, Rhodes, S, et al. Validity of the Agency for Healthcare Research and Quality clinical practice guidelines: how quickly do guidelines become outdated?. JAMA 2001;286:1461.

Shepard, M, Parker, M, DeClerque, N. The under-reporting of pressure sores in patients transferred between hospital and nursing home. J Am Geriatr Soc 1987;35:159.

Smith, DM, Winsemius, DK, Besdine, RW. Pressure sores in the elderly: can this outcome be improved?. J Gen Intern Med 1991;6:81.

Soloway, DN. Civil claims relating to pressure ulcers: a claimants' lawyer's perspective. Ostomy Wound Manage 1998;44:20.

Spector, WD, Fortinsky, RH. Pressure ulcer prevalence in Ohio nursing homes. J Aging Health 1998;44:20.

Spector, WD, Kapp, MC, Tucker, RJ, Sternberg, J. Factors associated with presence of decubitus ulcers at admission to nursing homes. Gerontologist 1988;28:830.

Takeda, T, Koyama, T, Izawa, Y, et al. Effects of malnutrition on development of experimental pressure sores. J Dermatol 1992;19:602.

ter Riet, G, Kessels, AG, Knipschild, PG. Randomized clinical trial of ascorbic acid in the treatment of pressure ulcers. J Clin Epidemiol 1995;48:1453.

Thomas, DR, Diebold, MR, Eggemeyer, LM. A controlled, randomized, comparative study of a radiant heat bandage on the healing of stage 3-4 pressure ulcers: a pilot study. J Am Med Dir Assoc 2005;6:46.

Thomas, DR, Goode, PS, Tarquine, PH, Allman, RM. Hospital-acquired pressure ulcers and risk of death. J Am Geriatr Soc 1996;44:1435.

Thomas, DR, Rodeheaver, GT, Bartolucci, AA, et al. Pressure ulcer scale for healing: derivation and validation of the PUSH tool. Adv Wound Care 1997;10:96.

Thomas, DR. Issues and dilemmas in the prevention and treatment of pressure ulcers: a review. J Gerontol A Biol Sci Med Sci 2001;56:M328.

Thomas, DR. Pressure ulcers. In: Geriatric Medicine, CK, Cassel (Ed), Springer, New York, 1997.

Thomas, DR. The promise of topical growth factors in healing pressure ulcers. Ann Intern Med 2003;139:694.

Treatment of Pressure Ulcers. Clinical Practice Guideline Number 15, AHCPR Publication no. 95-0652, December 1994.

Urinary incontinence in adults: acute and chronic management. Clinical Practice Guideline Number 2 (1996 Update), AHCPR Publication no. 96-0682, March 1996.

Vanderwee, K, Grypdonck, MH, De Bacquer, D, Defloor, T. Effectiveness of turning with unequal time intervals on the incidence of pressure ulcer lesions. J Adv Nurs 2007;57:59.

Versluysen, M. How elderly patients with femoral fracture develop pressure sores in hospital. Br Med J (Clin Res Ed) 1986;292:1311.

Wang, C, Schwaitzberg, S, Berliner, E, et al. Hyperbaric oxygen for treating wounds: a systematic review of the literature. Arch Surg 2003;138:272.

Whitney, JD, Salvadalena, G, Higa, L, Mich, M. Treatment of pressure ulcers with noncontact normothermic wound therapy: healing and warming effects. J Wound Ostomy Continence Nurs 2001;28:244.

Xakellis, G, Frantz, R, Arteaga, M, et al. A comparison of patient risk for pressure ulcer development with nursing use of preventive interventions. J Am Geriatr Soc 1992;40:1250.

Xakellis, GC, Chrischilles, EA. Hydrocolloid versus saline gauze dressings in treating pressure ulcers: a cost-effectiveness analysis. Arch Phys Med Rehabil 1992;73:463.

Xakellis, GC, Frantz, RA. The cost-effectiveness of interventions for preventing pressure ulcers. J Am Board Fam Pract 1996;9:79.

Yarkony, GM, Kirk, PM, Carlson, C, et al. Classification of pressure ulcers. Arch Dermatol 1990;126:1218.

Zappolo, A. Discharges from nursing homes. National Nursing Home Survey (Publication #PHS S81-1715). Hyattsville, MD: US Department of Health and Human Services, 1981.

Zeppetella, G, Paul, J, Ribeiro, MD. Analgesic efficacy of morphine applied topically to painful ulcers. J Pain Symptom Manage 2003;25:555.

Zeppetella, G, Ribeiro, MD. Morphine in intrasite gel applied topically to painful ulcers. J Pain Symptom Manage 2005;29:118.

Zinn, JS, Brannon, D, Weech, R. Quality improvement in nursing care facilities: extent, impetus, and impact. Am J Med Qual 1997;12:51.

ICU ROUNDS

Abraham, E. Coagulation abnormalities in acute lung injury and sepsis [comment]. Am J Respir Cell Mol Biol 2000;22:401.

Abraham, E, Laterre, PF, Garg, R, et al. Drotrecogin alfa (activated) for adults with severe sepsis and a low risk of death. N Engl J Med 2005;353:1332.

Absalom, A, Pledger, D, Kong, A. Adrenocortical function in critically ill patients 24 h after a single dose of etomidate. Anaesthesia 1999;54:861.

Adhikari, NK, Burns, KE, Friedrich, JO, et al. Effect of nitric oxide on oxygenation and mortality in acute lung injury: systematic review and meta-analysis. BMJ 2007;334:779.

Al-Saady, N, Bennett, D. Decelerating inspiratory flow wave form improves lung mechanics and gas exchange in patients on intermittent positive pressure ventilation. Intensive Care Med 1985;11:68.

Angus, DC, Clermont, G, Linde-Zwirble, WT, et al. Healthcare costs and long-term outcomes after acute respiratory distress syndrome: a phase III trial of inhaled nitric oxide. Crit Care Med 2006;34:2883.

Angus, DC, Linde-Zwirble, WT, Clermont, G, Ball, DE. Cost-effectiveness of drotrecogin alfa (activated) in the treatment of severe sepsis. Crit Care Med 2003;31:1.

Angus, DC, Linde-Zwirble, WT, Lidicker, J, et al. Epidemiology of severe sepsis in the United States: analysis of incidence, outcome, and associated costs of care. Crit Care Med 2001;29:1303.

Annane, D, Bellissant, E, Cavaillon, JM. Septic shock. Lancet 2005;365:63.

Annane, D, Sebille, V, Bellissant, E. Effect of low doses of corticosteroids in septic shock patients with or without early acute respiratory distress syndrome. Crit Care Med 2006;34:22.

Annane, D. Glucocorticoids for ARDS: just do it!. Chest 2007;131:945.

Annane, D. ICU physicians should abandon the use of etomidate!. Intensive Care Med 2005;31:325.

Anzueto, A, Baughman, RP, Guntupalli, KK, et al. Aerosolized surfactant in adults with sepsis-induced acute respiratory distress syndrome. Exosurf Acute Respiratory Distress Syndrome Sepsis Study Group. N Engl J Med 1996;334:1417.

Arnold, JH, Hanson, JH, Toro-Figuero, LO, et al. Prospective, randomized comparison of high-frequency oscillatory ventilation and conventional mechanical ventilation in pediatric respiratory failure. Crit Care Med 1994;22:1530.

Arnold, JH, Truog, RD, Thompson, JE, Fackler, JC. High-frequency oscillatory ventilation in pediatric respiratory failure. Crit Care Med 1993;21:272.

Artigas, A, Bernard, GR, Carlet, J, et al. The American-European consensus conference on ARDS, part 2. Ventilatory, pharmacologic, supportive therapy, study design strategies, and issues related to recovery and remodeling. Am J Respir Crit Care Med 1998;157:1332.

Aznar, J, Espana, F, Estelles, A, Royo, M. Heparin stimulation of the inhibition of activated protein C and other enzymes by human protein C inhibitor – influence of the molecular weight of heparin and ionic strength. Thromb Haemost 1996;76:983.

Bachli, EB, Vavricka, SR, Walter, RB, et al. Drotrecogin alfa (activated) for the treatment of meningococcal purpura fulminans. Intensive Care Med 2003;29:337.

Baudouin, SV. Exogenous surfactant replacement in ARDS – one day, someday, or never?. N Engl J Med 2004;351:853.

Benzing, A, Brautigam, P, Geiger, K, et al. Inhaled nitric oxide reduces pulmonary transvascular albumin flux in patients with acute lung injury. Anesthesiology 1995; 83:1153.

Bernard, G, Artigas, A, Carlet, J, et al. The American-European consensus conference on ARDS: definitions, mechanisms, relevant outcomes, and clinical trial coordination. Am J Respir Crit Care Med 1994;149:818.

Bernard, GR, Luce, JM, Sprung, CL, et al. High-dose corticosteroids in patients with the adult respiratory distress syndrome. N Engl J Med 1987;317:1565.

Bernard, GR, Vincent, JL, Laterre, PF, et al. Efficacy and safety of recombinant human activated protein C for severe sepsis. N Engl J Med 2001;344:699.

Bernard, GR. Acute respiratory distress syndrome: a historical perspective. Am J Respir Crit Care Med 2005;172:798.

Bersten, AD, Hersch, M, Cheung, H, Rutledge, FS, Sibbald, WJ. The effect of various sympathomimetics on the regional circulations in hyperdynamic sepsis. Surgery 1992;112:549.

Bloomfield, GL, Holloway, S, Ridings, PC, et al. Pretreatment with inhaled nitric oxide inhibits neutrophil migration and oxidative activity resulting in attenuated sepsis-induced acute lung injury. Crit Care Med 1997;25:584.

Bone, RC. Toward an epidemiology and natural history of SIRS (systemic inflammatory response syndrome). JAMA 1992;268:3452.

Bouachour, G, et al. Hemodynamic changes in acute adrenal insufficiency. Intensive Care Med 1994;20:138.

Bouros, D, Nicholson, AC, Polychronopoulos, V, du Bois, RM. Acute interstitial pneumonia. Eur Respir J 2000;15:412.

Brennan, JM, Blair, JE, Hampole, C, et al. Radial artery pulse pressure variation correlates with brachial artery peak velocity variation in ventilated subjects when measured by internal medicine residents using hand-carried ultrasound devices. Chest 2007;131:1301.

Brochard, L, Rauss, A, Benito, S, et al. Comparison of three methods of gradual withdrawal from ventilatory support during weaning from mechanical ventilation. Am J Respir Crit Care Med 1994;150:896.

Brochard, L, Rua, F, Lorino, H, Lemaire, F, Harf, A. Inspiratory pressure support compensates for the additional work of breathing caused by the endotracheal tube. Anesthesiology 1991;75:739.

Brower, RG, Lanken, PN, MacIntyre, N, et al. Higher versus lower positive end-expiratory pressures in patients with the acute respiratory distress syndrome. N Engl J Med 2004;351:327.

Brun-Buisson, C, Doyon, F, Carlet, J, et al. Incidence, risk factors, and outcome of severe sepsis and septic shock in adults: a multicenter prospective study in intensive care units. JAMA 1995;274:968.

Brunkhorst, FM, Engel, C, Bloos, F, et al. Intensive insulin therapy and pentastarch resuscitation in severe sepsis. N Engl J Med 2008;358:125.

Buchheit, J, Eid, N, Rodgers, GJ, et al. Acute eosinophilic pneumonia with respiratory failure: a new syndrome? Am Rev Respir Dis 1992;145:716.

Bursten, SL, Federighi, D, Wald, J, et al. Lisofylline causes rapid and prolonged suppression of serum levels of free fatty acids. J Pharmacol Exp Ther 1998;284:337.

Bursten, SL, Federighi, DA, Parsons, P, et al. An increase in serum C18 unsaturated free fatty acids as a predictor of the development of acute respiratory distress syndrome. Crit Care Med 1996;24:1129.

Bux, J, Sachs, UJ. The pathogenesis of transfusion-related acute lung injury (TRALI). Br J Haematol 2007;136:788.

Byrd R Jr, et al. Mechanical ventilation; accessed April 2009; http://emedicine.medscape.com/article/304068-overview

Calfee, CS, Eisner, MD, Ware, LB, et al. Trauma-associated lung injury differs clinically and biologically from acute lung injury due to other clinical disorders. Crit Care Med 2007;35:2243.

Casey, LC, Balk, RA, Bone, RC. Plasma cytokine and endotoxin levels correlate with survival in patients with the sepsis syndrome. Ann Intern Med 1993;119:771.

Chesnutt, AN, Matthay, MA, Tibayan, FA, et al. Early detection of type III procollagen peptide in acute lung injury. Pathogenetic and prognostic significance. Am J Respir Crit Care Med 1997;156:840.

Chiumello D, Pelosi P, Calvi E et al. Different modes of assisted ventilation in patients with acute respiratory failure. Eur Respir J 2002;20:925.

Choi, PT, Yip, G, Quinonez, LG, Cook, DJ. Crystalloids vs. colloids in fluid resuscitation: a systematic review. Crit Care Med 1999;27:200.

Chollet-Martin, S, Gatecel, C, Kermarrec, N, et al. Alveolar neutrophil functions and cytokine levels in patients with the adult respiratory distress syndrome during nitric oxide inhalation. Am J Respir Crit Care Med 1996;153:985.

Clark, M, Flick, M. Permeability pulmonary edema caused by venous air embolism. Am Rev Respir Dis 1984;129:633.

Clark, RH, Yoder, BA, Sell, MS. Prospective, randomized comparison of high-frequency oscillation and conventional ventilation in candidates for extracorporeal membrane oxygenation. J Pediatr 1994;124:447.

Clec'h, C, Fosse, JP, Karoubi, P, et al. Differential diagnostic value of procalcitonin in surgical and medical patients with septic shock. Crit Care Med 2006;34:102.

Cohen CA, Zagelbaum G, Gross D, et al. Clinical manifestations of inspiratory muscle fatigue. Am J Med 1982;73:308.

Colice, G, Matthay, M, Bass, E, Matthay, R. Neurogenic pulmonary edema. Am Rev Respir Dis 1984;130:941.

Cometta, A, Calandra, T, Gaya, H, et al. Monotherapy with meropenem versus combination therapy with ceftazidime plus amikacin as empiric therapy for fever in granulocytopenic patients with cancer. The International Antimicrobial Therapy Cooperative Group of the European Organization for Research and Treatment of Cancer and the Gruppo Italiano Malattie Ematologische Maligne dell'Adulto Infection Program. Antimicrob Agents Chemother 1996;40:1108.

Cone, LA, B Waterbor, R, Sofonio, MV. Purpura fulminans due to Streptococcus pneumoniae sepsis following gastric bypass. Obes Surg 2004;14:690.

Cook, D, Meade, M, Guyatt, G, et al. Trials of miscellaneous interventions to wean from mechanical ventilation. Chest 2001;120:438S.

Davidson, WJ, Dorscheid, D, Spragg, R, et al. Exogenous pulmonary surfactant for the treatment of adult patients with acute respiratory distress syndrome: results of a meta-analysis. Crit Care 2006;10:R41.

Dellinger, RP, Levy, MM, Carlet, JM, et al. Surviving Sepsis Campaign: international guidelines for management of severe sepsis and septic shock: 2008. Crit Care Med 2008;36:296.

Dellinger, RP, Zimmerman, JL, Taylor, RW, et al. Effects of inhaled nitric oxide in patients with acute respiratory distress syndrome: results of a randomized phase II trial. Inhaled Nitric Oxide in ARDS Study Group. Crit Care Med 1998;26:15.

Derdak, S, Mehta, S, Stewart, TE, Smith, T. High-frequency oscillatory ventilation for acute respiratory distress syndrome in adults: a randomized, controlled trial. Am J Respir Crit Care Med 2002;166:801.

Dhainaut, JF, Aird, W, Esmon, C. Introduction to the Fifth Margaux Conference on Critical Illness: protein C pathways: bedside to bench. Crit Care Med 2004;32:S193.

Doyle, RL, Szaflarski, N, Modin, GW, et al. Identification of patients with acute lung injury. Predictors of mortality. Am J Respir Crit Care Med 1995;152:1818.

Eichacker, PQ. Inhaled nitric oxide in adult respiratory distress syndrome: do we know the risks versus benefits? [editorial]. Crit Care Med 1997;25:563.

Ely, EW, Baker, AM, Dunagan, DP, et al. Effect on the duration of mechanical ventilation of identifying patients capable of breathing spontaneously. N Engl J Med 1996; 335:1864.

Esteban, A, Alia, I, Tobin, MJ, et al. Effect of spontaneous breathing trial duration on outcome of attempts to discontinue mechanical ventilation. Spanish Lung Failure Collaborative Group. Am J Respir Crit Care Med 1999;159:512.

Esteban, A, Frutos, F, Tobin, MJ, et al. A comparison of four methods of weaning patients from mechanical ventilation. Spanish Lung Failure Collaborative Group. N Engl J Med 1995;332:345.

Ettingshausen, CE, Veldmann, A, Beeg, T, et al. Replacement therapy with protein C concentrate in infants and adolescents with meningococcal sepsis and purpura fulminans. Semin Thromb Hemost 1999;25:537.

Fein, A, Lippman, M, Holtzman, H, et al. The risk factors, incidence and prognosis of the adult respiratory distress syndrome following septicemia. Chest 1983;83:40.

Fekety, R. Guidelines for the diagnosis and management of Clostridium difficile-associated diarrhea and colitis. American College of Gastroenterology, Practice Parameters Committee. Am J Gastroenterol 1997;92:739.

Ferguson, ND, Kacmarek, RM, Chiche, JD, et al. Screening of ARDS patients using standardized ventilator settings: influence on enrollment in a clinical trial. Intensive Care Med 2004;30:1111.

Fiastro, JF, Habib, MP, Shon, BY, Campbell, SC. Comparison of standard weaning parameters and the mechanical work of breathing in mechanically ventilated patients. Chest 1988;94:232.

Finfer, S, Bellomo, R, Boyce, N, et al. A comparison of albumin and saline for fluid resuscitation in the intensive care unit. N Engl J Med 2004;350:2247.

Forsythe, SM, Schmidt, GA. Sodium bicarbonate for the treatment of lactic acidosis. Chest 2000;117:260.

Fort, P, Farmer, C, Westerman, J, et al. High-frequency oscillatory ventilation for adult respiratory distress syndrome – pilot study. Crit Care Med 1997;25:937.

Fowler, A, Hamman, R, Good, J, et al. Adult respiratory distress syndrome: risk with common predispositions. Ann Intern Med 1983;98:593.

Francis, JS, Doherty, MC, Lopatin, U, et al. Severe community-onset pneumonia in healthy adults caused by methicillin-resistant Staphylococcus aureus carrying the Panton-Valentine leukocidin genes. Clin Infect Dis 2005;40:100.

Fridkin, SK, Hageman, JC, Morrison, M, et al. Methicillin-resistant Staphylococcus aureus disease in three communities. N Engl J Med 2005;352:1436.

Gallart, L, Lu, Q, Puybasset, L, et al. Intravenous almitrine combined with inhaled nitric oxide for acute respiratory distress syndrome. Am J Respir Crit Care Med 1998;158:1770.

Garnacho-Montero, J, Garcia-Garmendia, JL, Barrero-Almodovar, A, et al. Impact of adequate empirical antibiotic therapy on the outcome of patients admitted to the intensive care unit with sepsis. Crit Care Med 2003;31:2742.

Gattinoni, L, Brazzi, L, Pelosi, P, et al. A trial of goal-oriented hemodynamic therapy in critically ill patients. N Engl J Med 1995;333:1025.

Gattinoni, L, Pelosi, P, Suter, P, et al. Acute respiratory distress syndrome caused by pulmonary and extrapulmonary disease: different syndromes. Am J Respir Crit Care Med 1998;158:3.

Gattinoni, L, Pesenti, A, Torresin, A. Adult respiratory distress syndrome profiles by computed tomography. J Thorac Imag 1986;1:25.

Georgopoulos, D, Prinianakis, G, Kondili, E. Bedside waveforms interpretation as a tool to identify patient-ventilator asynchronies. Intensive Care Med 2006;32:34.

Gerlach, H, Keh, D, Semmerow, A et al. Dose-response characteristics during long-term inhalation of nitric oxide in patients with severe acute respiratory distress syndrome: a prospective, randomized, controlled study. Am J Respir Crit Care Med 2003;167:1008.

Gherini, S, Peters, RM, Virgilio, RW. Mechanical work on the lungs and work of breathing with positive end-expiratory pressure and continuous positive airway pressure. Chest 1979;76:251.

Ghosh, S, Latimer, RD, Gray, BM, et al. Endotoxin-induced organ injury. Crit Care Med 1993;21:S19.

Gibney, RT, Wilson, RS, Pontoppidan, H. Comparison of work of breathing on high gas flow and demand valve continuous positive airway pressure systems. Chest 1982;82:692.

Gibot, S, Cravoisy, A, Kolopp-Sarda, MN, et al. Time-course of sTREM (soluble triggering receptor expressed on myeloid cells)-1, procalcitonin, and C-reactive protein plasma concentrations during sepsis. Crit Care Med 2005;33:792.

Gibot, S, Kolopp-Sarda, MN, Bene, MC, et al. Plasma level of a triggering receptor expressed on myeloid cells-1: its diagnostic accuracy in patients with suspected sepsis. Ann Intern Med 2004;141:9.

Gibot, S, Le Renard, PE, Bollaert, PE, et al. Surface triggering receptor expressed on myeloid cells 1 expression patterns in septic shock. Intensive Care Med 2005;31:594.

Gil, A, Carrizosa, F, Herrero, A, et al. Influence of mechanical ventilation on blood lactate in patients with acute respiratory failure. Intensive Care Med 1998;24:924.

Gluck, E, Eubanks, DH. Mechanical Ventilation. In: Critical Care Medicine. Principles of Diagnosis and Management, Bone, RC, Parrillo, JE (Eds), Mosby, St Louis, 1995, p. 109.

Gong, MN, Thompson, BT, Williams, P, et al. Clinical predictors of and mortality in acute respiratory distress syndrome: potential role of red cell transfusion. Crit Care Med 2005;33:1191.

Greene, JH, Klinger, JR. The efficacy of inhaled nitric oxide in the treatment of acute respiratory distress syndrome. An evidence-based medicine approach. Crit Care Clin 1998;14:387.

Gutierrez, G, Palizas, F, Doglio, G, et al. Gastric intramucosal pH as a therapeutic index of tissue oxygenation in critically ill patients. Lancet 1992;339:195.

Hansen-Flaschen, JH. Dyspnea in the ventilated patient: a call for patient-centered mechanical ventilation. Respir Care 2000;45:1460.

Harbarth, S, Garbino, J, Pugin, J, et al. Inappropriate initial antimicrobial therapy and its effect on survival in a clinical trial of immunomodulating therapy for severe sepsis. Am J Med 2003;115:529.

Harvey, S, Harrison, DA, Singer, M, et al. Assessment of the clinical effectiveness of pulmonary artery catheters in management of patients in intensive care (PAC-Man): a randomised controlled trial. Lancet 2005;366:472.

Headley, AS, Tolley, E, Meduri, GU. Infections and the inflammatory response in acute respiratory distress syndrome. Chest 1997;111:1306.

Hebert, PC, Wells, G, Blajchman, MA, et al. A multicenter, randomized controlled clinical trial of transfusion requirements in critical care. N Engl J Med 1999;340:409.

Hochman, JS, et al. Current spectrum of cardiogenic shock and effect of early revascularization on mortality. Circulation 1995;91:873.

Hollenberg, SM, Ahrens, TS, Annane, D, et al. Practice parameters for hemodynamic support of sepsis in adult patients: 2004 update. Crit Care Med 2004;32:1928.

Horlander KT, et al. Acute respiratory distress syndrome, accessed August 2008: http://emedicine.medscape.com/article/362571-overview
http://www.rxlist.com/xigris-drug.htm

Hudson, LD, Milberg, JA, Anardi, D, Maunder, RJ. Clinical risks for development of the acute respiratory distress syndrome. Am J Respir Crit Care Med 1995;151:293.

Hybertson, BM, Bursten, SL, Leff, JA, et al. Lisofylline prevents leak, but not neutrophil accumulation, in lungs of rats given IL-1 intratracheally. J Appl Physiol 1997;82:226.

Ibrahim, EH, Sherman, G, Ward, S, et al. The influence of inadequate antimicrobial treatment of bloodstream infections on patient outcomes in the ICU setting. Chest 2000;118:146.

Imsand, C, Feihl, F, Perret, C, Fitting, JW. Regulation of inspiratory neuromuscular output during synchronized intermittent mechanical ventilation. Anesthesiology 1994;80:13.

Iribarren, C, Jacobs, DR Jr, Sidney, S, et al. Cigarette smoking, alcohol consumption, and risk of ARDS: a 15-year cohort study in a managed care setting. Chest 2000;117:163.

Iscimen, R, Cartin-Ceba, R, Yilmaz, M, et al. Risk factors for the development of acute lung injury in patients with septic shock: an observational cohort study. Crit Care Med 2008;36:1518.

Ito, Y, Manwell, SE, Kerr, CL, et al. Effects of ventilation strategies on the efficacy of exogenous surfactant therapy in a rabbit model of acute lung injury. Am J Respir Crit Care Med 1998;157:149.

Jackson, WL Jr. Should we use etomidate as an induction agent for endotracheal intubation in patients with septic shock?: a critical appraisal. Chest 2005;127:1031.

Jepsen, S, Herlevsen, P, Knudsen, P, et al. Antioxidant treatment with N-acetylcysteine during adult respiratory distress syndrome: a prospective, randomized, placebo-controlled study. Crit Care Med 1992;20:918.

Jubran, A, Grant, BJ, Laghi, F, et al. Weaning prediction: esophageal pressure monitoring complements readiness testing. Am J Respir Crit Care Med 2005;171:1252.

Jubran, A, Tobin, MJ. Pathophysiologic basis of acute respiratory distress in patients who fail a trial of weaning from mechanical ventilation. Am J Respir Crit Care Med 1997;155:906.

Jubran, A, Van de Graaff, WB, Tobin, MJ. Variability of patient-ventilator interaction with pressure support ventilation in patients with COPD. Am J Respir Crit Care Med 1995;152:129.

Katzenstein, AL, Myers, JL, Mazur, MT. Acute interstitial pneumonia. A clinicopathologic, ultrastructural and cell kinetic study. Am J Surg Pathol 1986;10:256.

Keel, JBP, Hauser, M, Stocker, R, et al. Established acute respiratory distress syndrome: benefit of corticosteroid rescue therapy. Respiration 1998;65:258.

Ketai, L, Grum, C. C3a and adult respiratory distress syndrome after massive transfusion. Crit Care Med 1986;14:1001.

Khan, H, Belsher, J, Yilmaz, M, et al. Fresh-frozen plasma and platelet transfusions are associated with development of acute lung injury in critically ill medical patients. Chest 2007;131:1308.

Kinch, JW, Ryan, TJ. Right ventricular infarction. N Engl J Med 1994;330:1211.

Kortgen, A, Niederprum, P, Bauer, M. Implementation of an evidence-based "standard operating procedure" and outcome in septic shock. Crit Care Med 2006;34:943.

Kotloff, RM, et al. Am J Respir Crit Care Med 2004;170:22.

Krishnan, JA, Moore, D, Robeson, C, et al. A prospective, controlled trial of a protocol-based strategy to discontinue mechanical ventilation. Am J Respir Crit Care Med 2004;169:673.

Kumar, A, Roberts, D, Wood, KE, et al. Duration of hypotension before initiation of effective antimicrobial therapy is the critical determinant of survival in human septic shock. Crit Care Med 2006;34:1589.

Laghi, F, Cattapan, SE, Jubran, A, et al. Is weaning failure caused by low-frequency fatigue of the diaphragm?. Am J Respir Crit Care Med 2003;167:120.

Laghi, F, D'Alfonso, N, Tobin, MJ. Pattern of recovery from diaphragmatic fatigue over 24 hours. J Appl Physiol 1995;79:539.

Laterre, PF, Abraham, E, Janes, JM, et al. ADDRESS (ADministration of DRotrecogin alfa [activated]in Early stage Severe Sepsis) long-term follow-up: one-year safety and efficacy evaluation. Crit Care Med 2007;35:1457.

Laterre, PF, Heiselman, D. Management of patients with severe sepsis, treated by drotrecogin alfa (activated). Am J Surg 2002;184:S39.

Laterre, PF, Wittebole, X. Clinical review: drotrecogin alfa (activated) as adjunctive therapy for severe sepsis – practical aspects at the bedside and patient identification. Crit Care 2003;7:445.

Laurent, T, Markert, M, Feihl, F, et al. Oxidant-antioxidant balance in granulocytes during ARDS. Effect of N-acetylcysteine. Chest 1996;109:163.

Lederle, FA, et al. Ruptured abdominal aortic aneurysm: the internist as diagnostician. Am J Med 1994;96:163.

Leibovici, L, Paul, M, Poznanski, O, et al. Monotherapy versus beta-lactam-aminoglycoside combination treatment for gram-negative bacteremia: a prospective, observational study. Antimicrob Agents Chemother 1997;41:1127.

Levi, M, Levy, M, Williams, MD, et al. Prophylactic heparin in patients with severe sepsis treated with drotrecogin alfa (activated). Am J Respir Crit Care Med 2007;176:483.

Levitt, JE, Vinayak, AG, Gehlbach, BK, et al. Diagnostic utility of B-type natriuretic peptide in critically ill patients with pulmonary edema: a prospective cohort study. Crit Care 2008;12:R3.

Levraut, J, Ciebiera, JP, Chave, S, et al. Mild hyperlactatemia in stable septic patients is due to impaired lactate clearance rather than overproduction. Am J Respir Crit Care Med 1998;157:1021.

Levy, MM, Fink, MP, Marshall, JC, et al. 2001 SCCM/ESICM/ACCP/ATS/SIS International Sepsis Definitions Conference. Crit Care Med 2003;31:1250.

Lewis, JF, Jobe, AH. Surfactant and the adult respiratory distress syndrome. Am Rev Respir Dis 1993;147:218.

Lim, CM, Jung, H, Koh, Y, et al. Effect of alveolar recruitment maneuver in early acute respiratory distress syndrome according to antiderecruitment strategy, etiological category of diffuse lung injury, and body position of the patient. Crit Care Med 2003;31:411.

Lintin, S, Isaac, P. Miliary tuberculosis presenting as adult respiratory distress syndrome. Intensive Care Med 1988;14:672.

Luce, JM. Pathogenesis and management of septic shock. Chest 1987;91:883.

Machala, W, Wachowicz, N, Komorowska, A, Gaszynski, W. The use of drotrecogin alfa (activated) in severe sepsis during acute pancreatitis – two case studies. Med Sci Monit 2004;10:CS31.

Macintyre, NR. High-Frequency Ventilation. In: Principles and Practice of Mechanical Ventilation, Tobin, MJ, (Ed), McGraw-Hill, New York, 1994, p. 455.

MacIntyre, NR. Respiratory function during pressure support ventilation. Chest 1986; 89:677.

Malerba, G, Romano-Girard, F, Cravoisy, A, et al. Risk factors of relative adrenocortical deficiency in intensive care patients needing mechanical ventilation. Intensive Care Med 2005;31:388.

Malhotra, A, Eikermann, M, Magder, S. Is brachial artery peak velocity variation ready for prime time?. Chest 2007;131:1279.

Manning, HL, Molinary, EJ, Leiter, JC. Effect of inspiratory flow rate on respiratory sensation and pattern of breathing. Am J Respir Crit Care Med 1995;151:751.

Manns, BJ, Lee, H, Doig, CJ, et al. An economic evaluation of activated protein C treatment for severe sepsis. N Engl J Med 2002;347:993.

Marini, JJ, Smith, TC, Lamb, VJ. External work output and force generation during synchronized intermittent mechanical ventilation: effect of machine assistance on breathing effort. Am Rev Respir Dis 1988;138:1169.

Marshall, J, Lowry, S. Evaluation of the adequacy of source control. In: Clinical Trials for the Treatment of Sepsis, Sibbald, WJ, Vincent, JL (Eds), Springer Verlag, Berlin, 1995, p. 329.

Marti-Carvajal, A, Salanti, G, Cardona, AF. Human recombinant activated protein C for severe sepsis. Cochrane Database Syst Rev 2007;CD004388.

Matthay, MA. The acute respiratory distress syndrome [editorial]. N Engl J Med 1996; 334:1469.

Matthay, MA, Pittet, JF, Jayr, C. Just say NO to inhaled nitric oxide for the acute respiratory distress syndrome [editorial]. Crit Care Med 1998;26:1.

McCloskey, RV, Straube, RC, Sanders, C, et al. Treatment of septic shock with human monoclonal antibody HA-1A. A randomized double-blind, placebo-controlled trial. Ann Intern Med 1994;121:1.

McCowen, KC, Malhotra, A, Bistrian, BR. Stress-induced hyperglycemia. Crit Care Clin 2001;17:107.

Meade, MO, Cook, RJ, Guyatt, GH, et al. Interobserver variation in interpreting chest radiographs for the diagnosis of acute respiratory distress syndrome. Am J Respir Crit Care Med 2000;161:85.

Meduri, GU, Belenchia, JM, Estes, RJ, et al. Fibroproliferative phase of ARDS. Clinical findings and effects of corticosteroids. Chest 1991;100:943.

Meduri, GU, Chinn, AJ, Leeper, KV, et al. Corticosteroid rescue treatment of progressive fibroproliferation in late ARDS. Patterns of response and predictors of outcome. Chest 1994;105:1516.

Meduri, GU, Golden, E, Freire, AX, et al. Methylprednisolone infusion in early severe ARDS: results of a randomized controlled trial. Chest 2007;131:954.

Meduri, GU, Headley, S, Golden, E, et al. Effect of prolonged methylprednisolone therapy in unresolving acute respiratory distress syndrome. JAMA 1998;280:159.

Mehta, S, Granton, J, MacDonald, RJ et al. High frequency oscillatory ventilation in adults: the Toronto experience. Chest 2004;126:518.

Mehta, S, Lapinsky, SE, Hallett, DC, et al. Prospective trial of high-frequency oscillation in adults with acute respiratory distress syndrome. Crit Care Med 2001;29:1360.

Micek, ST, Roubinian, N, Heuring, T, et al. Before-after study of a standardized hospital order set for the management of septic shock. Crit Care Med 2006;34:2707.

Michard, F, Boussat, S, Chemla, D, et al. Relation between respiratory changes in arterial pulse pressure and fluid responsiveness in septic patients with acute circulatory failure. Am J Respir Crit Care Med 2000;162:134.

Michard, F, Wolff, MA, Herman, B, Wysocki, M. Right ventricular response to high-dose almitrine infusion in patients with severe hypoxemia related to acute respiratory distress syndrome. Crit Care Med 2001;29:32.

Mikawa, K, Akamatsu, H, Maekawa, N, et al. Inhibitory effect of prostaglandin E1 on human neutrophil function. Prostaglandins Leukot Essent Fatty Acids 1994;51:287.

Milberg, JA, Davis, DR, Steinberg, KP, et al. Improved survival of patients with acute respiratory distress syndrome (ARDS): 1983-1993. JAMA 1995;273:306.

Miller, LG, Perdreau-Remington, F, Rieg, G, et al. Necrotizing fasciitis caused by community-associated methicillin-resistant Staphylococcus aureus in Los Angeles. N Engl J Med 2005;352:1445.

Modell, JH. Drowning. N Engl J Med 1993;328:253.

Monnet, X, Rienzo, M, Osman, D, et al. Esophageal Doppler monitoring predicts fluid responsiveness in critically ill ventilated patients. Intensive Care Med 2005; 31:1195.

Montgomery, A, Stager, M, Carico, C, et al. Causes of mortality in patients with the adult respiratory distress syndrome. Am Rev Respir Dis 1985;132:485.

Montgomery, AB, Stager, MA, Carrico, CJ, et al. Causes of mortality in patients with the adult respiratory distress syndrome. Am Rev Respir Dis 1985;132:485.

Moore, FA, Moore, EE, Read, RA. Postinjury multiple organ failure: role of extrathoracic injury and sepsis in adult respiratory distress syndrome. New Horiz 1993;1:538.

Moscucci, M, Bates, ER. Cardiogenic shock. Cardiol Clin 1995;13:391.

Moss, M, Bucher, B, Moore, FA, et al. The role of chronic alcohol abuse in the development of acute respiratory distress syndrome in adults. JAMA 1996;275:50.

Moss, M, Parsons, PE, Steinberg, KP, et al. Chronic alcohol abuse is associated with an increased incidence of acute respiratory distress syndrome and severity of multiple organ dysfunction in patients with septic shock. Crit Care Med 2003;31:869.

Muscedere, JG, Mullen, JB, Gan, K, et al. Tidal ventilation at low airway pressures can augment lung injury. Am J Respir Crit Care Med 1994;149:1327.

Nadel, S, Goldstein, B, Williams, MD, et al. Drotrecogin alfa (activated) in children with severe sepsis: a multicentre phase III randomised controlled trial. Lancet 2007;369:836.

Nicholas, TE, Doyle, IR, Bersten, AD. Surfactant replacement therapy in ARDS: White knight or noise in the system? Thorax 1997;52:195.

Niehoff, J, DelGuercio, C, LaMorte, W, et al. Efficacy of pulse oximetry and capnometry in postoperative ventilatory weaning. Crit Care Med 1988;16:701.

Nilsestuen, JO, Hargett, KD. Using ventilator graphics to identify patient-ventilator asynchrony. Respir Care 2005;50:202.

Nizami, IY, Kissner, DG, Visscher, DW, Dubaybo, BA. Idiopathic bronchiolitis obliterans with organizing pneumonia. An acute and life-threatening syndrome. Chest 1995;108:271.

Papazian, L, Bregeon, F, Gaillat, F, et al. Inhaled NO and almitrine bismesylate in patients with acute respiratory distress syndrome: effect of noradrenalin. Eur Respir J 1999; 14:1283.

Papazian, L, Roch, A, Bregeon, F, et al. Inhaled nitric oxide and vasoconstrictors in acute respiratory distress syndrome. Am J Respir Crit Care Med 1999;160:473.

Papazian, L, Thomas, P, Bregeon, F, et al. Open-lung biopsy in patients with acute respiratory distress syndrome. Anesthesiology 1998;88:935.

Parker, MM, Parrillo, JE. Septic shock. Hemodynamics and pathogenesis. JAMA 1983; 250:3324.

Parsons, P. Respiratory failure as a result of drugs, overdoses, and poisonings. Clin Chest Med 1994;15:93.

Patel, SR, Karmpaliotis, D, Ayas, NT, et al. The role of open-lung biopsy in ARDS. Chest 2004;125:197.

Paul, M, Benuri-Silbiger, I, Soares-Weiser, K, Leibovici, L. Beta lactam monotherapy versus beta lactam-aminoglycoside combination therapy for sepsis in immunocompetent patients: systematic review and meta-analysis of randomised trials. BMJ 2004;328:668.

Paul, M, Silbiger, I, Grozinsky, S, et al. Beta lactam antibiotic monotherapy versus beta lactam-aminoglycoside antibiotic combination therapy for sepsis. Cochrane Database Syst Rev 2006:CD003344.

Pepe, P, Potkin, R, Reus, D, et al. Clinical predictors of the adult respiratory distress syndrome. Am J Surg 1982;144:124.

Perkins, GD, McAuley, DF, Thickett, DR, Gao, F. The beta-Agonist Lung Injury Trial (BALTI): a Randomized Placebo-controlled Clinical Trial. Am J Respir Crit Care Med 2006;173:281.

Philit, F, Etienne-Mastroianni, B, Parrot, A, et al. Idiopathic acute eosinophilic pneumonia: a study of 22 patients. Am J Respir Crit Care Med 2002;166:1235.

Poeze, M, Solberg, BC, Greve, JW, Ramsay, G. Monitoring global volume-related hemodynamic or regional variables after initial resuscitation: what is a better predictor of outcome in critically ill septic patients?. Crit Care Med 2005;33:2494.

Pope-Harman, AL, Davis, WB, Allen, ED, et al. Acute eosinophilic pneumonia. A summary of 15 cases and review of the literature. Medicine 1996;75:334.

Practice parameters for hemodynamic support of sepsis in adult patients in sepsis. Task Force of the American College of Critical Care Medicine, Society of Critical Care Medicine. Crit Care Med 1999;27:639.

Randomized, placebo-controlled trial of lisofylline for early treatment of acute lung injury and acute respiratory distress syndrome. Crit Care Med 2002;30:1.

Rangel-Frausto, MS, Pittet, D, Costigan, M, et al. The natural history of the systemic inflammatory response syndrome (SIRS): a prospective study. JAMA 1995;273:117.

Raychaudhuri, B, Dweik, R, Connors, MJ, et al. Nitric oxide blocks nuclear factor-kappaB activation in alveolar macrophages. Am J Respir Cell Mol Biol 1999;21:311.

Reinhart, K, Bloos, F, Spies, C. Vasoactive drug therapy in sepsis. In: Clinical Trials for the treatment of sepsis, Sibbald, WJ, Vincent, JL (Eds), Springer Verlag, Berlin, 1995, p. 207.

Reuter, DA, Bayerlein, J, Goepfert, MS, et al. Influence of tidal volume on left ventricular stroke volume variation measured by pulse contour analysis in mechanically ventilated patients. Intensive Care Med 2003;29:476.

Rhodes, A, Bennett, ED. Early goal-directed therapy: an evidence-based review. Crit Care Med 2004;32:S448.

Rice, GC, Rosen, J, Weeks, R, et al. CT-1501R selectively inhibits induced inflammatory monokines in human whole blood ex vivo. Shock 1994;1:254.

Richard, C, Warszawski, J, Anguel, N, et al. Early use of the pulmonary artery catheter and outcomes in patients with shock and acute respiratory distress syndrome: a randomized controlled trial. JAMA 2003;290:2713.

Rivers, E, Nguyen, B, Havstad, S, et al. Early goal-directed therapy in the treatment of severe sepsis and septic shock. N Engl J Med 2001;345:1368.

Rocco, PR, Zin, WA. Pulmonary and extrapulmonary acute respiratory distress syndrome: are they different?. Curr Opin Crit Care 2005;11:10.

Rossaint, R, Falke, KJ, Lopez, F, et al. Inhaled nitric oxide for the adult respiratory distress syndrome. N Engl J Med 1993;328:399.

Rossaint, R, Gerlach, H, Schmidt-Ruhnke, H, et al. Efficacy of inhaled nitric oxide in patients with severe ARDS. Chest 1995;107:1107.

Rubenfeld, GD, Caldwell, E, Peabody, E, et al. Incidence and outcomes of acute lung injury. N Engl J Med 2005;353:1685.

Rubinstein, E, Lode, H, Grassi, C. Ceftazidime monotherapy vs. ceftriaxone/tobramycin for serious hospital-acquired gram-negative infections. Antibiotic Study Group. Clin Infect Dis 1995;20:1217.

Rudiger, A, Gasser, S, Fischler, M, et al. Comparable increase of B-type natriuretic peptide and amino-terminal pro-B-type natriuretic peptide levels in patients with severe sepsis, septic shock, and acute heart failure. Crit Care Med 2006;34:2140.

Russell, JA, Ronco, JJ, Dodek, PM. Physiologic effects and side effects of prostaglandin E1 in the adult respiratory distress syndrome. Chest 1990;97:684.

Safdar, N, Handelsman, J, Maki, DG. Does combination antimicrobial therapy reduce mortality in Gram-negative bacteraemia? A meta-analysis. Lancet Infect Dis 2004;4:519.

Sakuma, T, Okaniwa, G, Nakada, T, et al. Alveolar fluid clearance in the resected human lung. Am J Respir Crit Care Med 1994;150:305.

Sakuma, T, Suzuki, S, Usuda, K, et al. Preservation of alveolar epithelial fluid transport mechanisms in rewarmed human lung after severe hypothermia. J Appl Physiol 1996;80:1681.

Samama, CM, Diaby, M, Fellahi, JL, et al. Inhibition of platelet aggregation by inhaled nitric oxide in patients with acute respiratory distress syndrome. Anesthesiology 1995;83:56.

Sartori, C, Allemann, Y, Duplain, H, et al. Salmeterol for the prevention of high-altitude pulmonary edema. N Engl J Med 2002;346:1631.

Sasse, KC, Nauenberg, E, Long, A, et al. Long-term survival after intensive care unit admission with sepsis. Crit Care Med 1995;23:1040.

Sato, Y, Walley, KR, Klut, ME, et al. Nitric oxide reduces the sequestration of polymorphonuclear leukocytes in lung by changing deformability and CD18 expression. Am J Respir Crit Care Med 1999;159:1469.

Schramm, GE, Johnson, JA, Doherty, JA, et al. Methicillin-resistant Staphylococcus aureus sterile-site infection: the importance of appropriate initial antimicrobial treatment. Crit Care Med 2006;34:2069.

Schwarz AJ, et al. Shock; accessed February 2008; http://emedicine.medscape.com/article/908930-overview

Sessler, CN, Perry, JC, Varney, KL. Management of severe sepsis and septic shock. Curr Opin Crit Care 2004;10:354.

Shapiro, NI, Howell, MD, Talmor, D, et al. Implementation and outcomes of the Multiple Urgent Sepsis Therapies (MUST) protocol. Crit Care Med 2006;34:1025.

Shoemaker, WC, Appel, PL. Effects of prostaglandin E1 in adult respiratory distress syndrome. Surgery 1986;99:275.

Sibbald, WJ, Vincent, JL. Round table conference on clinical trials for the treatment of sepsis. Crit Care Med 1995;23:394.

Siegel, JP. Assessing the use of activated protein C in the treatment of severe sepsis. N Engl J Med 2002;347:1030.

Silverman, HJ, Slotman, G, Bone, RC, et al. Effects of prostaglandin E1 on oxygen delivery and consumption in patients with the adult respiratory distress syndrome. Results from the prostaglandin E1 multicenter trial. The Prostaglandin E1 Study Group. Chest 1990;98:405.

Skurnik, Y, Zhornicky, T, Schattner, A. Survival in miliary tuberculosis complicated by respiratory distress. Presse Med 1994;23:979.

Slutsky, AS. Mechanical ventilation. American College of Chest Physicians' Consensus Conference. Chest 1993;104:1833.

Sofer, S, Bar-Ziv, J, Scharf, S. Pulmonary edema following relief of upper airway obstruction. Chest 1984;86:401.

Spragg, RG, Lewis, JF, Walmrath, HD, et al. Effect of recombinant surfactant protein C-based surfactant on the acute respiratory distress syndrome. N Engl J Med 2004;351:884.

Spragg, RG, Lewis, JF, Wurst, W, et al. Treatment of acute respiratory distress syndrome with recombinant surfactant protein C surfactant. Am J Respir Crit Care Med 2003;167:1562.

Steinberg, KP, Hudson, LD, Goodman, RB, et al. Efficacy and safety of corticosteroids for persistent acute respiratory distress syndrome. N Engl J Med 2006;354:1671.

Suter, PM. Lung inflammation in ARDS – friend or foe?. N Engl J Med 2006;354:1739.

Tang, BM, Eslick, GD, Craig, JC, McLean, AS. Accuracy of procalcitonin for sepsis diagnosis in critically ill patients: systematic review and meta-analysis. Lancet Infect Dis 2007;7:210.

Taylor, RW, Zimmerman, JL, Dellinger, RP, et al. Low-dose inhaled nitric oxide in patients with acute lung injury. A randomized controlled trial. JAMA 2004;291:1603.

Thille, AW, Rodriguez, P, Cabello, B, et al. Patient-ventilator asynchrony during assisted mechanical ventilation. Intensive Care Med 2006;32:1515.

Third European Consensus Conference in Intensive Care Medicine. Tissue hypoxia: how to detect, how to correct, how to prevent. Societe de Reanimation de Langue Francaise. The American Thoracic Society. European Society of Intensive Care Medicine. Am J Respir Crit Care Med 1996;154:1573.

Tobin, MJ, Jubran, A, Laghi, F. Patient-ventilator interaction. Am J Respir Crit Care Med 2001;163:1059.

Tobin, MJ, Jubran, A. Weaning from mechanical ventilation. In: Principles and Practice of Mechanical Ventilation, Jubran, A, Tobin, MJ (Eds), McGraw Hill, New York, 2006, p.1185.

Tobin, MJ. Mechanical ventilation. N Engl J Med 1994;330:1056.

Treggiari, MM, Hudson, LD, Martin, DP, et al. Effect of acute lung injury and acute respiratory distress syndrome on outcome in critically ill trauma patients. Crit Care Med 2004;32:327.

Tugrul, S, Akinci, O, Ozcan, PE, et al. Effects of sustained inflation and postinflation positive end-expiratory pressure in acute respiratory distress syndrome: focusing on pulmonary and extrapulmonary forms. Crit Care Med 2003;31:738.

Verhoef, J, Hustinx, WM, Frasa, H, Hoepelman, AI. Issues in the adjunct therapy of severe sepsis. J Antimicrob Chemother 1996;38:167.

Villar, J, Perez-Mendez, L, Kacmarek, RM. Current definitions of acute lung injury and the acute respiratory distress syndrome do not reflect their true severity and outcome. Intensive Care Med 1999;25:930.

Villar, J, Perez-Mendez, L, Lopez, J, et al. An early PEEP/FIO2 trial identifies different degrees of lung injury in patients with acute respiratory distress syndrome. Am J Respir Crit Care Med 2007;176:795.

Vincent, JL, Angus, DC, Artigas, A, et al. Effects of drotrecogin alfa (activated) on organ dysfunction in the PROWESS trial. Crit Care Med 2003;31:834.

Vincent, JL, Bernard, GR, Beale, R, et al. Drotrecogin alfa (activated) treatment in severe sepsis from the global open-label trial ENHANCE: further evidence for survival and safety and implications for early treatment. Crit Care Med 2005;33:2266.

Walmrath, D, Grimminger, F, Pappert, D, et al. Bronchoscopic administration of bovine natural surfactant in ARDS and septic shock: impact on gas exchange and haemodynamics. Eur Respir J 2002;19:805.

Ware, LB, Matthay, MA. Clinical practice. Acute pulmonary edema. N Engl J Med 2005;353:2788.

Warren, HS, Suffredini, AF, Eichacker, PQ, Munford, RS. Risks and benefits of activated protein C treatment for severe sepsis. N Engl J Med 2002;347:1027.

Weinberger, B, Laskin, DL, Heck, DE, Laskin, JD. The toxicology of inhaled nitric oxide. Toxicol Sci 2001;59:5.

Wheeler, AP, Bernard, GR, Thompson, BT, et al. Pulmonary-artery versus central venous catheter to guide treatment of acute lung injury. N Engl J Med 2006;354:2213.

Wheeler, AP, Bernard, GR. Treating patients with severe sepsis. N Engl J Med 1999;340:207.

Wiedemann, HP, Wheeler, AP, Bernard, GR, et al. Comparison of two fluid-management strategies in acute lung injury. N Engl J Med 2006;354:2564.

Wilkes, MM, Navickis, RJ. Patient survival after human albumin administration. A meta-analysis of randomized, controlled trials. Ann Intern Med 2001;135:149.

Wunsch, H, Mapstone, J. High-frequency ventilation versus conventional ventilation for treatment of acute lung injury and acute respiratory distress syndrome. Cochrane Database Syst Rev 2004;CD004085.

Yang, SC, Yang, SP. Effects of inspiratory flow waveforms on lung mechanics, gas exchange, and respiratory metabolism in COPD patients during mechanical ventilation. Chest 2002;122:2096.

Zeni, F, Freeman, B, Natanson, C. Anti-inflammatory therapies to treat sepsis and septic shock: a reassessment. Crit Care Med 1997;25:1095.

Zwissler, B, Kemming, G, Habler, O, et al. Inhaled prostacyclin (PGI2) versus inhaled nitric oxide in adult respiratory distress syndrome. Am J Respir Crit Care Med 1996;154:1671.

PROCEDURES

American Family Physician, December 1, 2002 Cover Article: Office Procedures Diagnostic and Therapeutic Injection of the Elbow Region.

Arthrocentesis of the Knee. NEJM Videos in Clinical Medicine, http://content.nejm.org/cgi/content/short/354/19/e19

Barash P, Cullen, B, and Stoelting R. Clinical Anesthesia, 5th ed. Lippincott Williams & Wilkins, 2006, pp 595–643, 669–667.

Clinicalcases.org. V. Dimov, M.D., Clinical Assistant Professor of Medicine, Cleveland Clinic Lerner College of Medicine of Case Western Reserve University, Cleveland, Ohio; B. Altaqi, M.D., Assistant Clinical Professor of Medicine, University of Louisville, Kentucky

Diagnostic and Therapeutic Injection of the Elbow Region, American Family Physician, December 1, 2002

Dimov, V. Clinical Assistant Professor of Medicine, Cleveland Clinic Lerner College of Medicine of Case Western Reserve University, Cleveland, Ohio; Altaqi, B, Assistant Clinical Professor of Medicine, University of Louisville, Kentucky, http://www. clinicalcases.org/

Fundamentals of Endovascular Surgery From ACS Surgery: Principles & Practice, www.medscape.com/viewarticle/461026

Fundamentals of Endovascular Surgery, www.medscape.com/viewarticle/461026 ACS Surgery: Principles & Practice.

Iserson KV. High flow infusion techniques. In: Clinical Procedures in Emergency Medicine, 3rd ed., Robert JR, Hedges JR (eds.), Philadelphia: WB Saunders, 1998, p. 352.

NEJM Videos in Clinical Medicine. Arthrocentesis of the Knee, http://content.nejm.org/cgi/content/short/354/19/e19

Piccini and Nilsson: The Osler Medical Handbook, 2nd ed., 2006, http:www.mdconsult.com; last accessed August 4, 2009

Taylor R, Palagiri, A. Central Venous Catheterization: Concise Definitive Review. Crit Care Med. 2007;35(5):1390-1396.

Tintinalli, J. Emergency Medicine: A Comprehensive Study Guide, 6th ed. The American College of Emergency Physicians, 2008, pp. 1387–1389.

ETHICAL ISSUES

Advance Directives. Retrieved June 3, 2008, from Merck, 2007, http://www.merck.com/mmhe/sec01/ch009/ch009e.html

Appelbaum, PS. Assessment of patient's competence to consent to treatment. N Engl J Med 2007;357:1834-1840.

Aulisio, MP, Arnold, RM, Youngner, SJ. Health care ethics consultation: Nature, goals and competencies. Annals of Internal Medicine 2000;133(1):59-69.

Azar, AR, Gurrera, RJ, Karel, MJ, Moye, J. Neuropsychological predictors of decision-making capacity over 9 months in mild-to-moderate dementia. J Intern Med 2006;21(1):78-83.

Baranowski-Birkmeier, T, Johnson, RF, O'Donnell, JB. Advance directives in the medical intensive care unit of a community teaching hospital. Chest 107;1995:752-756.

Black, C, Schofield, P. Pain management in palliative care: a case study. J Can Nur 2005;19(3):12-17.

Campbell, ML, Curtis, JR, Haas, CE, et al.. Recommendations for end-of-life care in the intensive care unit: a consensus statement by the American Academy of Critical Care Medicine. Crit Care Med 2008;36:953-963.

Cherniak, EP. Implications of the use of DNR orders for the elderly. Internet Journal Law, Healthcare, Ethics 2003;1(2).

Cohen, S, Winter, B. ABC of intensive care: withdrawal of treatment. Br Med J 1999;319:306-308.

Edwards, KA. Informed Consent. Retrieved June 3, 2008, from University of Washington School of Medicine, 2008, http://depts.washington.edu/bioethx/topics/consent.html

Ethics Committee and Ethics Consultation. Retrieved June 12, 2008, from University of Washington School of Medicine, http://www.depts.washington.edu/bioethx/topics/ethics.html

Fallon, M, O'Neill, B. ABC of palliative care: principles of palliative care and pain control. Br Med J 1997;315:801-804.

Haas, LJ, Leiser, JP, Magill, MK, Sanyer, ON. Management of the difficult patient. Am Fam Physician 2005;72:10.

HIPPA privacy rule and public health. Retrieved June 3, 2008, from CDC, 2003, http://www.cdc.gov/mmwr/preview/mmwrhtml/su5201al.htm

Informed Consent. Retrieved June 3, 2008 from American Medical Association, 2008, http://www.ama-assn.org/ama/pub/category/4608.html

Jecker, NS, Jonsen, AR, Schneiderman, LJ. Medical futility: response to critiques. Annals of Internal Medicine 1996;125:669-674.

Orentlicher, D. The legalization of physician-assisted suicide. New England Journal Medicine 335;1996:663-667.

Patient Confidentiality. Retrieved June 3, 2008 from American Medical Association, 2007, http://www.ama-assn.org/ama/pub/category/4610.html

Phillips, BJ. Determining DNR status. Internet Journal Law Healthcare Ethics 2005;2(2).

Steinmetz, D, Tabenkin, H. The difficult patient as perceived by family physicians. Fam Pract 18;2001:495-500.

Truog, RD. Tackling medical futility in Texas. N Engl J Med 2007;357(2):1-3.

RISK MANAGEMENT

Apker J, Mallak LA, Gibson, SC. Communicating in the "gray zone": perceptions about emergency physician-hospitalist handoffs and patient safety. Acad Emerg Med 2007; 14:884-94.

Becker, C. Hospitalist's role at center of racketeering lawsuit. Modern Physician Online, 2007;Aug 6. (published online)

Croskerry P, Wears RL. Patient safety in emergency medicine. In: Markovchick VJ, Pons PT (Eds). Emergency Medicine Secrets, 3rd ed. Philadelphia, PA, Hanley & Belfus, 2003, pp. 29-36.

Goldman, L, Pantilat, SZ, Whitcomb, WF. Passing the clinical baton: 6 principles to guide the hospitalist. Am J Med. 2001;111(9B):36S-39S.

Government Accounting Office. Improving the Efficiency of Hospital-Based Emergency Care: Hospital-Based Subcommittee Report. Washington, DC, U.S. General Accounting Office, 2003, pp. 101-27.

Kunz v. Little Company of Mary Hosp., 373 Ill.App.3d 615.

Lurie, JD, Miller, DP, Lindenauer PK, Wachter RM, Sox HC. The potential size of the hospitalist workforce in the United States. Am J Med 1999;106:441-5.

Pantilat, SZ, Alpers, A, Wachter, RM. A new doctor in the house: ethical issues in hospitalist systems. JAMA 1999;282:171-4.

Pham, HH, Devers, KJ, Kuo, S, Berenson R. Health care market trends and the evolution of hospitalist use and roles. J Gen Intern Med 2005;20:101-7.

Pham, HH, Devers, KJ, May, JH, Berenson R. Financial pressures spur physician entrepreneurialism. Health Aff (Millbank) 2004;23:70-81.

Plauth, WH, Pantilat, SZ, Wachter, RM, Fenton CL. Hospitalists' perceptions of their residency training needs: results of a national survey. Am J Med 2001;111:247-54.

Wachter, RM, Goldman L. The hospitalist movement 5 years later. JAMA 2002;282:487-94.

Index

Note: Page numbers followed by an f indicate pages with figures.